Contributions to Psychology and Medicine

Contributions to Psychology and Medicine

Stuart Biddle   Nanette Mutrie

Psychology of Physical Activity and Exercise

A Health-Related Perspective

With 75 Figures

Springer-Verlag
London   Berlin   Heidelberg   New York
Paris   Tokyo   Hong Kong
Barcelona   Budapest

Stuart Biddle BEd, MSc, PhD
School of Education, University of Exeter,
Exeter EX1 2LU, UK

Nanette Mutrie DPE, MEd, PhD
Department of Physical Education and
Sports Science,
University of Glasgow, Glasgow
G12 8LT, UK

Advisor
J. Richard Eiser BA, PhD
Department of Psychology,
Washington Singer Laboratories,
University of Exeter,
Exeter EX4 4QG, UK

British Library Cataloguing in Publication Data
Biddle, Stuart
   Psychology of physical activity and exercise.
   1. Physical fitness. Psychology
   I. Title II. Mutrie, Nanette, *1953*– III. Series 613.7019
   ISBN 3-540-19621-8

Library of Congress Cataloging-in-Publication Data
Biddle, Stuart.
Psychology of physical activity and exercise / Stuart Biddle &
   Nanette Mutrie
      p. cm.–(Contributions to psychology and medicine)
   Includes bibliographical references.
   ISBN 3-540-19621-8. – ISBN 0-387-19621-8
   1. Exercise–Psychological aspects. 2. Exercise therapy–
   Psychological aspects. I. Mutrie, Nanette, 1953– . II. Title
   III. Series.
   QP301.B473 1991
   613.7'1'019–dc20   90-26576
                                                        CIP

Printed in Germany
First published 1991

The use of registered names, trademarks etc. in this publication does not imply, even in the
absence of a specific statement, that such names are exempt from the relevant laws and
regulations and therefore free for general use.

Product liability: The publisher can give no guarantee for information about drug dosage and
application thereof contained in this book. In every individual case the respective user must
check its accuracy by consulting other pharmaceutical literature.

Typeset by Photo·graphics, Honiton, Devon
2128/3830-543210 Printed on acid-free paper
ISBN 3-540-19621-8 Springer-Verlag Berlin Heidelberg New York
ISBN 0-387-19621-8 Springer-Verlag New York Berlin Heidelberg

Dedicated to
Dorothy V. Harris
(1931–1991)

Preface

This book was conceived in a pub on the Great West Road in West London. Not a very appropriate location for the planning of a book on healthy pursuits! However, the occasion was a social meeting at the annual conference of BASS (British Association of Sports Sciences, not the beer!), held in 1987 at the West London Institute. At this conference we had arranged a special symposium "Exercise and Health Psychology". This was a new topic for BASS and one that we felt required greater exposure to a group predominantly interested in competitive sport behaviours. Having addressed the major topics of exercise adherence, psychological antecedents of exercise, and the benefits of exercise to mental health in this symposium, we realised that there was a need for a British book in this area. It seemed easy enough to agree on the need for such a book, but it took several years to organise our thoughts into a manuscript. Although there are a number of books on sports psychology, as well as numerous journals, relatively little has been published in book form on the psychology of physical activity and exercise. We hope this book fills a gap. It is aimed primarily at researchers and students studying the psychology of exercise and health, as well as interested professionals in medicine, teaching, health education and promotion, and related fields.

This book presents review material in three main areas. First, it reviews the psychological antecedents of participation in physical activity and exercise, including the important issues of the adoption and maintenance of exercise. Second, the psychological outcomes of exercise are considered, including the proposed mental health outcomes for both clinical and "normal" populations. Finally, the book covers the applied issues of intervention strategies for both individuals and institutions.

All books suffer from a time lag. This one is no exception and with the literature on the psychology of exercise expanding at an ever-increasing rate we anticipate that new developments and insights will be with us soon and possibly will answer many of the questions we pose. However, this is one of the first books to address in a comprehensive way the psychological antecedents, consequences and applied interventions of health-related exercise and physical activity. We hope it stimulates further thought and action in both psychology and exercise.

We owe a great debt to our mentor Professor Dorothy V. Harris. Sadly, she died in January 1991, just prior to the publication of this book. It is a strange but happy coincidence that we have come together to write this book having both graduated from the Pennsylvania State University, but at different times, under the guidance of Prof. Harris. Her courses on "sport" psychology included material beyond the confines of the competitive arena and she considered it important to address issues of exercise participation long before exercise and health became fashionable topics for study. Her courses and encouragement gave us the impetus to research and write in this area.

As everyone knows, writing is not an easy task. We would like to thank the family, friends and colleagues who have helped us complete this book for their time, encouragement, initial comments, and "being there".

Thanks are extended to the following people for making helpful comments on earlier drafts of chapters: Dr. Neil Armstrong (University of Exeter), Dr. Ken Fox (University of Exeter), Andy Smith (Kerland Sports Services), Gareth Stratton (Liverpool Polytechnic), and Dr. Jim Whitehead (University of North Dakota).

We would also like to thank Michael Jackson and Wendy Darke of Springer-Verlag for their motivating "encouragement" (prodding!) as the manuscript unfolded slowly. Finally, we would like to thank the series advisor, Professor Dick Eiser, for his advice and support.

Exeter   Stuart Biddle
Glasgow   Nanette Mutrie
January 1991

Contents

x Contents

Section A

INTRODUCTION AND RATIONALE

1

Physical Activity and Exercise: An Introduction

The apparent benefits of physical activity were recognised by some of the earliest civilisations, yet it is only relatively recently that we have begun to understand the complex interaction between physical activity, physical fitness, and mental and physical health. Even now, a lack of agreement over research methods and definitions of key terms has hampered the production of an unequivocal consensus in some areas. Nevertheless, it could be stated with some confidence that the latter part of the twentieth century has been a period of unprecedented concern about human health, particularly from a preventive point of view. One is reminded of the story of a young man on a river bank who, exhausted from dragging out five struggling people from the river, asked a passer-by what should be done if more were found in the river. The passer-by suggested he went upstream to stop the person throwing people in from the bridge! Certainly the preventive medicine message is clearer and stronger now than it was a few years ago.

Knowledge of how human evolution has proceeded has led researchers to suggest that current lifestyles may be unsuitable for the maintenance of optimal health. Despite the interest shown by people in health, and in particular the relationship between healthy bodies and minds expressed by civilisations such as the ancient Greeks (see Ryan 1984), it is only very recently in the time-span of human development that a clearer understanding of the mechanisms of health and disease has evolved. Blair (1988), for example, suggests that four evolutionary periods are important in understanding the relationship between physical activity and health.

The pre-agricultural period (up until about 10 000 years ago) was characterised by hunting and gathering activities. Exercise levels were high and diet was low in fat. The agricultural period (from 10 000 years ago until about the beginning of the nineteenth century) was also characterised by reasonably high levels of physical activity and relatively low-fat diets, although the fat content probably increased during this time.

The industrial period (1800–1945) saw the development of the "industrialised society" with the accompanying problems of over-crowding, poor diet, poor public health measures and inadequate medical facilities and care. Infectious diseases were responsible for a high proportion of premature deaths. However, this trend became reversed in the "nuclear/technological" period, which Blair (1988) identified as being from 1945 until the present. The major improvement in public health measures and medical advances meant that infectious diseases were becoming less common in "advanced" societies. However, health problems were merely shifted in terms of causes and outcomes. The major causes of premature mortality have now become "lifestyle related"; for example, risk factors for coronary heart disease include cigarette smoking, lack of physical activity, and a diet high in saturated animal fats (see Powell 1988; Powell et al. 1986). Other major health risks are cancers and accidents, particularly those involving motor vehicles.

In short, humans have now adopted lifestyles in industrialised countries that were quite unknown until very recently in terms of human evolution. This is not to say, of course, that "health" has necessarily deteriorated: far from it in some cases, although the terms used to define and measure health can differ. Life-span itself has increased dramatically (see Fig. 1.1). Similarly, other indicators of physical and mental health have shown improvements, although Malina (1988) says that these are largely restricted to the "developed" countries. Yet, alongside apparently positive changes, we have experienced a period of unprecedented cultural change. Malina (1988, p. 10) states:

> In the short period of time since the Neolithic, and the negligible changes in our physical structure over the past 30 000 years or so, several questions immediately surface. For example, how long can rapid cultural change be tolerated on essentially the same biological base? Or, in another perspective, are we biologically equipped for one kind of lifestyle, but forced by cultural circumstances to live another? Does the increased prevalence of degenerative diseases such as cardiovascular disease and some cancers signal problems with the human machine?

The change in lifestyle, particularly in the latter part of the twentieth century, has brought its own health problems. Some writers have referred to a selection of these as "hypokinetic diseases", or health problems caused by or related to a lack of physical activity (see Kraus and Raab 1961). Such hypokinetic problems can include coronary heart disease (CHD), obesity, low back pain, osteoporosis, hypertension and diabetes. The

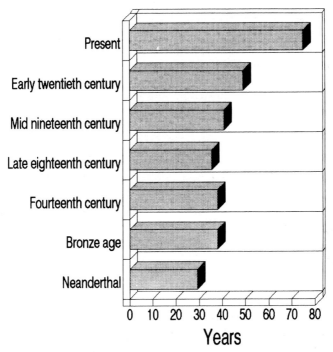

Figure 1.1. Estimated life expectancy in human evolution (Adapted from Malina 1988.)

evidence linking patterns of physical activity with such health measures is increasing rapidly and will be reviewed in brief later in this chapter.

Objectives of this Book

The focus of this book is twofold: physical activity and psychology, but from a health-related perspective. The changing face of health in western industrialised countries is partly associated with current levels of physical activity, although physical activity is but one part of the health issue.

This book outlines the major psychological influences and outcomes associated with regular involvement in physical activity, including structured exercise. The major objective is to summarise the literature on the psychology–physical activity interface with the view to helping health professionals and other interested parties, understand better (a) the issues of starting and maintaining health-related physical activity, and (b) the psychological outcomes of regular physical activity. It is recognised that psychology is but *one* aspect of a complex interaction of factors, including biological, social, economic and political forces, acting on the individual and society in determining activity levels. While competitive sport will receive some attention, the primary focus in this discussion is on habitual physical activity and exercise in its widest sense. There is a large and developing literature on the psychology of competitive sport, where the main interest is on the antecedents and consequences of the competitive sport experience (see Gill 1986; Silva and Weinberg 1984), and on the enhancement of sport performance. A wider view is taken in this book because a public health perspective is adopted. From this point of view, the major concern is about the health and well-being of the community rather than any one individual. As Powell (1988, p. 16) states "the public health importance of various conditions is judged by their impact on the vitality of society as a whole rather than on any individual". However, adopting a psychological approach makes it difficult always to separate the individual and the society, although strategies aimed at promoting individual behaviour change will be discussed later.

Clarification of Terms

Increasing interest is being shown in the exercise and sports sciences, and links are now being made between various medical and non-medical disciplines in relation to physical activity, but the terminology adopted in the study of health and physical activity has not always been consistent. This section will give operational definitions and clarifications to key words and terms and will be based mainly on the work of Bouchard et al. (1990) and Caspersen et al. (1985).

Health and Well-being

A definition of health usually encompasses the phrase "not merely the absence of disease". Indeed, health is multifactorial in nature and includes dimensions of the physical, mental and social, and some might argue the "spiritual". Bouchard et al. (1990) point out that it encompasses a continuum with positive and negative end points. High positive health is sometimes referred to as "wellness" or high-level well-being. This could be characterised by positive physical and emotional well-being with a high capacity for enjoying life and challenges, and possessing adequate coping strategies in the face of difficulties. Although the word "wellness" does not sit happily with the English language, high-level wellness, in our opinion, is an appropriate way of describing "good health" or positive well-being.

Patton et al. (1986) outline two models of health – an "illness model" and a "wellness model". They suggest that an illness model merely describes an intervention aimed at reducing or eliminating the illness whereas a wellness model attempts to describe the *movement* from "sickness" to a point further along the "wellness" continuum.

The negative end of the health/wellness continuum refers to morbidity, that is to say ill-health usually with a known pathology, and mortality (Bouchard et al. 1990).

Physical Activity, Exercise and Sport

Physical Activity

Physical activity, as defined by Caspersen et al. (1985), involves the three following elements: (a) movement of the body produced by the skeletal muscles, (b) resulting energy expenditure which varies from low to high, and (c) a positive correlation with physical fitness.

This last statement has been the point of some debate in recent years and will be discussed later in the chapter.

Sometimes physical activity is referred to as "habitual physical activity" (HPA) (see Mercer 1989). Perhaps of more interest to researchers in the field of physical and health education is the role HPA plays in leisure-time activities. From a psychological point of view it is important that factors related to the choice of HPA in leisure time are identified (see Chap. 2).

Exercise

A subset of activities within HPA includes exercise and sport. Caspersen et al. (1985, p. 127) define exercise with reference to a number of factors. Their first two points also define physical activity and are that body movement is produced by skeletal muscles and that the resulting energy expenditure varies from low to high. In addition, exercise is "very positively correlated with physical fitness", is "planned, structured and repetitive bodily movement", and its objective is to maintain or improve physical fitness.

Although these definitions will be used in a broad sense in this book, the distinction between HPA and exercise is not always so clear-cut. Caspersen et al. suggest that the objective of exercise is to maintain or improve physical fitness, yet the reasons people become physically active, be it in exercise, sport or other pursuits, are complex and dynamic. Similarly, there will be situations where HPA and exercise overlap, such as with the individual who cycles to work for the dual purposes of getting to work and maintaining personal fitness. Other people may cycle for recreation at weekends but not be interested in the physical fitness outcomes. Bouchard et al. (1990) define exercise as leisure-time physical activity. This is a good starting point and should be used alongside the more specific factors of Caspersen et al. (1985). In this book, exercise will usually refer to more structured leisure-time physical activity, such as participation in jogging, swimming, "keep-fit" activities, and recreational sports.

Sport

Philosophers have argued long and hard over the word sport, but for our purposes we define it as a sub-component of exercise whereby the activity is rule-governed, structured and competitive and involves gross motor movement characterised by physical strategy, prowess and chance (see Rejeski and Brawley 1988). The competitive nature of sport has sometimes been difficult to clarify. Indeed, the Sports Councils in Great Britain have jurisdiction over activities that are non-competitive (e.g. keep-fit and yoga), and "Sport for All" campaigns have often included a wider range of activities than "traditional" competitive sports (see Wankel 1988). It is common to hear the phrase "mass sport" on the European mainland to describe what is more usually termed physical recreation by the British.

Physical and Physiological Fitness

Bouchard et al. (1990) suggest that "fitness" is an elusive concept. For example, they propose a distinction between "physical fitness" and "physiological fitness", whereas other workers (e.g. Caspersen et al. 1985; Corbin and Lindsey 1988) distinguish between "health-related" and "skill-related" aspects of fitness.

Physical fitness refers to the ability of the individual to perform muscular work. Caspersen et al. (1985, p. 129) define it as "a set of attributes that people have or achieve that relates to the ability to perform physical activity". This suggests that physical fitness is partly related to current physical activity levels ("attributes that people *achieve*") and partly a function of heredity ("attributes that people *have*"; see Bouchard 1988, 1990; Schull 1990). In addition, Bouchard et al. (1990) refer to "physiological fitness" in terms of the effectiveness of the biological systems of the body in matters such as blood pressure, fat distribution and stress tolerance.

In recent years it has become more usual to refer to health-related and skill-related components of physical fitness (Caspersen et al. 1985; Corbin and Lindsey 1988; Pate 1988). The skill-related aspects of fitness are associated with athletic ability and are sometimes referred to as "motor fitness". The components are agility, balance, coordination, power, reaction time and speed. There is no evidence linking the development of such qualities to "health" outcomes, such as the reduction of risk for chronic disease. However, they may have more indirect or less tangible health benefits such as through the development of independence for older people. Generally speaking though, they are separated from health-related components of fitness and epidemiological evidence supports such a distinction. The skill-related aspects of fitness are important, of course, for sport and other activities relying on motor skills and abilities.

The health-related components of physical fitness are usually listed as cardiovascular (cardiorespiratory or cardiopulmonary) fitness, muscular strength and endurance, muscle flexibility, and body composition (Caspersen et al. 1985; Corbin and Lindsey 1988). The addition of stress management has sometimes been advocated (Biddle 1988a). The development of these components of health-related fitness (HRF) have been related to specific "health" or disease outcomes. Indeed, Pate (1988) has argued that "physical fitness" should be defined solely in terms of the health-related aspects by stating that the following two criteria should be met in such a definition. First, fitness should refer to the functional capacities required for comfortable and productive involvement in day-to-day activities, and second, it should "encompass manifestation of the health-related outcomes of high levels of habitual activity" (Pate 1988, p. 177). The health outcomes of the components of HRF will be discussed more fully later.

Given the public health perspective adopted in this book, the types and forms of exercise and physical activity that have been reviewed in relation to psychological principles and research are generally health-related. The development and control of motor skill activities, and associated psychological aspects, are described elsewhere (e.g. Magill 1989; Schmidt 1986). Similarly, competitive sport, except where it sheds some light on the wider public health aspects of exercise and physical activity, is not covered in detail, but is described by other authors (e.g. Bird and Cripe 1986; Carron 1980; Cox 1985; Gill 1986; Iso-Ahola and Hatfield 1985; Silva and Weinberg 1984). As already stated, however, it is not always clear-cut when sport becomes exercise or vice versa. The focus of this book, though, is not on high-level competitive sport or the psychological factors affecting such performances.

Policy and Position Statements on Exercise, Physical Activity, Fitness and Health

The changing trends in morbidity and mortality discussed briefly in the opening section of this chapter are reflected in the growing number of organisations producing position statements and policy documents on health-related behaviours, including exercise. Two of the largest projects undertaken in this respect emanate from the World Health Organization and the Department of Health and Human Services in the United States.

Health for All 2000

The World Health Organization (WHO) published its targets for "health for all" in their European region in 1985. The 1986 revision of their book

Targets for Health for All (WHO 1986, p. 1) "set out the fundamental requirements for people to be healthy, to define the improvements in health that can be achieved by the year 2000 for the peoples of the European Region of WHO, and to propose action to secure these improvements". Broadly, WHO list four dimensions of health outcomes they wish to achieve. These are equity in health, adding "life to years", adding "health to life", and adding years to life. Specifically, 38 targets have been outlined for achievement by the year 2000. The targets which are of particular interest to exercise researchers are summarised in Table 1.1.

Such broad statements are only likely to be effective when placed in a more specific national and regional context and with more precise goals. Nevertheless, the importance of such statements should be recognised as indicative of a greater role for preventive health practices in the latter part of this century.

Health Objectives for the American Nation

A more specific set of goals was established by the Department of Health and Human Services (DHHS) of the United States' government (DHHS

Table 1.1. Selected WHO "Health For All" Targets up to the Year 2000 that are Particularly Relevant to Exercise Science

Target Number and Target

9. **Diseases of the Circulation**: by the year 2000, mortality in the Region[a] from diseases of the circulatory system in people under 65 years of age should be reduced by at least 15%.

13. **Healthy Public Policy**: by 1990, national policies in all Member States[b] should ensure that legislative, administrative and economic mechanisms provide broad intersectoral support and resources for the promotion of healthy lifestyles and ensure effective participation of the people at all levels of such policy-making.

15. **Knowledge and Motivation for Healthy Behaviour**: by 1990, educational programmes in all Member States should enhance the knowledge, motivation and skills of people to acquire and maintain health.

16. **Positive Health Behaviour**: by 1995, in all Member States, there should be significant increases in positive health behaviour, such as balanced nutrition, non-smoking, appropriate physical activity and good stress management.

32. **Research Strategies**: before 1990, all Member States should have formulated research strategies to stimulate investigations which improve the application and expansion of knowledge needed to support their "health for all" developments.

[a] Region: Europe.
[b] Member states: the 33 European countries who are members of WHO.

1980). Initially, the DHHS set 223 "health objectives for the nation" by the year 1990. As with the WHO targets these included a number of objectives unrelated to physical activity. However, the DHHS did set eleven objectives for 1990 which were concerned specifically with exercise and physical fitness (see DHHS 1980; Dishman 1988a; Powell et al. 1986). A review of these objectives in 1985 revealed a mixed pattern of success, and Powell et al. (1986, p. 15) reported that although considerable progress had been made, "much remains to be learned, and most segments of society would benefit from increased levels of physical activity". For example, data indicated that two of the 11 objectives would be achieved by 1990, four were unlikely to be achieved, two had insufficient data to make a prediction, one was not quantifiable, and the other two appeared to be partly achievable (Dishman 1988a).

Consequently, a revision of the 1990 objectives was made in a "midcourse review". New proposals (DHHS 1986) suggested that 36 exercise and fitness objectives should be stated for the year 2000. Of particular importance from the point of view of the psychological approach are the following two objectives (Dishman 1988a, p. 435): "By 2000, the relationship between participation in various types of physical activities during childhood and adolescence and the physical activity practices of adults will be known. ... By 2000, the behavioural skills associated with a high probability of adopting and maintaining a regular exercise programme will be known".

The latter objective, of course, is central to this book and will be addressed throughout. The objective dealing with the carry-over from childhood to adulthood is an important issue in need of further research and is discussed later (Chap. 10).

Position Statements

A number of position statements have emerged that address the issues of exercise and physical fitness, particularly with respect to children. This probably reflects the growing concern over the current levels of activity in children (Armstrong 1990).

One of the first statements, however, dealt with adults. The American College of Sports Medicine (ACSM 1978) produced the standard guidelines for the development of fitness in healthy adults. This has now been revised and extended into a new position paper (ACSM 1990). The ACSM is currently working on another statement concerning the amount of physical activity necessary to derive health benefits, since the 1990 statement is only about the development and maintenance of physical fitness. However, the statement is primarily a set of physiological guidelines and only makes passing reference to the need to identify factors that will maintain participation. As stated elsewhere in this book, such guidelines may be inappropriate for promoting adherence, at least in the initial stages of exercise. This requires further study, however. Nevertheless, the ACSM (1990) statement is comprehensive in its coverage for a paper of this type and is supported by 174 references.

The ACSM has also made a statement about the physical fitness of children and youths (see ACSM 1988 and Chap. 10 of this volume). There are eight specific recommendations, including the development of appropriate school programmes for physical education that emphasise lifetime exercise habits, enhanced knowledge about exercise, and positive behaviour change; the encouragement of a greater role in the development of their children's levels of activity by parents, community organisations and health-care professionals; the adoption of a scientifically sound approach to fitness testing in schools whereby the emphasis is placed on health-related aspects assessed in relation to acceptable criteria rather than normative comparison; and, finally, award schemes for fitness to encourage individual exercise behaviour and achievement rather than superior athletic ability (see Chaps 4 and 10).

A similar statement on children was issued by the English Sports Council, in conjunction with the Health Education Authority, and covered the topics of the physical growth and development of the child, promotion of health and prevention of disease, body weight, children with special needs, and ten recommendations for the future (Sports Council and Health Education Authority 1988). From the standpoint of this book, the most important recommendation was that more research was required on the development of effective strategies for promoting exercise habits in children. Currently, little is known about children and exercise from a psychological point of view, although a few studies are now emerging (see Dishman 1989; Dishman and Dunn 1988).

A position statement has also emerged from a joint working party of the British Association of Sports Sciences, the Health Education Authority, and the Physical Education Association of Great Britain and Northern Ireland. This working party produced a summary of consensus knowledge on children, physical activity and health and called for the new "national curriculum" in Britain, to support the role of health-related activity in physical education curricula in schools (Health-related physical activity in the National Curriculum 1990).

More comprehensive statements on exercise and health are now available. These include the workshop on epidemiologic and public health aspects of physical activity and exercise, arranged by the American Centres for Disease Control in 1984 and now published as a special issue of *Public Health Reports* (1985 vol. 100, issue 2); the National Institute of Mental Health workshop in 1984 which addressed the issue of the proposed relationship between exercise and mental health with a view to producing a consensus statement (see Morgan and Goldston 1987), and finally, the comprehensive volume stemming from the 1988 international conference in Toronto, Canada on exercise, fitness and health (Bouchard et al. 1990).

In summary, there is no shortage of guidance on aspects of physical activity, exercise and health, yet these statements are strongly oriented towards biological adaptation rather than long-term behaviour change. As argued elsewhere in this book, there is now a need to investigate the physiological guidelines for fitness and health in terms of the ability of humans to sustain such behaviour patterns.

Health-related Outcomes of Physical Activity, Exercise and Fitness

It is not the purpose of this section to give a comprehensive review of the health-related outcomes of physical activity as this can be found elsewhere (Bouchard et al. 1990). However, it is important to identify the links between physical activity and health that have been proposed recently. The relationship between activity, exercise and fitness will be discussed later.

Exercise and Chronic Disease

Coronary Heart Disease

Much of the literature dealing with the health outcomes of physical activity and exercise has been associated with chronic diseases and health risks such as coronary heart disease (CHD), diabetes, osteoporosis, and obesity.

Most interest, if the volume of research is indicative, has been focussed on the proposed link between the risk of CHD and physical activity. CHD is known to be a major health problem in many industrialised countries. For example, Barker and Rose (1990) report that in England and Wales CHD is the leading cause of mortality in males and females and is the condition leading to the second highest number of hospital admissions after cancers. Cardiovascular disorders rank second in terms of certified days lost at work. Countries of the United Kingdom are very high in the international league table for premature deaths from CHD, with 1985 estimates putting the total cost of CHD for the National Health Service at just under £400 000 000 (Wells 1987).

Powell et al. (1987) selected 43 studies having the criterion of sufficient data to calculate a relative risk or "odds ratio" for CHD at varying levels of physical activity. They concluded (Powell et al. 1987, italics added):

> The inverse association between physical activity and incidence of CHD is consistently observed, especially in the better designed studies; this association is appropriately sequenced, biologically graded, plausible and coherent with existing knowledge. Therefore, the observations reported in the literature support the inference that physical activity is inversely and *causally* related to the incidence of CHD.

The strength of their conviction about the nature of the CHD– activity relationship is noteworthy as this is the first time that such respected researchers have stated their belief that the relationship is causal. Indeed, more conservative researchers remain unconvinced of the power of this relationship and are reluctant to give physical inactivity more than the usual "secondary" risk factor status. However, Powell et al. (1987, p. 283) say "the relative risk of inactivity appears to be similar in magnitude to that of hypertension, hypercholesterolemia, and smoking".

The bulk of the evidence associating CHD and physical inactivity has been accumulated with epidemiological methods. These involve the quantification of health-related behaviours and disease in the population. Specifically, epidemiology attempts to establish the magnitude of the health problem, the causes and modes of transmission, the scientific basis for prevention, and evaluation of the effectiveness of preventive or curative measures (Caspersen 1989). The emergent field of "physical activity epidemiology" can now be identified (see Caspersen 1989; Paffenbarger 1988; Powell 1988; Walter and Hart 1990).

The initial CHD–physical activity studies investigated activity at work, with the studies of Morris in Britain and Paffenbarger in the USA forming the basis of a demonstrated link (see Morris et al. (1953, 1966); and Paffenbarger et al. (1978; 1986) for reports of specific epidemiological studies, and Morris et al. (1987), Paffenbarger (1988), Paffenbarger and Hyde (1988) and Paffenbarger et al. (1990) for recent reviews).

Although initial epidemiological studies can be criticised for problems of self-selection, as was the case with the early studies by Morris and co-workers, the establishment of a plausible cause–effect relationship is possible but requires a number of criteria to be satisfied first, such as temporal sequencing, consistency, specificity, and a dose–response relationship (see Paffenbarger 1988). The weight of evidence now appears to support such a relationship between physical inactivity and CHD risk. The mechanisms of such a relationship still remain open to debate, although the multifactorial nature of CHD risk suggests that exercise may be able to affect a number of these factors, including obesity, blood lipid profiles, and hypertension.

The nature and type of exercise necessary to affect CHD risk positively has also been debated. Morris's work has tended to support the notion that aerobic activity of a relatively vigorous nature (e.g., brisk walking, cycling etc) is the key to reduced CHD risk. He has suggested that the activity should be of the intensity requiring energy expenditure of 7.5 kcal/min sustained for three periods of 20 minutes per week. Alternatively, Paffenbarger and his coworkers stress total leisure-time energy expenditure rather than exercise intensity *per se*. Paffenbarger's study of Harvard alumni showed that those who expended less than 2000 kcal/week in leisure time were significantly more at risk of premature mortality from CHD than those who expended more than 2000 kcal/week (see Paffenbarger 1988; Paffenbarger et al. 1990).

These results question whether it is physical fitness developed through intense aerobic activity or habitual physical activity that is critical in the reduction of CHD risk. In reviewing his own studies, Morris et al. (1987, p. 15) concluded that:

> The main finding in the present studies is that habitual vigorous aerobic exercise for sustained periods, involving the movement of large muscle masses, is the only exercise factor which is consistently and substantially associated with a lower incidence of coronary heart disease. This type of exercise improves "physical fitness" and its principal components, aerobic power or $\dot{V}O_2$ max; and even more, aerobic capacity, stamina and endurance fitness, which means the capacity to function for prolonged periods at a high proportion of $\dot{V}O_2$ max whatever the level of that may be.

This summary suggests that Morris has some faith in the physical fitness hypothesis for CHD protection. However, his studies provided measures of activity rather than fitness, so his suggestion that fitness provides the protection for CHD has yet to be substantiated, at least in his research.

Although the epidemiological studies of both work and leisure-time activity and CHD tend to support the physical activity hypothesis, a large-scale prospective study of healthy men and women has supported the hypothesis that fitness is related to lowered CHD risk (Blair et al. 1989a). Specifically, Blair et al. (1989a) split their sample into five fitness categories based on scores on a maximal treadmill test. Age-adjusted all-cause death rates showed significantly greater risk for the lower fitness groups. This is illustrated in Fig. 1.2. where the higher fitness group (5) is represented by the relative risk of 1.0.

It appears, therefore, that both physical fitness (at least cardiovascular fitness) and habitual physical activity are inversely related to CHD risk in adults, although the magnitude of each remains to be determined. Fig. 1.3 depicts Cureton's (1987) model for the likely relationships between physical activity, cardiorespiratory fitness and health. Cureton (1987) recognises that while activities that increase cardiovascular fitness can also have health benefits, so could activities which do not result in a fitness gain. It should also be recognised that the lines in Fig. 1.3 do not represent causal links, but mere relationships. For example, the "link" between physical activity and cardiorespiratory fitness is problematic, particularly with children (see Armstrong et al. 1990b), due to the strong influence of heredity in cardiorespiratory fitness. However, Cureton (1987, p. 316) states:

> The distinction between health and physical fitness outcomes of exercise is a critical one, and it is important to conceptualise clearly the causal relationships among physical activity, cardiorespiratory fitness and health outcomes . . . Physical activity has been shown experimentally to directly affect both cardiorespiratory fitness and health outcomes (disease risk

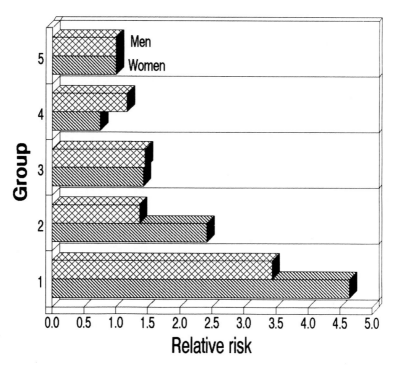

Figure 1.2. Relative risk for age-adjusted all-cause death rates per 10 000 person-years by physical fitness group, indicating the importance of low physical fitness as a risk factor (adapted from Blair et al. 1989a) Most fit group is the reference category with a relative risk of 1.0. All other groups are expressed in relation to this. (1 = low fitness group).

factors and other health behaviours). The mechanisms underlying these effects are undoubtedly different however.

Other Health Outcomes

Hypertension

Recent reviews suggest that exercise can favourably affect hypertension (Fentem et al. 1988; Hagberg 1990; Powell 1988). Specifically, moderate aerobic exercise can reduce diastolic and systolic blood pressures by about 10 mm Hg, although Powell (1988) reports lower values. Nevertheless, if such reductions were made in large sections of the population, significant public health benefits would accrue. The use of resistance training methods with hypertensives has usually been seen to be contra-indicated. However, recent evidence suggests that light resistance training may bring health

Figure 1.3. Proposed relationships between physical activity, cardiorespiratory fitness and health. (From Cureton (1987). Reprinted with permission from *Research Quarterly for Exercise and Sport*, 58: 316. *Research Quarterly* is a publication of the American Alliance for Health, Physical Education, Recreation and Dance, 1900, Association Drive, Reston, VA 22091, USA.)

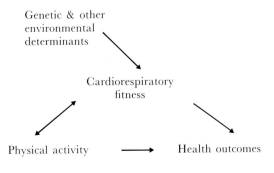

benefits to populations prone to cardiac and coronary disease, although there is little research in this area as yet (Goldberg 1989; Kelemen 1989; Stewart 1989). However, the issue of adherence to exercise among hypertensives requires further study (see Martin and Calfas 1989).

Obesity

Fentem et al. (1988) report that 7% of the adult population in the UK are severely obese. Apart from the known health risks of such obesity, it can present psychological problems for individuals in a society that values thinness. However, despite the apparently simple concept that body fat will be stored when energy consumption exceeds energy expenditure, the relationship between exercise and body fat is complex (Bray 1990; Fox 1991; Thompson et al. 1982). Nevertheless, the use of exercise in the control of levels of body fat is supported despite the small caloric expenditure associated with exercise in comparison with normal dietary intake (Bray 1990; Brownell and Stunkard 1980; Epstein and Wing 1980; Fentem et al. 1988; Garfinkel and Coscina 1990; Thompson et al. 1982). However, some researchers have argued that measurement of body composition has hindered progress in the assessment of weight control techniques (Eisenman 1986). For a comprehensive review of the techniques used in the assessment of body composition, see Brodie (1988).

Diabetes

The potential positive effects of exercise on diabetes are well documented (Fentem et al. 1988), although there are very few experimental studies which use exercise as an independent variable. In addition, the relationship between exercise and metabolic control is complex (Vranic and Wasserman 1990). Berg (1986) reports that even prior to the discovery of insulin in

1921, exercise was recommended in the treatment of diabetes. Indeed, the "treatment triad" of diet, insulin and exercise is a frequent term in protocols for the control of diabetes (Cantu 1982).

Diabetes is a metabolic disorder which may have its origins in childhood or adulthood. Type I (insulin-dependent) diabetes is less common than Type II (non-insulin-dependent), but exercise has potential benefits for both types. Berg (1986) identifies the following benefits: improved blood sugar control, reduced likelihood of hypoglycaemia during exercise, enhanced efficiency of fat metabolism, reduced requirement for insulin for Type I diabetics and reduced amount or elimination of insulin required to control blood sugar in Type II diabetics, and reduced body weight. Glucose tolerance decreases with increased age and obesity, and exercise has been shown to slow this effect (Fentem et al. 1988).

Osteoporosis

The excessive loss of mineral content in bone, often resulting in fractures, is the condition known as osteoporosis. It is common in older people, particularly women after the menopause. At this time, loss of bone mineral increases from about 1% per year to 2%–3% (Smith et al. 1990). Fentem et al. (1988) report that physical activity is correlated with bone density and that bone density can be improved with exercise. Weight-bearing activities, such as walking, are considered the most appropriate for reducing the risk of osteoporosis, although the optimal frequency and intensity of exercise for the prevention of osteoporotic fractures have not yet been determined (Smith et al. 1990). It is possible that severe training schedules experienced by athletes may actually increase the likelihood of osteoporosis. For example, Harrison and Chow (1990) report that women marathon runners are at increased risk of amenorrhea. Evidence suggests that such women have lower bone mass and are more likely to suffer stress fractures. Clearly, more research is required on the optimal quantity of exercise for osteoporosis.

Low Back Pain

It has been reported that over 80% of adults will suffer from back pain at some time in their lives, although only about 10% will seek medical attention. Approximately 10% of certified days of absence from work in England and Wales in 1982/3 were attributed to back pain, and the annual cost to the National Health Service has been estimated at over £150 000 000 (Wells 1985).

Despite the widespread recommendation of improving the strength, endurance and flexibility of muscles for the prevention of low back pain and the rehabilitation of sufferers (e.g. Patton et al. 1986), there is little evidence that muscle fitness prevents this problem (Nachemson 1990;

Powell 1988). Nevertheless, there is evidence of a weak relationship between a generally healthy lifestyle, including moderate exercise of the lumbar region of the spine, and lack of pain in the lower back (Nachemson 1990). Usually, exercises that improve the strength and flexibility of muscles of the pelvic girdle are recommended although more research is required to assess their beneficial effect across different conditions of low back pain.

Immune Function

The relationship between exercise and all-cause mortality has been demonstrated by Paffenbarger et al. (1986). Although the clearest evidence for a relationship between mortality and low levels of physical activity and exercise is for CHD, there is some evidence linking low levels of exercise with cancer. However, the complexities of the numerous forms and aetiologies of cancers provides researchers with a difficult problem in identifying any clear links with exercise. Nevertheless, Calabrese (1990) reports that an inverse relationship has been identified between exercise and cancer of the colon, although a number of methodological problems exist.

Linked with the cancer and exercise issue is the wider concern for the relationship between immune function and physical activity (Calabrese 1990; Mackinnon 1989). Although plausible hypotheses can be stated for a positive link between activity and enhanced immune function, such as the effect of exercise on lowering levels of stress from emotional causes, Calabrese (1990, p. 577) concludes that although exercise and immune function may or may not be related "it appears premature to discount totally the role of immunologic adaptation from exercise and training in altering host defences to infections for malignancies".

Mental Health

The link between exercise and mental health has been supported, if only anecdotally, for centuries. However, only recently have data been accumulated on the complex processes involved. This subject is discussed at some length in Chaps 6, 7 and 8.

Risks of Exercise

Although the evidence supports quite clearly the generally beneficial health effects of exercise, there are some aspects of physical activity and exercise that may be contra-indicated for some groups, or situations in which a particular health risk is elevated during exercise.

The most commonly cited risks of exercise are sudden cardiac death and musculoskeletal injury (Siscovick 1990). Although the risk of sudden cardiac death is elevated during exercise, the balance of cardiac benefit and risk as a result of being an exerciser is positive. Siscovick et al. (1984) reported that men who exercised vigorously for more than 20 min each week had an overall risk of primary cardiac arrest only 40% of their sedentary counterparts. It appears, therefore, that the temporary rise in risk during exercise is outweighed by the long-term effects of exercise on cardiac risk.

Koplan et al. (1985) report that knowledge on the musculoskeletal risks of exercise is not extensive, although clinical studies have been conducted on swimming, running, cycling, calisthenics and racket sports and have identified a number of injuries. Epidemiological methods have not generally been employed until more recently. For example, Blair et al. (1987a) reported three population studies on the rates of running injuries. In their first study, Blair et al. found that 24% of runners reported an injury during the previous year and the rate increased with body weight and weekly distance run. In their second study, they compared runners with non-runners at a preventive medicine clinic and found that only knee injuries were significantly higher in runners. Finally, a worksite population study found that risk of injury was associated with a number of factors, including increased age and body mass index.

Koplan et al. (1985) suggest that a lack of agreement on the risks of exercise to musculoskeletal integrity is hampered by a lack of clear definitions, poor characterisation of subgroups in studies, lack of control subjects, selection bias, a lack of a time perspective, and a lack of risk–benefit comparisons.

Some mental health problems have been identified with exercise, such as eating disorders or dependence on exercise. These are discussed more fully in Chaps 6, 7 and 8.

Participation Patterns in Exercise

The proposed health outcomes of physical activity suggest that considerable public health benefits could be achieved with the adoption and maintenance of appropriate exercise habits, although some risks are also evident. However, the impact on public health is dependent on the number of people taking part. The identification of participation patterns is important in any effort to plan public health initiatives in exercise.

The problems in determining the activity levels of the population should not be underestimated. The measurement of physical activity becomes less reliable as techniques more suited to large-scale surveys are used. In a review of physical activity assessment in epidemiological research, LaPorte et al. (1985) identified over 30 different techniques. For large-scale population-based research, however, the use of some variation on survey recall of activity is inevitable. However, physiological indicators, such as heart rate, can be measured in smaller samples and have been used with success with children (see Armstrong 1990).

The estimates of activity levels of the population, therefore, will partly be dependent on the method used. Similarly, the criteria defining the quantification of "activity" are likely to be inversely related to the activity levels reported. In other words, the more stringent the criterion adopted for classifying people as "active", the fewer people will be classified as active. This accounts for Stephens et al.'s (1985) finding, in their analysis of eight national leisure-time physical activity surveys, that estimates of physical activity levels in the population varied from 15% to 78%. They concluded, however, that in North America approximately 20% of the population take part in leisure-time physical activity of sufficient intensity and frequency that cardiovascular benefits are likely to result, while 40% may be considered to be sedentary. The other 40% would appear to be moderately or intermittently active, with the possibility of some health benefits. These figures are supported by the British survey of over 9000 adults conducted by Cox et al. (1987).

The problem with statistics such as those produced by Stephens et al. (1985) is that the health/fitness benefits are usually stated in terms of cardiovascular fitness only. Other forms of exercise, such as lifting or stretching, have been known to have health-related benefits, but are often more difficult to quantify.

Stephens (1987) investigated whether North American adults are more active now than they were in the past. He used three sources of data: national probability surveys, national non-probability surveys, and trend data on leisure-time physical activity indicators, such as the purchase of sports and exercise magazines and sports equipment. In his conclusion, he stated (p. 102) "that there are no truly satisfactory statistical sources for judging trends in adult leisure-time activity". However, despite the methodological problems encountered, he concluded that there had been an increase in activity during the 1970s and 1980s, and identified the following factors: (a) women had increased activity levels more than men, (b) adults over 50 years of age had increased activity more than younger adults, and (c) the increase in activity is not confined to low or moderately intense activities. It was also reported that the following findings were "suspected": (a) the rate of increase was most pronounced in the 1970s, (b) some activities had seen a decline in participation, (c) the trend towards greater activity can be traced back to the 1960s, and (d) the more vigorous activities, such as jogging, had shown the greatest increase in participation.

In response to Stephens (1987), Ramlow et al. (1987) suggested that it was also important to consider the full "epidemiologic spectrum" of physical activity since they argued that Stephens had failed to take into account the changing patterns of activity that occur with disability and/or ageing. Demographic trends show an increase in the proportion of old people in society. Similarly, they show that the number of "activity limited" individuals (e.g., diseased, disabled, obese) has increased in the USA from just over 20% in 1966 to over 30% in 1981. Ramlow et al. (1987, p. 113) conclude by saying: "If it were possible to take the 14% of the US population who have impaired activity and raise their activity levels *up* to that of sedentary white collar workers, this very likely would have greater public health impact than attempting to transform sedentary workers into 10K [kilometre] runners".

This is an important statement about the measurement of physical activity in population studies. The whole epidemiological spectrum must be considered. However, to date the majority of data come from North America. The "National Fitness Survey", launched in England in 1990, should go some way to redressing this imbalance.

Evidence on the physical activity patterns of British children is now emerging. Armstrong et al. (1990a) studied the continuous heart rate of 266 children aged 11–16 years over 12-h periods on three consecutive weekdays and one Saturday. The measurements of heart rate do not provide a direct measure of physical activity but one of relative stress placed on the cardiopulmonary system.

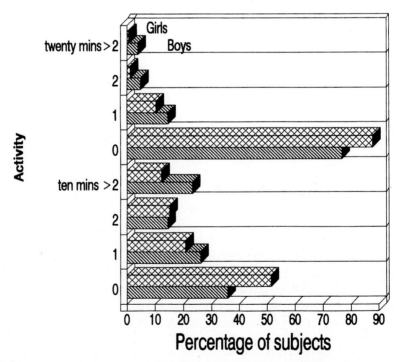

Figure 1.4. Number of sustained periods of heart rate above 139 beats/min during weekday monitoring of boys and girls. (Armstrong et al. 1990a.)

The results showed that the children experienced few sustained periods of vigorous physical activity. Fig. 1.4 shows the number of 10- and 20-min periods of heart rate above 139 beats/min for weekdays. As can be seen, few children have high levels of activity, and the girls are less active than the boys.

Conclusion

This chapter has introduced the topics of physical activity, exercise, fitness and health. Background information on definitions, interrelationships, exercise and chronic disease, and activity patterns is important in setting the scene for the psychological concepts that follow. Physical activity is a biological process although, as will be argued in the rest of this book, it is influenced by a multitude of biological and non-biological factors, and the basic concepts of activity and health therefore require a biological perspective to achieve some context.

The current opinion is that appropriate physical activity can have significant health benefits for all sectors of the population. The rest of this book will consider a number of psychological factors likely to influence the participation of individuals in this particular health-related behaviour, as well as the likely psychological outcomes from exercise.

Section B

PSYCHOLOGICAL ANTECEDENTS OF EXERCISE

2

Exercise Adoption and Maintenance

The evidence presented in Chap. 1 shows that appropriate physical activity can have beneficial effects on physical and mental health. However, these benefits are, of course, dependent on the extent to which an individual adheres to the appropriate behaviour that is thought (or known) to bring about such effects. Unfortunately, the evidence suggests that people do not adhere to health-related behaviours very well, and that physical exercise is no exception. Consequently, the issue of adherence to exercise programmes, as well as less structured "free-living" physical activity, is an important one if the health benefits of exercise are to be achieved by larger numbers of people.

Adherence in Medical Settings

The initial research work into adherence and health-related behaviours centred on measuring the ability of patients to comply with a prescribed medical treatment, such as a course of tablets or attendance at a treatment centre. This has been referred to as "secondary prevention" (Benfari et al. 1981). In addition, researchers have been interested in the adherence rates to behaviours that are associated with risk reduction rather than disease management or cure. This is "primary prevention" (Benfari et al. 1981) and may be a more relevant perspective for the exercise scientist, although there are cases of exercise being used in secondary prevention, such as in coronary rehabilitation programmes.

Benfari et al. (1981) suggest that the two perspectives (primary and secondary) present different situations as far as adherence is concerned.

For example, it could be argued that the responsibility for behaviour change in a primary, risk-reduction situation resides more with the individual, whereas curative, secondary regimes may be perceived more as being controlled by someone else, such as a physician.

Although this distinction may indeed be important, it is more difficult to assess adherence to a health-related behaviour that has been adopted freely by an individual without any intervention from a health professional. When such individuals are assessed, self-report estimates of adherence are often exaggerated.

The medical literature has reported relatively low adherence across a number of settings, and this includes people being treated for potentially dangerous diseases. Usually, fewer than half the patients adhere to the prescription for 80% of the time, although the range of adherence rates can be quite large (Mathews and Steptoe 1988).

Recognition of the Problem

Many of the recently published public health documents have stated aims and objectives that are behavioural, as well as physiological, in nature. For example, the American Department of Health and Human Services (DHHS 1980) health objectives for the USA for 1990 have shown poor adherence rates. A subsequent review, discussed in Chap. 1, has shown that only two of the 11 physical fitness and exercise objectives are likely to be met in the projected time span (see Dishman 1988a; Powell et al. 1986). One of the new objectives set for the year 2000 is that the skills required for an increased probability of adopting and maintaining a regular exercise programme will be identified.

The purpose of this chapter, therefore, is to look at the psychological factors related to participation in health-related exercise with particular reference to the adoption and maintenance of exercise behaviours. What do we currently understand about the psychological correlates or determinants of exercise adoption and maintenance and what do we need to know for more effective planning and intervention? This chapter will discuss motivational issues, including participation motives and reasons for drop-out, self-motivation and other personality variables, reinforcement in exercise and behaviour modification studies, the influence of group exercise settings, and the assessment of exercise adherence. Although it is recognised that factors influencing the *adoption* of exercise may differ from those influencing *maintenance* (Dishman et al. 1985), both will be discussed in this chapter. Differences will be highlighted, however, where research suggests this is necessary.

A number of more detailed theoretical models that could help in the understanding and explanation of the adoption and maintenance of exercise are discussed in subsequent chapters, as well as applied intervention strategies for both individuals and organisations.

Motivation, Participation and Drop-out

To state that "motivation" is an important part of exercise adherence might appear to be stating the obvious. However, the psychological study of motivational processes is vast. This necessitates knowing more precisely which motivational factors are likely to be important and how they may be influential.

Descriptive Approaches to Participation and Drop-out

Participation Motives

One of the simplest forms of analysis has been to ask exercisers why they participate. This method, while having potentially high ecological validity, has some difficulties and the results are likely not to generalise very well across activities. This is because the reasons stated may be highly specific to the activity chosen or be related to environmental and/or life-cycle factors. Research on participation motivation has also rarely tested for response bias. The specificity of motives stated may have greater ecological validity if they refer to "free-living" activity rather than structured exercise programmes. Dishman (1987) is also critical of using self-report data in isolation, without examining how they interact with other factors. For example, an individual may express strongly positive intentions to exercise for reasons of fitness and health yet have environmental factors which work equally strongly against him or her being able to exercise.

British data have not been widely reported in the published literature whereas North American studies of children's sport motives are more familiar to psychologists interested in sport and exercise (Gould and Horn 1984). However, Heartbeat Wales (1987) have reported figures suggesting that health-related reasons are important for "taking up sport". The use of the word "sport" may be a problem here, as it may be perceived by respondents to exclude non-competitive leisure-time physical activities, such as jogging and other "fitness" pursuits. Nevertheless, the figures do suggest that fitness, weight loss and general health maintenance are important incentives. Summary data are shown in Fig. 2.1.

The Canada Fitness Survey (1983a) data also support the view that reasons for being active are strongly health-related. Of the Canadian adults asked, 60% reported that to "feel better" was a "very important" reason for being active (see Fig. 2.2).

Clough et al. (1988) investigated the motives of nearly 500 participants

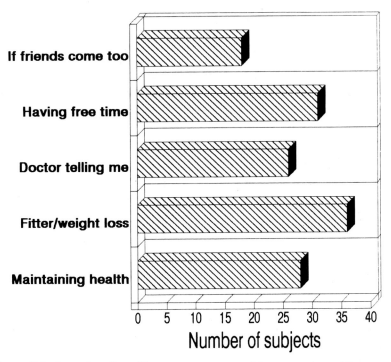

Figure 2.1. Incentives for taking up sport reported by respondents 16 years and older in Wales. (Adapted from Heartbeat Wales 1987.)

in a marathon in Scotland. A questionnaire included 70 reasons for running, from which six factors were derived by means of a factor analysis. These factors were named: well-being, social, challenge, status, addiction and health/fitness.

Challenge, health/fitness and well-being were found to have the greatest influence on running behaviour in this sample. Clough et al. (1988) suggest that these clusters of motives are very similar to motivations that are central to other leisure pursuits, as illustrated in Fig. 2.3. In particular, well-being, social, challenge, and status are common motives for taking up and maintaining leisure pursuits. However, this study did not identify whether these motives were related solely to maintaining participation or whether they also were influential in starting running.

An investigation by Barrell et al. (1988) did try to separate reasons for starting running and reasons for taking part. Their study of British non-elite runners revealed eight main motivation factors for taking part in a half or full marathon. These were: personal challenge, personal satisfaction, physical fitness, enjoyment, curiosity, family and friends, media, and charity. The factors identified with taking up running for the first time were: challenge, physical fitness, to feel better, enjoyment, to lose weight,

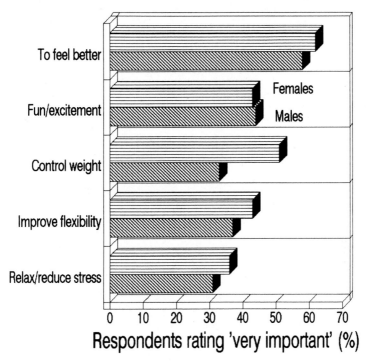

Figure 2.2. Percentage of males and females in Canada strongly supporting selected "reasons for being active". (Adapted from Canada Fitness Survey 1983a.)

to train for other sports, and family and friends. Although there are some differences here, the results showed that runners had very similar reasons for taking up the activity in the first place and for entering a structured running event. Overall, the strongest factors in taking up running were challenge, fitness, and to feel better and the strongest factors for entering a half or full marathon event were challenge, satisfaction, and fitness.

These results from British surveys are similar to one reported in Australia (Summers et al. 1983). In their survey of a sample of participants from the 1980 Melbourne marathon, they found that participants reported that physical fitness, feelings of achievement, challenge, feeling better and enjoyment were strongly felt outcomes from running, whereas the main reasons for attempting a marathon were challenge and achievement. Negative consequences were also perceived, especially having less free time, disrupting family commitments, and suffering physical injury or muscle soreness.

Biddle and Bailey (1985) investigated single-sex exercise classes in England and found men reporting participation motives that strongly reflected health and fitness whereas women strongly endorsed cathartic and social factors. This could partly reflect the activity classes themselves

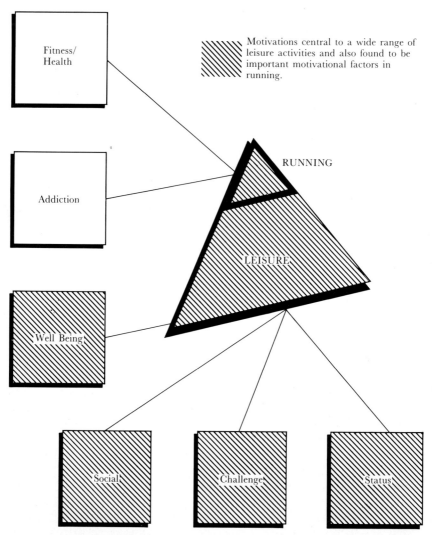

Figure 2.3. Motivations for running in the context of leisure motivation. (From Clough et al. 1988; reprinted with permission.)

and the nature of exercises offered, which differed between the two groups. Similarly, female participants in the Melbourne marathon study were also found to have higher social/affiliation motives than males (Summers et al. 1983).

Ashford and Biddle (1990), in a survey of community sports centres in an English city, found that males were significantly more motivated towards excellence, aggression, achievement, competition, skill learning, and excitement than females, although these differences were attenuated with age. For example, participants over 25 years of age were much more likely to report motives associated with health and relaxation than were younger subjects.

In short, participation motives for exercise appear to be diverse but certainly include physical fitness and well-being. However, the reply is dependent on the degree of introspection of the respondent (Shephard 1985). It is also likely to be related to the time of questioning such that the reasons for adopting exercise may change with time as the respondent's experience of exercise develops. The distinction between exercise *adoption* and *maintenance*, therefore, may be an important one and has been made by authors in the past. For example, Dishman et al. (1985) suggest that while health factors may be important in the *initiation* of an exercise programme, they are unlikely to *sustain* involvement. Adherence may be related to more immediate sensations of enjoyment and well-being. This will be discussed in more detail later, but suffice it to say here that exercise promoters have a problem in keeping people involved until such time that more pleasurable reinforcers are evident. Initial bouts of exercise, however well planned and carefully monitored, can sometimes create feelings of discomfort, stiffness and embarrassment.

Ceasing Participation

Dropping out of exercise may not be an "all or none" phenomenon but a process that may change throughout the life cycle (Collins 1987; Sonstroem 1988), yet the most commonly cited reasons for quitting are lack of time and inconvenience, although no evidence has been produced that demonstrates exercise drop-outs have any less time than adherers (Shephard 1985).

Gould (1987) summarises the reasons for withdrawal from childrens' sport programmes as conflicts of interest, lack of playing time, lack of success, limited improvement in skills, lack of fun, boredom, and injury. Competitive stress and dislike of the coach have also been cited as reasons.

Most of the research into withdrawal from physical activity has tended to focus on sport settings, and in particular on children (see Gould 1987, Gould and Horn 1984). However, Lee and Owen (1985a) studied the reasons why people discontinued physical activity after a structured aerobic fitness course. Over 50% of participants (n = 193) ceased participation and they yielded 287 reasons for discontinuing their involvement. The major reasons appeared to be time constraints, medical problems, such as injury or illness, being unmotivated or lazy, and situational/practical factors such as expense, travelling distance and class times.

Although gender differences have been reported (Ashford and Biddle 1990; Biddle and Bailey 1985), this is not invariably so. This is likely to depend on other factors too. However, Canada Fitness Survey (1983a) did find that women were more likely to state that their reasons for being active were related to weight control, flexibility, relaxation, companionship and "doctor's orders" than men, whereas men were more likely to be interested in activity as a way of challenging their abilities.

Of equal importance to gender differences is the way motives and reasons for drop-out may vary as a function of stage of the life cycle. Mihalik et al. (1989) studied the extent to which participation in sport "expanded" and "contracted" across the life-span. Using data from the 1983 Nationwide Recreation Survey in the United States (n = 6720), Mihalik et al. (1989) were particularly interested in the extent to which participation in sports activities across the life-span were marked by "deletion" (contraction) or "addition" (expansion). The results showed that in the expansion category an increase was found for the 18–21- and 22–28-year-old groups whereas a decrease was found for the 29–36-year-olds. The middle years showed an increase in the rate of deletion but this was reversed after age 51 years. In short, the life-cycle stages, such as early family commitments and grown children leaving home, may be important factors in the decision to adopt, maintain or cease participation.

Boothby et al. (1981) also investigated reasons for ceasing participation in sports activities. They conducted in-depth interviews with 254 adults in the north-east of England and used the technique of content analysis to cluster the numerous reasons reported for ceasing participation into fewer categories. Their results showed that from over 1000 activities reported, more than 80% of respondents had given up at least one sports activity. There were 815 separate reasons for quitting, which were reduced to 43 main types of reasons. The most frequently cited categories were loss of interest, lack of facilities, physical problems (such as lack of fitness or disability), leaving a youth organisation, moving away from the area, and not having spare time. In short, the reasons reflected either some aspects of the individual (e.g., disability) or a change in the relationship between the individual and the environment (e.g., change in social networks).

Comparisons of Adherers and Drop-outs

A number of studies have attempted to differentiate exercise adherers from non-adherers on the basis of psychological and other variables (see Dishman 1987, 1988a). For example, data from the Ontario Exercise Heart Collaborative Study showed that adherence to a post-coronary exercise programme was related to the convenience of the exercise facility, perceptions of the exercise programme, and family/lifestyle factors (Andrew and Parker 1979, Andrew et al. 1981). In particular, spouse support was a significant predictor of adherence.

One of the earliest attempts to characterise the exercise "drop-out" was reported by Massie and Shephard (1971). They found that both physiological and psychological factors at entry to a fitness programme differed between adherers and drop-outs such that drop-outs tended to be overweight, but stronger, were more likely to smoke (a finding supported by Andrew et al. 1981), and were more extroverted. Other studies have also reported physiological differences between adherers and drop-outs at entry to a programme, and factors such as muscle fibre type (Ingjer and Dahl 1979), functional capacity (Blumenthal et al. 1982), and body composition (Dishman 1981) have been significant. In all cases the most likely explanation is that biological factors which make exercise a more difficult (or less reinforcing) experience will predict drop-out. For example, exercisers with greater amounts of body fat will experience more discomfort in exercise, and may also experience some embarrassment.

A Psychobiological Model

Perhaps the most widely cited study of the discriminating power of physiological and psychological variables in predicting adherence to exercise is that of Dishman and Gettman (1980). In this study the researchers investigated the predictive utility of both psychological and biological variables in a prospective design. A 20-week exercise programme was used whereby all subjects were assessed at entry on a variety of psychological measures, including self-motivation ("Self-Motivation Inventory" (SMI); Dishman et al. 1980; Dishman and Ickes 1981) (the SMI will be discussed in more detail later in this chapter), physical activity attitudes (Kenyon 1968), health locus of control (Wallston and Wallston 1978) and physical estimation and attraction (Sonstroem 1978). Biological variables assessed were metabolic capacity (predicted oxygen consumption), body weight and percentage body fat.

The results reported by Dishman and Gettman (1980) showed that both psychological and biological factors predicted adherence after 20 weeks. This led the authors to propose a "psychobiological model" of adherence. Specifically, adherers and drop-outs could be significantly discriminated from each other on the basis of body fat, self-motivation and body weight. Further analysis showed that just under 80% overall (81.4% for adherers and 73.9% for drop-outs) could be classified correctly as adherers or drop-outs based on their scores on these three variables. A multiple regression analysis showed that these factors accounted for 45% of the variance in adherence.

A partial replication of the Dishman and Gettman (1980) study was carried out by Ward and Morgan (1984) who studied 100 men and women in a prospective investigation over 32 weeks of an exercise programme. Complete data were provided by 76 subjects on seven biological variables: height, weight, blood pressure, per cent body fat, flexibility, muscular endurance, and aerobic capacity. In addition, assessment was made of self-motivation and mood (Profile of Mood States; McNair et al. 1971).

Ward and Morgan (1984) analysed the adherence patterns at three time periods: 10, 20 and 32 weeks. After 32 weeks they tested the accuracy of predicting adherence with the regression equation developed by Dishman and Gettman (1980). The overall prediction accuracy was 71% for adherers and 25% for drop-outs, showing that the psychobiological model held up quite well for adherers but not for drop-outs. Using discriminant analysis, Ward and Morgan could accurately classify 76% of subjects as adherers or drop-outs at 10 weeks, and 75% at 20 and 32 weeks. The nature of the discriminating variables did change for each time period, supporting the notion of adherence as a *process* rather than an "all-or-none" phenomenon (Sonstroem 1988). SMI scores were not significant discriminators between adherers and drop-outs at any of the three time periods in the Ward and Morgan (1984) study, however.

Although a psychobiological model retains some intuitive appeal, it has not been possible to support it fully since the Dishman and Gettman (1980) research. While psychological and physiological variables may interact to predict participation, which variables become important may differ across exercise settings. For example, adherence to a high-intensity aerobic endurance programme is likely to require high self-motivation and favourable physiological factors such as a high percentage of Type I ("slow twitch") muscle fibres and a low body fat score. However, this may not be true for other exercise regimes or habitual physical activity of a "free-living", unstructured nature. Similarly, the psychobiological model was only developed on 66 subjects and is, therefore, in need of validation with larger and more diverse samples (Sonstroem 1988).

Perceived Benefits and Barriers

The research reported on exercise adherence so far has centred on perceptions of the benefits of exercise and barriers to exercise. However, until recently, studies have been handicapped by a lack of consistent measurement technology. Sechrist et al. (1987) and Steinhardt and Dishman (1989) have recently developed, independently, psychometric scales for the measurement of exercise barriers and benefits.

Initial psychometric work by Steinhardt and Dishman (1989) revealed through factor analysis that the three major factors representing exercise benefits were "psychologic", "body image", and "health". Competition, fun and social factors were also identified when a second sample was analysed. Factors representing barriers were time, effort, obstacles, and "limiting health". Not all of these factors were robust across student and worksite samples. However, for the students, subscales significantly predicted supervised running and free-living physical activity at several time intervals. Similarly, the scales, in conjunction with socio-demographic data, predicted membership and participation in a worksite health/fitness programme. Unfortunately, analyses were not reported separately for each gender. One might expect gender differences, and this requires further investigation. The same criticism can be levelled at the Sechrist et al. (1987) study.

In a similar psychometric exercise, Sechrist et al. (1987) found that responses of 650 adults on barriers and benefits of exercise formed five factors on benefits and four on barriers. The benefit factors were labelled life enhancement, physical performance, psychological outlook, social interaction and preventive health, whereas the barriers were labelled exercise milieu, time expenditure, physical exertion, and family encouragement. The scales of Steinhardt and Dishman (1989) and Sechrist et al. (1987) now require further testing with diverse samples. However, so far they do seem to reflect the reported outcomes and barriers from descriptive epidemiological surveys such as the Canada Fitness Survey (1983a).

Personality and Individual Difference Factors

One approach to the study of exercise adherence has been to attempt to identify stable characteristics of the exerciser. Although some studies have found that certain personality variables distinguish between adherers and non-adherers (Blumenthal et al. 1982; Massie and Shephard 1971; Young and Ismail 1977), there remains a lack of consistency across studies. However, the notion that a persistent, committed or self-motivated individual will be more likely to persevere with exercise, particularly more intense forms, holds intuitive appeal.

Self-motivation

Dishman and his co-workers have reported research which suggests that "self-motivation" is an important factor in adherence (see Dishman and Gettman 1980, Dishman et al. 1980; Dishman and Ickes 1981). Initial psychometric research led to the development of the "Self-Motivation Inventory" (SMI), a 40-item questionnaire measuring (Dishman 1982, p. 242) "a generalised, nonspecific tendency to persist in habitual behaviour regardless of extrinsic reinforcement and is thus largely independent of situational influence".

Although the SMI was found to correlate with social desirability and ego-strength, a study investigating adherence to a rowing training programme demonstrated that the SMI score was the most important in terms of predicting adherence, and did so independently of social desirability and ego-strength. Similarly, Dishman and Gettman (1980), as already reported, found that self-motivation was a clear discriminator between exercise adherers and drop-outs.

Recent British data on the SMI has been reported by Robertson and Mutrie (1989). They contacted 110 subjects who had previously taken a fitness assessment at Glasgow University. A postal questionnaire was sent out five months after this initial assessment, and this questionnaire included the SMI. Non-adherers were classified as those who were no longer exercising for three sessions of 20 min per week. Only the SMI results will be reported here.

For females who returned the questionnaire (n = 36, 17 of whom were non-adherers), adherers had a significantly higher score (m = 142.4, sd = 15.5) than non-adherers (m = 125.7, sd = 11.7, $p < 0.05$), as predicted by previous research (Dishman and Gettman 1980). However, the trend was reversed for males with adherers (m = 126.7, sd = 12.7) scoring lower on the SMI than non-adherers (m = 135.1, sd = 21.1), although the difference was not significant (see Fig. 2.4). One explanation for these results could be the high variability of the data although why such variability occurred is not known. More needs to be known about the way the SMI is interpreted by people from outside the American culture.

Wankel et al. (1985) tested the utility of the SMI and motivational interventions in predicting adherence to exercise. In their first study, Wankel et al. (1985) investigated the singular and combined effects of self-motivation and a decision-balance sheet technique on adherence. The decision-balance sheet technique involves participants listing the anticipated

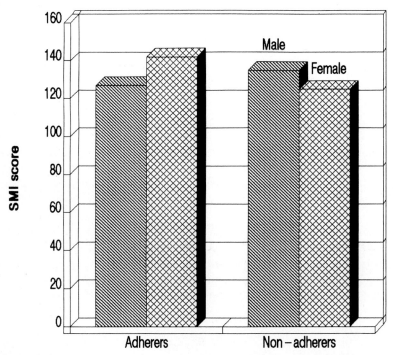

Figure 2.4. Self-motivation scores of males and females reported by Robertson and Mutrie (1989).

gains and losses of involvement in an activity programme and has been successful in helping people to maintain activity levels (Wankel and Thompson 1977). Fifty-two adult females volunteering for a community fitness programme were studied. The SMI was administered to all subjects and two groups were then created: "high" and "low" self-motivation (split either side of the mean score). Subjects were paired on the basis of SMI score similarity and then allocated either to a control or to an experimental group. The experimental intervention was the decision-balance sheet procedure. Attendance over three classes was studied and used as the dependent variable in a 2 (high/low SMI) by 2 (treatment/control) design. The results are illustrated in Fig. 2.5.

Results showed a significant effect for treatment such that the experimental subjects' attendances were significantly better than those of the controls. There was no significant effect for self-motivation or a significant interaction between SMI and the interventions.

A follow-up study by Wankel et al. (1985) used a similar design. This time they assessed 186 females enrolled on an aerobic dance programme. After administration of the SMI three groups were created: high, medium and low self-motivation groups. The motivational treatment in this study was "structured social support material". This consisted of a booklet

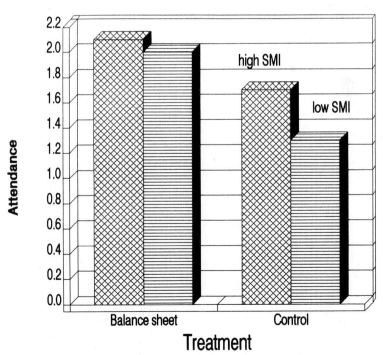

Figure 2.5. Self-motivation, decision-balance sheet intervention and adherence, with maximum possible attendance being 3. (Adapted from Wankel et al. 1985, study I.)

outlining a variety of information and strategies relevant to adherence and motivation, and subjects were also given personal attendance and social support charts for self-monitoring. As before, only half the subjects in each of the SMI groups received the experimental intervention, thus creating six groups in a 3 (SMI group) by 2 (treatment/control) design. The dependent variable was attendance over the final nine weeks of a ten-week class. The results are shown in Fig. 2.6.

Results revealed a trend for social support (p < 0.06) but not for SMI (p > 0.05). There was no significant interaction.

Wankel et al.'s data, therefore, suggest that short-term adherence rates appear to be unaffected by self-motivation. This conclusion is not surprising nor is it a necessary criticism of the self-motivation construct. It is quite likely that if self-motivation does exist, particularly as a relatively permanent trait, it will be influential in predicting long-term adherence rather than attendance over a few sessions, as used by Wankel et al. (1985). Indeed, the initial validation of the SMI used a 32-week period. One could argue that the first study reported by Wankel et al. uses a time period (3 exercise sessions) that is not particularly meaningful. Adherence (or mere attendance) will be influenced by many possible factors unrelated to motivation. The motivational interventions reported were successful and reflect the utility

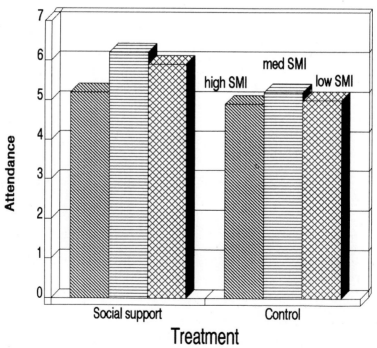

Figure 2.6. Self-motivation, social support material and adherence, with maximum possible attendance being 9. (Adapted from Wankel et al. 1985, study II.)

of such approaches to adherence. However, the effects were relatively weak and require investigating over longer time periods.

Olson and Zanna (1982), in a descriptive study of adherers and drop-outs from Canadian fitness clubs over a three-month period, found that adherers had significantly higher SMI scores than occasional attenders or drop-outs.

Self-motivation, and the use of the SMI, remains an intuitively appealing area of adherence. However, although the results may appear to be equivocal as to the importance of self-motivation in exercise, it is likely that environmental factors also need to be considered. Despite the original definition suggesting that self-motivation was "largely independent of situational influence" (Dishman 1982, p. 242), the effects for self-motivation are likely to be seen when the situation is relatively unfavourable from a motivational perspective and few extrinsic motivators are in evidence. This requires testing in a longitudinal design extending the methodology of Ward and Morgan (1984) who studied adherence at different time intervals.

In her cogent review of behavioural management techniques in exercise, Knapp (1988, p. 220) suggests that the exact nature of the behavioural tendency to persevere is not clearly defined but "it may be useful to hypothesise that self-motivation is a learned set of skills and habitual responses that function to assist individuals to adhere to activities that are not adequately cued and reinforced by the environment or that may even be punished".

Knapp goes on to suggest, as proposed in the preceding discussion, that the influence of self-motivation "is thus more likely to be observed in situations where cuing and reinforcement are not sufficient by themselves to maintain a behaviour to which an individual is committed".

Similarly, if self-motivation, as measured by the SMI, is a relatively stable, yet socially learned, trait (Dishman 1987), more needs to be known about how such a trait is learned, to what extent it can be modified, and how it changes over the life cycle.

Apart from the initial papers reporting the SMI (Dishman et al. 1980; Dishman and Ickes 1981), there has been little psychometric validation of the instrument. Heiby et al. (1987), however, report cross-validation data, obtained by using male and female members of a marathon club. They found that SMI scores were positively correlated with self-reports of prior exercise experience. They also found that those with high SMI scores also tended to employ self-reinforcement/reward strategies more often. However, the correlations from these analyses were modest.

Another methodological issue associated with the SMI is that of its factor structure. Dishman and Ickes (1981) report 10 factors extracted from an analysis of the responses of 401 subjects. Although each of the factors had a moderate to high internal consistency, the total scale had a very high internal consistency ($\alpha = 0.91$), thus suggesting that one common factor also underpinned the entire questionnaire – i.e., self-motivation. Nevertheless, future studies might fruitfully investigate the factor structure of the SMI and the possibility of particular factors being more important than others in the exercise adherence process. The 10 factors identified by Dishman and Ickes (1981) were effort commitment, goal striving, reliability and dependability, diligence, lethargy and laziness, apathy, perseverance and persistence, determination, willpower, and organisation. Our own preliminary investigations of a modified SMI for children have revealed factors pertaining to laziness, challenge and achievement, and effort. However, further psychometric work is required before one can understand the nature of self-motivation in children. Preliminary use of the modified scale found that it was not predictive of habitual physical activity levels in children (Biddle and Armstrong 1990b).

Finally, although the SMI has been used primarily to predict adherence to supervised or structured exercise programmes, little is known about its role in unsupervised or habitual "free-living" activity. Dishman and Steinhardt (1988), however, did report significant ($p < 0.05$) correlations between SMI scores and self-administered 7-day recall of physical activity ($r = 0.33$ and 0.25) and a 7-day diary ($r = 0.19$ and 0.42) in two American college samples. Further work along these lines is required, particularly in finding out how self-motivation may be related to different forms of exercise in "free-living" contexts. This should be a research priority, given that the greatest public health benefits from exercise are likely to come from increased activity levels beyond the confines of fitness clubs and other supervised settings.

Exercise Commitment

A related construct to self-motivation is that of "commitment". Carmack and Martens (1979) provided preliminary data on the psychometric properties of a "Commitment to Running Scale" (CRS) and showed that runners reporting higher levels of commitment tended also to report greater running distances, higher perceived addiction to running, and greater discomfort if a run was missed. Future work is required, however, to know whether a particular direction of influence is at work here. For example, are runners more committed because of the success achieved in completing greater distances (which Carmack and Martens reported were likely to lead to better psychological states anyway), or does the higher commitment lead to longer runs?

An extension of the concept of commitment to running was provided by Corbin and colleagues (Corbin et al. 1987b) who developed a modification of the CRS so that it became applicable to a wide range of physical activities. This led to the "Commitment to Physical Activity (CPA) Scale". Preliminary psychometric data are presented by Corbin et al. (1987b) although the same group of researchers also argue elsewhere (Nielsen et al. 1984) that both activity-specific modifications of the CPA scale, as well as the CPA scale itself, have their uses and they draw the analogy with general and specific locus of control measures. Corbin et al. (1987b) report a significant difference in CPA scores between groups differing in activity levels. However, further work is required in differentiating commitment from self-motivation at psychometric and behavioural levels, if such a difference actually exists. The CPA scale may be more of a general attitude scale than one measuring motivation *per se*.

Goal Orientations

So far, the adherence research that we have reported has tended to focus on descriptive studies of motives and reasons for drop-out, comparisons between adherers and drop-outs, and personality variables such as self-motivation. Recently, however, attention has been directed at the meaning attached to a particular behaviour and the motivational consequences of such perceptions. In short, some researchers have suggested that a fruitful avenue for understanding motivated behaviour is to utilise Personal Investment (PI) Theory (Maehr and Braskamp 1986).

PI Theory states that the behaviours associated with motivation are collectively referred to as "personal investment". In other words, for exercise, exercise motivation is inferred from exercise behaviours, i.e., personal investment in exercise. Secondly, PI Theory states that one must focus on the nature of choices and decisions made by people (e.g. which type of exercise). Third, what meaning does the individual attach to the situation and behaviour in question? The meaning, according to Maehr and Braskamp (1986), comprises three interrelated components: personal incentives, sense of self, and perceived options.

"Personal incentives" refer to the motivational focus of an individual and are similar to participation motives discussed earlier. Maehr and Braskamp (1986) identify both intrinsic and extrinsic personal incentives. Intrinsic incentives tend to focus either on doing better than others, or understanding and mastering a task for its own sake. Extrinsic incentives might include pleasing others (social solidarity) or gaining an extrinsic reward (e.g., money).

The "sense of self" component of the theory refers to perceptions of competence, self-reliance (such as a belief that one can motivate oneself), goal-directedness (self-ascribed tendency to set goals), and social identity (characteristics of significant other people). Finally, "perceived options" refers to the behavioural alternatives that the individual perceives to be available. For example, this might include barriers to exercise as well as likely perceived positive outcomes.

As far as exercise adherence is concerned little has been written about the PI theory until very recently, with the work of Duda and colleagues now being more prominent (Duda 1988, 1989; Duda and Tappe 1988, 1989a, b). One of the central themes of the theory is the meaning individuals attach to the situation in terms of personal incentives. For example, it has been suggested that people may hold different goals in physical activity and as such define "success" in different ways, such as in terms of winning or self-improvement. These goals have been identified in a number of contexts and with various labels and are summarised in Table 2.1. Some researchers have suggested that self-improvement (mastery) goals will promote persistence and effort in the face of difficulties, whereas ego-involved goals, particularly for those low in perceived ability, may lead to decreased motivation, and even helplessness, in the face of failure (Dweck and Leggett 1988). The extent to which this can be applied to exercise has yet to be demonstrated.

Most of the research in physical activity has centred on sport, where the two major goals of ego and task mastery orientations appear to be prominent (see Duda 1989; Roberts 1984). However, Duda (1989) has also posed the question whether people participating in recreational exercise might also hold similar goals. Although the goal of task mastery appears to be used in exercise, the research so far has been unclear about the prominence of an ego-oriented goal. In fact, exercise goals appear to be more diverse, with Duda and Tappe (1988) reporting personal incentives related to mastery, competition, social affiliation, recognition from others, health benefits, coping with stress and physical fitness. Where ego-involved exercise goals have been found, they have been held more strongly by males than females (Duda 1989). In a study of middle-aged men and women, Duda and Tappe (1988) found that the incentives of recognition by others,

Table 2.1. Major Goal Orientations Identified by Different Researchers

Goal	Description	Alternative labels
Ego orientation (Maehr and Nicholls 1980; Maehr and Braskamp 1986)	Bettering others; winning; avoiding demonstrating low ability in relation to others	Performance goal (Dweck and Leggett 1988) Outcome goal (Burton 1989) Competitive goal (Ames and Ames 1984)
Task mastery orientation (Maehr and Nicholls 1980; Maehr and Braskamp 1986)	Understanding; self-improvement; experiencing adventure and novelty	Learning goal (Dweck and Leggett 1988) Performance goal (Burton 1989) Individualistic goal (Ames and Ames 1984)
Social approval (Maehr and Nicholls 1980; Maehr and Braskamp 1986)	Pleasing others	Co-operative goal (Ames and Ames 1984)

physical fitness, and coping with stress all predicted current physical activity levels. Similarly, the mastery incentive was the major predictor of future intentions for physical activity.

PI Theory and goal orientations pose intriguing possibilities for the understanding of exercise involvement. However, further work is required in recreational and health behaviours before conclusions can be drawn. What is currently known, however, points to the need to recognise that people will be differentially motivated in exercise and may define success in many different ways.

Motivational Orientations

Statements about exercise adherence often refer to the need to develop or enhance intrinsic motivation. However, research with children suggests that the intrinsic-extrinsic continuum may be more complex than originally thought. For example, Harter (1981) has identified five motivational orientations which she measured with children in class-room settings. These were used by Weiss et al. (1985) in the development of their "Motivational Orientation in Sport Scale" (MOSS). The five motivational factors are challenge, curiosity, mastery, judgement and criteria. Challenge refers to the intrinsic motivation of seeking a challenge or seeking easy work; curiosity refers to wanting to satisfy one's own curiosity and interest versus wanting to please the teacher/coach or obtain good grades in assessments; mastery refers to the preference for seeking out solutions to problems in contrast to being dependent on others for help in problem-solving. Harter and Connell (1984) found that these three factors clustered to form an "intrinsic mastery motivation" factor. Additionally, judgement refers to whether the child feels capable of making judgements about what to do in physical education and sports or whether the opinion of the teacher is needed. Criteria refers to whether the child has some internal sense of whether he or she has succeeded or whether external sources of evaluation are required. These two variables, judgement and criteria, were found to cluster together and have been labelled "autonomous judgement" since they seem to be referring to "cognitive-informational" structures of the child; that is to say, the ways the child might think about making decisions.

These constructs have only been studied with children and may not be applicable to adults. However, preliminary evidence on children's exercise (Biddle and Armstrong 1990b) has shown that they may be important motivational determinants of habitual physical activity, as measured by heart rate telemetry. Biddle and Armstrong (1990b) found that intrinsic mastery motivation was positively and significantly correlated with activity for 11- and 12-year-old boys, but not for girls, whereas autonomous judgement correlated significantly and negatively with activity for girls but not for boys. The latter result shows that the girls were more extrinsic in their orientation. Overall, the activity of boys was related to intrinsic motivation whereas the activity of girls was related, in a weaker fashion, to extrinsic motivation.

Such results require further investigation on two main counts. First, more needs to be known about different intrinsic/extrinsic motivational states in children and adults, and second, further research is required to see if such gender differences are robust. Further discussion on the measurement of intrinsic motivation can be found later in the chapter.

Reinforcement Strategies and Behaviour Modification Studies in Exercise Adherence

This section will focus on behaviour modification studies that have specifically addressed the issue of exercise adherence. There will be discussion of the role of positive affect, feelings of well-being, and exercise enjoyment as potential reinforcers of exercise behaviours. More detail is given in Chap. 9.

Behaviour Modification Strategies and Adherence

Martin et al. (1984) conducted a number of studies that investigated behavioural strategies in the acquisition and maintenance of walking and jogging. Many of the strategies involved goal-setting, a strategy that has been reported to have had considerable success in encouraging particular behaviours in a number of settings including sport and exercise (Harris and Harris 1984; Locke et al. 1988; Mento et al. 1987; Naylor and Ilgen 1984). The practical application of such strategies is also discussed in Chap. 9.

Overall, despite some methodological problems and small sample sizes, Martin et al. (1984) showed that the use of flexible goal-setting and instructor praise and feedback during exercise could be supported in promoting exercise adherence.

Keefe and Blumenthal (1980) report the results of behaviour modification interventions on three overweight adult males with a history of poor exercise adherence. A combination of stimulus control (warming-up, exercising at the same time and place, goal-setting) with self-reinforcement was used. After nine months of a walk/jog programme, significant gains in aerobic performance and decrease in body fat were achieved. The exercise habit was successfully maintained and the three subjects reported that self-reinforcement became less important with time as the exercise itself increased in reward value. This is an important point and one that will be discussed later in relation to exercise intensity and the effects of exercise on mental health.

Atkins et al. (1984) studied adherence to a walking programme in patients suffering from chronic obstructive pulmonary disease (COPD).

Five experimental groups were created: behaviour modification, cognitive modification, cognitive-behaviour modification, an attention control group, and a no-treatment control group. The results clearly supported the use of the intervention strategies; the experimental groups had a significantly higher weekly walking rate than the two control groups from week 4 to week 12 of the programme. The cognitive-behaviour modification strategy proved to be the most effective.

Similar results were also obtained for exercise tolerance and feelings of well-being, suggesting that such interventions, either singly or in combination, may provide the impetus for both improved exercise performance and intrinsic reinforcement through improved feelings of well-being. Exercise may then become self-reinforcing.

Self-monitoring has been a common technique used in behaviour modification. Oldridge and Jones (1983) investigated its effectiveness on the rates of exercise adherence of cardiac rehabilitation patients in Canada, with 120 post-myocardial infarction (MI) patients who were split into control and experimental groups. The control group received a standard twice-weekly exercise programme whereas the experimental group received help with self-management strategies. Specifically, these patients signed an agreement to participate in the exercise programme for 6 months and also took part in regular self-monitoring with self-report diaries. These included the recording of self-monitored heart rates at various times during exercise, activity levels, weight loss, and smoking habits. Drop-out was defined as non-attendance at eight consecutive sessions. The results showed that within 6 months the experimental group had an adherence rate of 54% compared with the control group's 42%. This was found to be non-significant. However, some of the experimental group refused to sign the 6-month agreement and they were found to have significantly lower adherence rates. This may reflect differences in self-motivation or commitment (Corbin et al. 1987b; Dishman et al. 1980).

The use of reinforcement, behaviour management and modification strategies, therefore, can be an effective way of initiating exercise in some groups. However, the results illustrated here demonstrate the need for strict experimental control for a clearer understanding of which techniques, if any, are the most beneficial. Similarly, two important questions about exercise techniques require investigation:

1. How successful are these techniques in maintaining participation over long periods of time (i.e. greater than 1 year)?
2. Which individuals require such techniques more than others?

Given evidence on the possible undermining effects of extrinsic rewards on intrinsic motivation (see Chap. 4 and Deci and Ryan 1985; Vallerand et al. 1987), behaviour modification strategies that use primarily extrinsic rewards must be monitored carefully.

Group Factors and Adherence

The tendency in exercise adherence research has been to concentrate on individual psychological or biological factors that may predict adherence or drop-out. Rarely has research focussed on group factors such as exercise leadership or group dynamics. This is despite the widely held view that such social psychological factors may be crucial in successful adherence strategies. For example, Franklin (1988) suggests that poor exercise leadership, a lack of group camaraderie or spirit, and spouse/peer disapproval are all factors likely to predispose people to drop out of group exercise programmes. Consequently, Franklin suggests that strategies designed to increase adherence should include the encouragement of group participation, the recruitment of spouse support for the programme (see Andrew and Parker 1979; Oldridge 1988; Taylor et al. 1985), and the provision of qualified, enthusiastic exercise leaders. Despite the reliable finding that spouse support is important in adherence to post-coronary exercise rehabilitation programmes (Oldridge 1982, 1984, 1988), few research studies have been conducted on the nature of such interactions and the type of support that may be required. This is also true of group dynamics, exercise leaders and adherence.

King and Frederiksen (1984) studied the effects of different social strategies on the initiation of jogging in sedentary women. Fifty-eight subjects were assigned to one of four conditions:

1. Group only: members were encouraged to jog with at least one other team member during the study. They were also exposed to a variety of team building and group cohesion exercises in an effort to develop social support within the group and they were led through discussions on the different forms of exercise.

2. Relapse only: members of this group were told of the relapse effect in exercise (see later in this chapter and Chap. 9). Cognitive strategies were taught and rehearsed both singly and in a group.

3. Group and relapse: subjects in this group received both of the interventions just described.

4. Control: subjects were asked to jog alone and were led in discussions on the different forms of exercise.

All subjects were then given a set of cards on which to record their jogging frequency for the following 5 weeks. Adherence was operationally defined as the number of cards returned.

The results of this study showed that the group-only and relapse-only conditions were significantly higher in the number of cards returned than the other two groups. At a 3-month follow-up it was found that the relapse-only group was superior.

These results are unsurprising as far as the two intervention groups are concerned. However, the failure of the combined relapse and group strategy is not so easily explained. It may be related to the fact that this group reported less group cohesion than the other two. This raises the important issue of group cohesion and social attractiveness of exercise groups.

Group cohesion and attention. Although some people have claimed that group cohesion is important for exercise motivation (Franklin 1988), evidence is hard to come by and, while it appears quite logical that good staff support in supervised programmes should promote adherence, systematic evaluation has not been forthcoming. Nevertheless, some research studies are now addressing some of these issues. However, definitive guidelines will not be available until we have further information.

Weber and Wertheim (1989) investigated the influence of staff attention on the adherence patterns of new recruits to a community gymnasium in Australia. Fifty-five women were randomly allocated to one of three groups: control, self-monitoring of gym attendance, and self-monitoring plus extra staff attention. Over a 12-week period it was found that the attendance was highest for the self-monitoring group and lowest for the control group, the difference being significant. However, the attendance of the self-monitoring plus staff attention group, although slightly better than the control, was not significantly superior. The intervention based on the exercise leader, therefore, was not successful over and above that of self-monitoring (see Martin et al. 1984). It may be that trying to identify one set of successful leadership behaviours in health-related exercise will prove as unfruitful as in other contexts, including sport, due to the complex interaction between personal and environmental factors (see Carron 1988). Nevertheless, exercise leaders will almost certainly be important individuals in helping exercisers maintain participation. Unfortunately, yet again the training and education of exercise leaders is almost exclusively in the biological sciences with little attention paid to interpersonal skills or understanding exercise adherence.

The study of group dynamics, cohesion and individual adherence to group activities, such as exercise, may be a fruitful line for research. To this end Carron et al. (1988) continued their research programme on group cohesion in sport (Widmeyer et al. 1985) by investigating cohesion and adherence in fitness and recreation, as well as sport, contexts. Carron et al. (1988) looked at fitness class adherers and non-adherers as well as elite sport adherers and non-adherers. These 4 groups were assessed using the Group Environment Questionnaire (GEQ) (Widmeyer et al. 1985) which is an instrument yielding scores on four subscales: individual attraction to the group-task (ATG-T), individual attraction to the group-social (ATG-S), group integration-task (GI-T), and group integration-social (GI-S). Slight modification was made to the GEQ to allow it to be administered to the fitness groups, since the original scale was written for sport groups. Analysis of the fitness group scores showed that two of the GEQ variables significantly discriminated adherers from non-adherers. Specifically, adherers had higher scores on both ATG subscales thus showing that drop-outs were less personally attracted to the group's task and to the group as a social unit.

Considerably more work is required, however, in understanding the nature and extent of social psychological variables of the group and exercise adherence. For example, the type of exercise may be crucial. Studies on diverse activities such as distance running, weight training, and aerobic exercise-to-music may reveal different results. Similarly, the type of participant and exercise leader are important ingredients in this type of research. Although it is usual to encourage sedentary people to take part in exercise with a partner or in groups, much more needs to be known before specific advice about the nature of such group factors and exercise adherence can be made. For example, it is now common for exercise-to-music classes to consist of more than 50 people. We know little about the motivational effects of being in such a large group, the concomitant lack of instruction and attention, or whether these are unimportant given enjoyable exercises and motivating music. Alternatively, the anonymity of exercising in a large group may be perceived as a positive feature for some people. Group size, therefore, requires further investigation. Similarly, although a group environment may be perceived positively in the short term, longer term adherence to exercise may suffer if individual behavioural skills are not taught or learned, particularly if the exercise group ceases after a period of time.

Reinforcement Through Positive Affect

A rationale for increasing activity levels in all sections of the population is usually made on biological grounds, particularly because of the potential for affecting CHD risk. This is wholly appropriate in many cases and can provide a most convincing argument for reversing the sedentary lifestyles that are thought to exist. It has also been the case that the *promotion* of exercise has been made using the same biological rationale. However, it is most unlikely that individual activity levels will increase in the long term simply because people are fearful of disease later in life. Humans tend to subscribe to much more hedonistic principles, although health/disease factors may also be important for some people, and more likely as a long-term, more abstract, goal. Dishman et al. (1985, p. 166) stated that "feelings related to well-being and enjoyment seem more important to maintaining activity than concerns about health". This section, therefore, will deal with two main themes: exercise enjoyment, and exercise and mental health, in the context of reinforcement of exercise behaviours. The issue of exercise and mental health will be dealt with in more detail in Chaps 6, 7 and 8. Here the discussion will centre on the possible links between the mental health outcomes of exercise and the motivational effects these could have.

Exercise Enjoyment. Little has been written about the nature of the enjoyment of sport or exercise. However, survey research has shown that feelings of enjoyment and "well-being" are important factors in the decision to be active (see Canada Fitness Survey (1983a); Fig. 2.2). Health and well-being feature prominently in Fig. 2.2 as reasons for being active. However, "fun and excitement" is also included as a separate category and is rated in second place overall. It seems likely, therefore, while positive health factors and feelings of well-being and enjoyment will be important reinforcers and motivators of exercise behaviour, disease prevention factors may not be. Persuading people to undertake a particular health action for reasons of disease prevention alone has often failed (see Eiser and van der Pligt 1988).

The sparse literature on the nature of enjoyment in physical activity contexts has been focussed almost exclusively on competitive sport and, therefore, may not be applicable to recreational participation in health-related exercise (Wankel and Kreisel 1985). Scanlan and Lewthwaite (1986), in a study of 76 young male wrestlers aged 9–14 years, proposed a model of sport enjoyment and this is illustrated in Fig. 2.7.

The model allows for a classification of predictors of sport enjoyment based on the two dimensions of achievement/non-achievement and intrinsic/extrinsic. The four quadrants are explained by Scanlan and Lewthwaite (1986, p. 33) as follows:

1. Achievement-intrinsic: "predictors related to personal perceptions of competence and control, such as the attainment of mastery goals and perceived ability".

2. Achievement-extrinsic: "predictors related to personal perceptions of competence and control that are derived from other people".

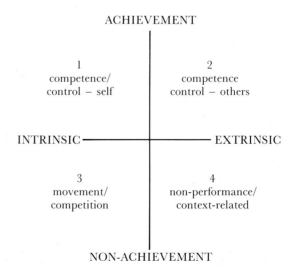

Figure 2.7. A model of sport enjoyment proposed by Scanlan & Lewthwaite (1986). (From "Social psychological aspects of competition for male youth sport participants: IV. Predictors of enjoyment" by T.K. Scanlan and R. Lewthwaite (1986) *Journal of Sport Psychology*, 8: 33. Reprinted with permission of Human Kinetics Publishers.)

ACHIEVEMENT

1
competence/
control – self

2
competence
control – others

INTRINSIC ———————————— EXTRINSIC

3
movement/
competition

4
non-performance/
context-related

NON-ACHIEVEMENT

3.   Non-achievement-intrinsic: "Predictors related to (a) physical activity
      and movement such as sensations, tension release . . . and (b)
      competition such as excitement".

4.   Non-achievement-extrinsic: "Predictors related to non-performance
      aspects of sport such as affiliating with peers".

This model now requires testing with a larger and more representative
sample of sports participants as well as in health-related contexts. It would
appear that area 3 on the model may have some relationship with exercise
and feelings of well-being.

Wankel (1985) reported results from an interview and questionnaire
study with 111 participants and drop-outs from an employee fitness
programme. The participants, as expected, were found to have high levels
of enjoyment and positive feelings about the programme. One of the
problems with this study, however, is that the data were collected 8–
10 months after the start of the programme. Although Wankel (1985)
believes that "truthful" replies were given, the results could have been
rationalisations of decisions already made.

The concept of "enjoyment" remains elusive. However, Csikszentmihalyi
(1975) studied a range of activities participated in for apparently intrinsic
reasons and sought to explain the factor of enjoyment. He labelled the
activities "autotelic", meaning "self goals" or "self purpose" and suggested
that supreme states of enjoyment ("flow") were possible when the demands
of such activities were met by the individual's capabilities. A mismatch
was likely to lead to feelings of boredom, worry or anxiety, and
Csikszentmihalyi (1975, p. 36) says: "In the flow state, action follows upon
action according to an internal logic that seems to need no conscious
intervention by the actor. He experiences it as a unified flowing from one
moment to the next, in which he is in control of his actions, and in which
there is little distinction between self and environment, between stimulus
and response, or between past, present and future. Flow is what we have
been calling the 'autotelic experience' ".

Whether "flow" is the same as intrinsic motivation is yet to be determined.
Flow, as described by Csikszentmihalyi, may be a "higher order" state of
consciousness with strong reinforcing powers.

Csikszentmihalyi's work, however, is the closest we get to an understanding
of intrinsic enjoyment states, yet a great deal more needs to be
known about this process in the exercise context. Wankel (1988) relates
Csikszentmihalyi's work to sport and exercise by suggesting that some
runners have reported high levels of enjoyment and mental well-being after
initial periods of discomfort. The challenge for exercise leaders, therefore,
appears to be in matching individual preferences to the demands of the
activity. It is quite likely that the traditional guidelines for the improvement
of fitness laid down by the American College of Sports Medicine (ACSM
1986, 1990) are too severe for the majority of the population to tolerate

with enough comfort to promote intrinsic motivation and enjoyment. If fitness leaders are to match the capabilities of the participant with the activity itself, such physiological guidelines may not be helpful in the initial stages (see Dishman 1988b). Indeed, Rejeski and Kenney (1988) suggest that exercisers should move through three stages in promoting adherence to exercise. The first is referred to as the starter phase, and the emphasis is placed on gentle adaptation to new exercise but with active *discouragement* of fitness improvements. The growth phase follows, in which the focus is on fitness improvement, along the lines of traditional exercise prescription for fitness. Finally, the maintenance phase occurs when continued involvement is encouraged at a level sufficient to maintain levels of functioning and fitness. Of course, not all participants will necessarily want fitness improvements and their involvement may be for other reasons. This also needs taking into account by exercise leaders and promoters. Elaboration on "stage models" in adherence can be found in Kristeller and Rodin (1985).

Exercise and Mood States. A great deal has been written about the proposed "mental health" benefits of exercise and further discussion of this can be found in Chaps 6, 7 and 8. However, the research in this area has usually investigated the emotional and cognitive consequences resulting from involvement in an exercise programme, such as reductions in state anxiety or depression, or elevations in self-esteem and feelings of well-being. However, few studies have investigated the *motivational* benefits of such changes in affect. As already stated, mental health benefits may not be perceived by a large number of exercisers in the initial phases of involvement. These people are likely to cease participation prior to being reinforced by positive mental states. A clear research priority, therefore, is to look into the long-term motivational benefits of changes in mental health resulting from, or associated with, exercise.

Exercise Intensity and Reinforcement. The standard physiological guidelines for exercise prescription (ACSM 1990) have already been questioned on the grounds of suitability for exercise adherence (Dishman 1988b). However, until recently, little was known about the reactions of exercisers to different intensities of exercise. Steptoe and co-workers, however, have studied this and their results are reported in three papers (Moses et al. 1989; Steptoe and Bolton 1988; Steptoe and Cox 1988).

Steptoe and Cox (1988) studied the effect of acute aerobic exercise on mood, with female medical students aged 18 to 23 years. Four 8-min trials of exercise were carried out by each subject with two at a "high" intensity (2 kg/100 W) and two at a "low" intensity (0.5 kg/25 W). These conditions were subdivided by being accompanied by either music or a metronome. Subjects were also classified as "fit" or "unfit" based on their heart rate response to exercise. Mood was assessed before and after each trial.

The results showed that the sound manipulation was unrelated to post-exercise mood, but exercise intensity was. Specifically, the high-intensity condition produced elevated levels of tension-anxiety, while the low-intensity condition produced elevated levels of vigour and exhilaration. These mood changes were largely unaffected by physical fitness levels.

This study was partially replicated by Steptoe and Bolton (1988). Female students were studied in conditions of both high (100 W) and low (25 W) exercise intensity but this time no music was used. Mood states were assessed before and after 15-min exercise bouts on a cycle ergometer. The results showed that, for those in the low intensity condition, anxiety reduced significantly from pre-exercise levels when assessed at 6 and 12 minutes into the exercise period. This is shown in Fig. 2.8.

Increases in tension-anxiety scores from the Profile of Mood States (POMS) for the high-intensity group were also found, thus supporting Steptoe and Cox (1988). Similarly, a study by Moses et al. (1989) demonstrated that reductions in anxiety-tension after a 10-week aerobic exercise programme were evident only for the group participating in moderate exercise intensity, compared with subjects in the high-intensity condition, in the attention-placebo group and those in the waiting list group.

The results from Steptoe and co-workers show that positive mood changes are evident only with lower exercise intensities. This is an important finding

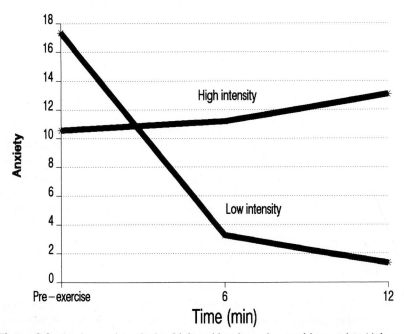

Figure 2.8. Anxiety ratings during high and low intensity aerobic exercise. (Adapted from Steptoe and Bolton 1988.)

for exercise adherence and strongly supports the notion of carefully graded exercise experiences for novices. Steptoe and Bolton (1988, pp. 104–105) conclude by saying that "it may be that particular schedules can be devised that lead to immediate positive mood responses, and that these will in turn promote greater uptake and adherence to exercise programmes".

Similarly, Moses et al. (1989, p. 60) conclude by suggesting that if the results of their research are shown to be robust, "they may have important implications for the way in which training programmes should be devised for the general public". However, one is tempted to avoid the word "training" at all when it comes to promoting exercise adherence as it is likely to evoke negative perceptions of high exercise intensity. Nevertheless, the research by Steptoe and his colleagues provides some interesting pointers for future research on mental health, reinforcement and exercise adherence.

Of note in the study by Steptoe and Bolton (1988) was the result that for feelings of vigour there was an interaction between fitness level and exercise intensity such that positive changes in vigour were experienced only by the high-fitness subjects in the high-intensity condition. This contradicts Steptoe and Cox (1988). The relationship between exercise tolerance, preferences for different exertional levels, and mood states requires further study and may hold some important clues to the issue of exercise adherence.

Exertion Perceptions and Preferences. The standard prescription of exercise involves setting and regulating the frequency, intensity, duration and mode of exercise (ACSM 1990). The duration and frequency of exercise, for example, could present major behavioural barriers to participation if the prescription demands high frequency and long duration. Regardless of the physiological training effects, from a behavioural standpoint the initial bouts of exercise should not demand excessive time commitment from the participant yet should, nevertheless, establish a regular routine.

An important factor already mentioned is the intensity of the exercise bout. The rating of "effort sense" (ratings of perceived exertion, RPE) has received considerable attention as a result of the work of Gunnar Borg and the use of his RPE scales (see Bar-Or and Ward (1989) and Williams and Eston (1989) for recent reviews on children and adults). Effort ratings have been obtained in field and laboratory settings with exercising subjects by the verbal reporting of a number read from a scale representing the continuum of effort from minimal to maximal. Williams and Eston (1989) suggest that while the use of effort ratings has often been reported as a reliable index of the metabolic cost of exercise, about 30% of the variance between RPE and physiological parameters remains unexplained. This suggests that further investigation is warranted into the psychological mechanisms of effort perceptions.

Personality research suggests that pain tolerance differs between introverts and extroverts, with the latter group demonstrating higher tolerance

(Eysenck 1967). Similarly, Type A personalities have been thought to overestimate exercise tolerance, because of their high motivation and suppressed RPE scores, although Graham et al. (1989) found that RPE was not predicted by Type A, as measured by the Jenkins Activity Survey. Also, it has been suggested that individuals high in public self-consciousness may report lower RPEs in an effort to present a more favourable social image, but again recent research is equivocal on this (Tieman et al. 1989). Hardy et al. (1986) did find that RPEs were lower when a subject exercised with another person present. This was also found to be true when the co-acting exerciser exhibited non-verbal signs that the exercise intensity was low.

Individual differences in RPE have also been reported when subjects differing in sex-role perception have been studied. Social psychologists have often used psychometric scales to measure the extent to which subjects, in describing themselves, endorse predominantly masculine characteristics, predominantly feminine characteristics, or a mixture of both (Bem 1974). When both characteristics are equally strongly endorsed, subjects are described as androgynous and are thought to have a propensity for flexible sex-role behaviour in the light of gender-related cues.

Rejeski and his co-workers have studied this issue in relation to exercise intensity. Based on his social psychophysiological model of effort perception, Rejeski (1981) has proposed that exercise tolerance may partly be related to past experience with fatigue and the social context of the behaviour. This suggests that those with limited experience of exercise fatigue or those who are inhibited by the social situation of physical exercise (e.g., those who believe that the exercise is sex-role "inappropriate") will inflate effort ratings. This was supported by Hochstetler et al. (1985), whose female subjects ran on the treadmill for 30 min at 70% of $\dot{V}O_{2max}$; they recorded RPEs and a number of related physiological variables at every 5-min period. Three groups were created as a result of psychometric assessment of sex-role orientation: masculine-typed, feminine-typed and androgynous. Results showed that greater RPEs were reported by the feminine-typed subjects compared with the other two groups (Fig. 2.9). Also, the feminine-typed group reported greater unease and less self-assurance prior to the run than the other groups. However, some methodological problems were evident with this study. The feminine group was found to have a lower $\dot{V}O_{2max}$ than the androgynous subjects. Although the groups exercised at the same relative workload, this difference meant that the absolute workload was lowest for the feminine group. The post-exercise affect scores, which showed greater psychological distress for the feminine subjects, may be partly a function of having lower perceptions of physical fitness although this point is purely speculative and there are no further data on it.

Rejeski and Sanford (1984) studied the RPEs during cycle ergometry of feminine-typed females. However, in addition to subjects pedalling for 20 min at 80% $\dot{V}O_{2max}$, they were shown a video of a model participating

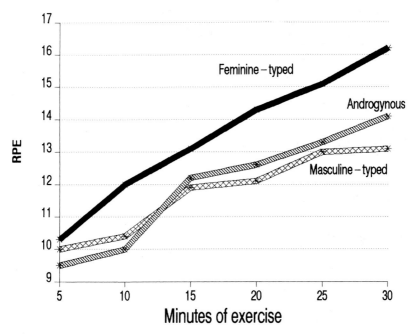

Figure 2.9. Effort ratings and sex-role perception. (From "The influence of sex-role orientation on ratings of perceived exertion" by S.A. Hochstetler, W.J. Rejeski and D.L. Best (1985) *Sex Roles* 12: 830. Reprinted with permission of Plenum Publishing Corporation.)

in the task. The model was either showing signs of exercise tolerance or intolerance. The results showed that higher RPEs were reported by subjects who were shown the intolerant model, again suggesting the importance of social cues in perceptions of exercise intensity. It is not possible to ascertain the extent to which this reaction is unique to feminine females. Similarly, Kenney et al. (1987) reported lower RPEs for subjects who had undertaken a "distress management training programme", which included learning appropriate coping strategies.

These studies point to a wider perspective on exercise prescription and adherence (Rejeski 1985; Rejeski and Kenney 1988). Instead of rigid compliance to physiological guidelines, it may be appropriate to consider affective and cognitive factors too. For example, Dishman (1988b) points to the use of exertion *preferences* in addition to exertion *perceptions* in the prescription of exercise. It may, as Hardy and Rejeski (1989) suggest, be important not just to look at *what* one feels during exercise but *how* one feels. In other words, similar RPEs may have different *meanings* for different individuals.

Hardy and Rejeski (1989) report the use of a "Feeling Scale" (FS) to assess affective reactions during exercise. After initial psychometric work, these researchers investigated the use of the FS with 30 undergraduate males. Subjects pedalled cycle ergometers at 30%, 60% and 90% of $\dot{V}O_{2max}$ in three successive 4-min stages. RPE and FS were moderately correlated such that increased exercise intensity related to increasingly negative feelings. These correlations increased in strength with exercise intensity. The results show that feelings about exercise intensity are not identical to perceptions of effort loading, although the two constructs become more similar with increasing workloads. In short, exercise leaders should be taking into consideration the perception of effort *and* the feelings associated with such effort if their goal is to promote adherence.

From the point of view of promoting physical activity it is important to resolve some of these issues. In particular, it is our view that the physiologically-driven guidelines for optimal fitness development through appropriate exercise prescription (e.g., ACSM 1986, 1990), may need to be reviewed from a *behavioural* point of view. Dishman (1988b, p. 53) suggests that "the optimal volume of exercise for promoting adherence and health outcomes remains to be identified. Not only may rigid prescriptions be too behaviourally challenging for some, they may not be biologically necessary".

Relapse from Exercise

Adherence to exercise is not a simple process and, as stated already, is not an "all or none" or "either/or" phenomenon (Sonstroem 1988). After adopting exercise people are likely to maintain this habit to varying degrees, drop out at different points in the life cycle and then, in some cases, start again. The early attempts at investigating adherence ignored the important point that people's adherence to exercise will vary by degree. This process has been reviewed earlier in the chapter through reference to the study by Mihalik et al. (1989).

The process of adherence may bear some resemblance to the relapse effect studied in other health contexts. For example, Marlatt (1985) proposes a "relapse prevention" model in an effort to explain the lack of adherence to abstinence to addictions associated with alcohol, smoking and other drugs. These are high frequency, undesired behaviours whereas exercise, Knapp (1988) notes, is a low frequency yet desired behaviour. The extent to which a parallel can be drawn between the two, therefore, remains to be seen (see Chap. 9).

Marlatt (1985, p. 3) identifies "relapse" as a "breakdown or setback in a person's attempt to change or modify any target behaviour", and refers to relapse in terms of a voluntary self-control situation rather than compulsory behaviour change such as in some institutions. Fig. 2.10 illustrates Marlatt's relapse prevention (RP) model in the context of exercise.

The high-risk situation is the threat to self-control that could produce relapse. Marlatt (1985) has identified negative emotional states, interpersonal conflict, and social pressure as the three primary high-risk situations

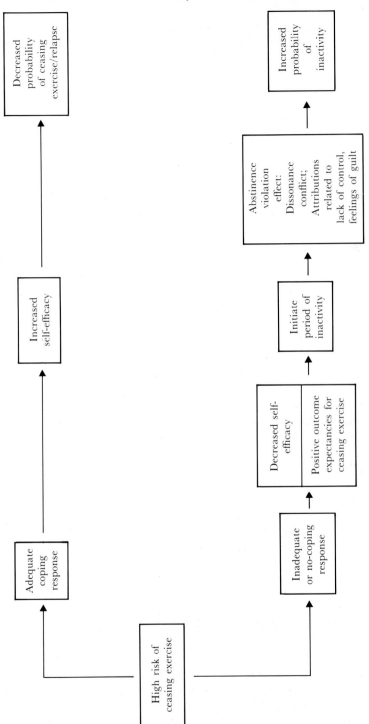

Figure 2.10. Marlatt's "relapse prevention model" applied to exercise. (Adapted from Marlatt 1985.)

for individuals with addiction problems. Whether these lead to relapse will, however, depend on the adequacy of the individual's coping skills and response. The high-risk situation for exercise might involve extra work pressures, thus producing a perception of reduced time for exercise, or the raising of costs in using an exercise facility. The probability of relapse from this situation is reduced if the individual adopts an adequate coping response (e.g., time-management skills) and perceives maintained or increased levels of self-efficacy or confidence (see Chap. 5). However, a lack of a coping response may lead to difficulties in maintaining the exercise habit.

Marlatt proposes that a lack of a coping response will lead to a decrease in self-efficacy and a positive expectation of the effects of relapse. In the case of drug abuse, this is where the pleasurable effects are high-lighted and, in the case of exercise, where rest from physical exertion may be seen as a positive outcome. The model then proposes that a relapse will occur and, from our perspective, exercise will cease. This could lead to what has been termed the "abstinence violation effect" (AVE) where the individual may display feelings of guilt or self-blame. This effect will depend on the degree of cognitive dissonance, or conflict, and the type of attributions for the failure to continue the desired behaviour. For example, attributions reflecting negative personal characteristics and feelings of helplessness and lack of control will increase the probability of a sustained relapse. Knapp (1988) suggests that people in such situations require flexible goal-setting and cognitive restructuring.

The relapse prevention approach has not received much attention in the exercise science literature. One of the studies reported by Martin et al. (1984) attempted to investigate relapse in exercise but suffered from methodological problems. However, King and Frederiksen (1984) employed successfully a relapse preparation training procedure and demonstrated its efficacy, alongside social support procedures, in increasing and maintaining frequency of jogging sessions in a small sample of previously sedentary college women. Support for the relapse prevention approach has also come from Belisle et al. (1987) (see Chap. 9). However, more needs to be known about the mechanisms of relapse in exercise as the behaviour itself is substantially different from the addictive behaviours which the relapse model was designed to explain.

Future Directions of Research into Exercise Adherence

This chapter has introduced the problems associated with the adoption and maintenance of physical activity. The convincing evidence that now exists for the beneficial effects of exercise is of limited use if adoption and adherence rates remain low. It is suggested, therefore, that one of the greatest challenges facing researchers in the exercise sciences is to identify

POPULATION SEGMENTS

RACE, ETHNICITY,
SEX, SOCIOECONOMIC
STATUS, EDUCATIONAL
LEVEL, AGE

×

PHYSICAL ACTIVITY

×

DETERMINANTS
OR
CORRELATES

PSYCHOLOGICAL
e.g., motivation
self-perceptions

BIOBEHAVIOURAL
e.g., perceived exertion
activity history

SOCIAL-ENVIRONMENTAL
e.g., education
access to facilities

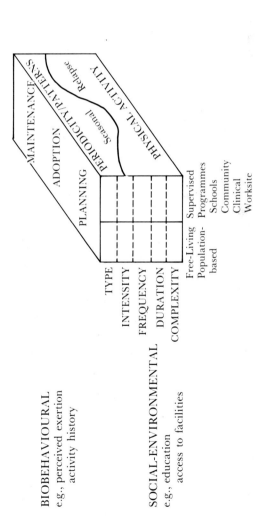

TYPE
INTENSITY
FREQUENCY
DURATION
COMPLEXITY

Free-Living Supervised
Population- Programmes
based   Schools
             Community
             Clinical
             Worksite

PLANNING
ADOPTION
MAINTENANCE
PERIODICITY/PATTERNS
Seasonal Relapse
PHYSICAL ACTIVITY

Figure 2.11. A "Life-span Interaction Model" for exercise adherence. (Adapted from Dishman (1990).)

the major determinants and/or correlates of habitual physical activity across the life-span. This is a stated goal for the Department of Health and Human Services in the USA. However, as numerous authors have already stated, exercise adherence research has suffered from an atheoretical approach (Dishman 1988a, 1990; Sonstroem 1988).

Key Issues in the Psychology of Exercise Adherence

Despite over a decade of sustained interest in the problem of exercise adherence, there remains a great deal to be learnt. A summary model, shown in Fig. 2.11, has been presented by Dishman and Dunn (1988) and expanded by Dishman (1990). The model suggests that progress will only be made by looking across disciplines and including psychological, biobehavioural and social-environmental determinants of physical activity. Fig. 2.11 lists possible key determinants, and how these will be likely to interact with aspects of physical activity itself, such as the type of activity, its frequency, intensity, complexity and duration, and may differ between free-living and supervised types of exercise. Seasonal changes and relapse may also have to be considered. Finally, Dishman (1990) suggests that different sections of the population will have to be considered, such factors as age, educational level and race being taken into account.

This model is merely a guide to help structure the complex area of physical activity determinants and more detail can be found in Dishman (1990). Future research is required on aspects of the model, and in particular the interactions between parts of the model. Up to now, we appear to know rather more about exercise adherence of adults in supervised settings, and in particular in clinical settings, than, say, children in free-living spontaneous activity situations (Biddle and Armstrong 1990b; Chubb 1990).

3

Beliefs and Attitudes

It is quite logical to think that people's behaviour is influenced by their beliefs in the benefits or advantages of certain things. To some extent, both education in general and health education campaigns in particular are clearly aimed at changing beliefs (or at least "knowledge") in the attempt to bring about change in behaviour. Unfortunately, changes in awareness, beliefs and knowledge far from guarantee changes in behaviour. The link between beliefs and behaviour has occupied social psychologists for many years in health research.

A number of theoretical models have been proposed that attempt to explain the role of beliefs and attitudes in human behaviour. The purpose of this chapter, therefore, is to outline the major integrating theories in both health beliefs and attitudes, and to report research findings that have a bearing on exercise behaviours.

Although beliefs and attitudes are treated separately in this chapter, the two concepts are closely linked. Beliefs refer primarily to knowledge, thoughts and perceptions; attitudes are also about these things, but in addition are associated with feelings, values and behaviours, whether actual or intended.

Beliefs

The Health Belief Model

Theoretical Origins

The question of why people do, or do not, seek health care has been an important one for health psychologists, and for other social scientists (Rosenstock and Kirscht 1979). Indeed, the field was initially typified by diverse findings and an apparently irreconcilable set of behavioural predictors until, in the 1950s, a group of American social psychologists attempted to integrate the work on health behaviours. Until this time the explanations for peoples' health behaviours were based on medical, economic, social, demographic, motivational, organisational and many other perspectives. Such diversity led these researchers to develop an integrated model, The Health Belief Model (HBM) (Becker et al. 1977a; Maiman and Becker 1974; Rosenstock 1974).

The HBM developed from Kurt Lewin's "field theory" and an expectancy-value approach to motivation and behaviour. Lewin's phenomenological perspective advocated that behaviour was influenced by both the individual's characteristics and the environment. The expectancy-value approach can be seen to have been influential in contemporary psychology through attribution theory, achievement motivation, self-efficacy, locus of control and other approaches (see Weiner 1980).

Behaviour, according to an expectancy-value approach, will be influenced by the value placed on the behaviour or outcome, and the expectation, or estimate of likelihood, that a given action will produce the desired result. Task difficulty will be likely to interact, however, since success at a difficult task will produce high positive value, whereas failure at an easy task will have a high negative value attached to it. Similarly, some tasks are more highly valued than others by some individuals, and exercise is clearly a case in point.

Lewin's "field theory" stated that we exist in a "life space" or regions of both positive and negative value, and forces attract and repel us from these. Illness, for example, is a region of negative value and hence we are motivated to avoid it most of the time. Value on its own, however, will not always determine behaviour. Very difficult tasks which could elicit great satisfaction in success, and minimal dissatisfaction in failure, are not always attempted. This could be due to the low expectation of success we are likely to have in such situations, thus showing that expectancy can modify the influence of value.

The Model

Based on this theoretical perspective, the HBM was devised in an attempt to predict health behaviours, primarily in response to low rates of adoption and adherence of preventive health care behaviours. Becker et al. (1977a) stated that the HBM was adopted as an organising framework for four main reasons:

1. the model has potentially modifiable variables
2. the model is derived from well-known psychological and behavioural theory
3. although the HBM was first developed to account for preventive health behaviours, it has also been employed successfully to account for "sick-role" and "illness" behaviours. ("Sick-role" behaviours are primarily associated with seeking treatment or a remedy for illness, whereas "illness" behaviours are primarily associated with seeking advice or help on the nature and/or extent of the illness (Kasl and Cobb 1966))
4. the HBM is consistent with other health behaviour models (see Becker et al. 1977a)

The HBM has subsequently been applied to a wide variety of health behaviours, including asthma (Becker et al. 1978), dietary behaviour (Becker et al. 1977b; O'Connell et al. 1985), breast self-examination (Champion 1985), sex education (Eisen and Zellman 1986), attendance at a blood pressure screening clinic (King 1982), alcoholism treatment (Rees 1985; Rees and Farmer 1985), tuberculosis screening (Wurtele et al. 1982), and exercise (Biddle and Ashford 1988; Lindsey-Reid and Osborne 1980; Olson and Zanna 1982; Noland and Feldman 1984, 1985; O'Connell et al. 1985; Slenker et al. 1984; Tirrell and Hart 1980).

The model hypothesises that people will not seek (preventive) health behaviours unless: (a) they possess minimal levels of health motivation and knowledge, (b) they view themselves as potentially vulnerable, (c) they view the condition as threatening, (d) they are convinced of the efficacy of the "treatment", and (e) they see few difficulties in undertaking the action.

These factors can be modified by socio-economic and demographic factors, as well as "cues to action", such as media campaigns or the illness of a close friend or relative. The HBM is illustrated in Fig. 3.1 and a subsequent, more detailed, model based on the HBM, for the prediction and explanation of individual health-related behaviours is shown in Fig. 3.2.

Health and Illness Research. Although the focus of this book is on exercise as a health-related behaviour, the majority of the HBM research has involved illness, sick-role or preventive behaviours other than exercise. Indeed, Rosenstock (1974, p. 333) stated that "it should be noted explicitly that the Model has a clearcut avoidance orientation". The extent to which this can be applied to exercise without modifications, therefore, remains to be seen and will be discussed later.

Janz and Becker (1984), after a decade of systematic research using the HBM, published a state-of-the-art review. They reported (Janz and Becker 1984, p. 1) that "the HBM has continued to be a major organising

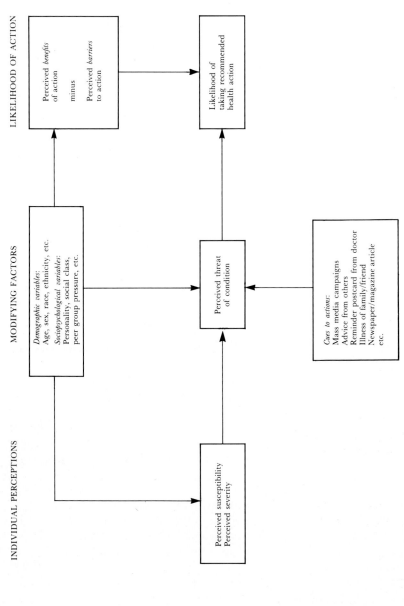

Figure 3.1. The original Health Belief Model. (Modified from "Selected psychosocial models and correlates of individual health-related behaviours" by M.H. Becker et al. (1977) *Medical Care*, 15 (5): 30.)

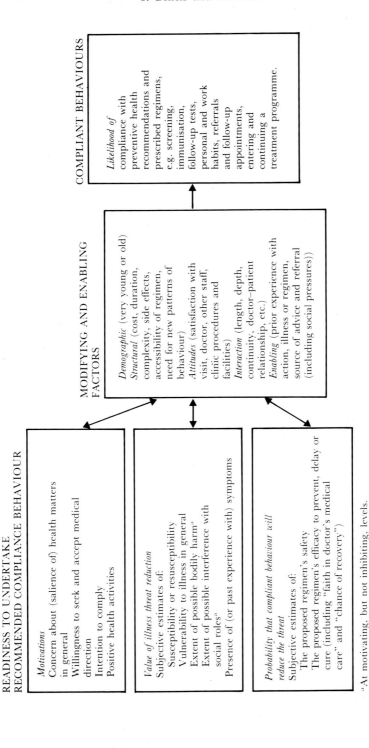

Figure 3.2. The expanded Health Belief Model. (From "Selected psychosocial models and correlates of individual health-related behaviours" by M.H. Becker et al. (1977) *Medical Care*, 15 (5): 39. Reprinted with permission of J.B. Lippincott Co.)

framework for explaining and predicting acceptance of health and medical care recommendations". They concluded that:

1. there was substantial support for the model across more than 40 studies
2. the HBM is the most extensively researched model of health-related behaviours
3. prior to 1974, "perceived susceptibility" (to illness) was the most significant predictor and powerful dimension of the model. However, the variable of "perceived barriers to action" had not been used in many of the studies
4. post-1974 research showed that "perceived barriers" was the most consistently powerful predictor
5. beliefs associated with susceptibility appeared to be more important in preventive health behaviours
6. beliefs in the perceived benefits of action seemed more important in sick-role and illness behaviours
7. despite the variability of measuring instruments, the HBM has remained robust across a wide variety of settings and with a wide variety of research techniques

Exercise Research. Despite its illness-avoidance orientation, the HBM has been used as a framework for investigating exercise behaviours. Lindsay-Reid and Osborn (1980) studied 124 sedentary male fire-fighters in Canada. A prospective design was used whereby health beliefs were measured at the beginning of an exercise programme and also 6 months later. Scores on three health belief indices were elicited: heart disease risk index (HDRI), illness probability index (IPI), and benefits index (BI). Fig. 3.3 shows the percentage of exercise adherers and non-adherers (at 3 months) scoring below the mean score on the three health belief indices. The number of exercisers reporting low perceptions of risk of heart disease (HDRI) and illness probability (IPI) was significantly more than non-exercisers.

Lindsay-Reid and Osborn (1980) concluded that those who adhered to the exercise programme tended to have beliefs associated with reduced susceptibility of CHD and general illness, contrary to the HBM. Feelings associated with illness susceptibility, therefore, were not motivating for this sample in terms of adopting and maintaining physical activity.

The results of this prospective study were supported in a cross-sectional retrospective street survey by Biddle and Ashford (1988). In their first study of 433 adults, they analysed the health beliefs, knowledge and attributions concerning cardiovascular health of aerobic exercisers and non-exercisers. These two groups were found to be quite different, exercisers being higher in knowledge, health motivation, and perceptions of control, and reporting that they had done more in the past to maintain their cardiovascular health. Non-exercisers, on the other hand, reported greater

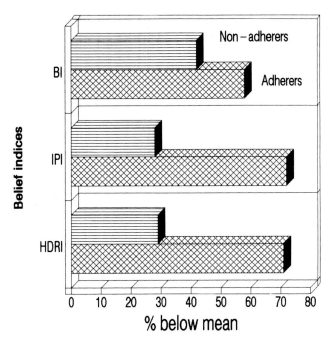

Figure 3.3. Health belief indices and exercise adherence. (Adapted from Lindsay-Reid and Osborn 1980.) BI = benefits index; IPI = illness probability index; HDRI = heart disease risk index.

perceptions of vulnerability to general and cardiac ill-health.

In a second study of 468 subjects, Biddle and Ashford (1988) found similar results. Specifically, they reported that exercisers were higher in exercise intention, importance and benefits, and also had stronger beliefs in exercise control, were more likely to have been active in the past, and were more likely to have modified other health habits. Non-exercisers had higher perceptions of general health vulnerability.

These two sets of results suggest that perceptions of vulnerability to ill-health are related to *inactivity* rather than to positive health behaviours as predicted by the HBM. This may be the result of thinking that exercise is something to be done "when well" and that some forms of exercise may be hazardous, particularly for certain groups. Some support was found for this in the second study reported by Biddle and Ashford (1988) where subjects under 40 years of age felt that exercise was safer and had a stronger intention to exercise. Of course it is true that exercise when "ill" is not advised, but the longer-term public health benefits of physical activity for people of all ages and disabilities is now well documented (Powell 1988; see Chap. 1).

Tirrell and Hart (1980) investigated the HBM and its relationship with adherence to a walking programme for patients who had recently undergone

coronary bypass surgery. Overall adherence was associated with fewer
barriers to exercise, knowledge of the exercise programme, and perceived
efficacy of the programme. Beliefs in susceptibility and severity, as well as
a composite measure of the HBM, were unrelated to exercise compliance.

Similarly, Slenker et al. (1984) reported in their study of joggers and
non-exercisers that the single most powerful predictor of jogging was the
barriers variable. This included time, other responsibilities, and the weather.
Fig. 3.4 illustrates the relative contribution of the variables to jogging
behaviour with the columns representing the R^2 change value in a multiple
regression analysis. This shows that barriers account for almost 40% of
jogging behaviour, while the other variables add much smaller amounts to
this.

A comprehensive social psychological study of exercise adherence
conducted by Olson and Zanna (1982) included the measurement of health
beliefs. Specifically, 60 new members of four fitness clubs in Toronto,
Canada were studied for 3 months. The HBM was used as the basis for
measuring health beliefs. Susceptibility, seriousness and the efficacy of
exercise in prevention were assessed in each of four health "problems" –
heart, lungs, blood pressure and obesity.

Consistent with findings by Lindsay-Reid and Osborn (1980) and Biddle
and Ashford (1988), but inconsistent with the HBM, Olson and Zanna

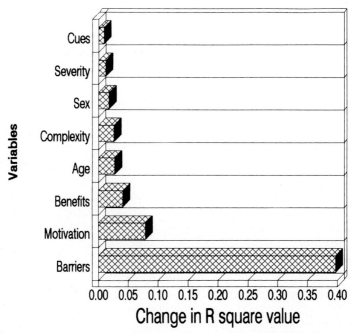

Figure 3.4. Predictors of exercise behaviour, showing R^2 change values from
multiple regression analysis. (Adapted from Slenker et al. (1984).)

(1982) found that exercisers ("regular attenders") considered heart, blood pressure and respiratory problems to be less serious (at the time of joining the club) than other subjects. However, these results are less clear, due to some interesting and consistent gender differences. As illustrated in Fig. 3.5, male adherers reported greater susceptibility to problems associated with heart, lungs and obesity than male non-adherers, whereas female adherers reported less susceptibility to these health problems than female non-adherers.

These results show that the HBM illness-avoidance orientation predicts exercise involvement for men, whereas the results reported by some of the earlier studies, many of which contradict the HBM, seem more consistent with the results for women. Given the greater incidence of heart disease in men than women (National Forum for Coronary Heart Disease Prevention 1988), it is possible that men may be more motivated by seeing exercise as an appropriate preventive health behaviour. However, this is inconsistent with some of the previously cited studies. Similarly, given the social pressure on women to maintain or lose body fat, one would have predicted that female exercisers would report greater susceptibility to obesity problems. This is, as shown in Fig. 3.5c, contrary to the results found by Olson and Zanna (1982). Clearly, some clarification is required if exercise behaviours and health beliefs are to be more clearly understood in the future.

O'Connell et al. (1985) used the HBM as a framework for predicting exercise and dietary behaviours of obese and non-obese adolescents. For obese children, these researchers found that the variable "cues to exercise" was a significant predictor of exercise behaviour. These cues included poor muscle tone, peer pressure, and poor health. No variables predicted exercise for non-obese adolescents.

HBM: Conclusions and Critique. From the evidence presented here on exercise and the HBM, it is clear that the supportive findings reported by Janz and Becker (1984) do not necessarily hold true for exercise behaviours. Although isolated variables, such as barriers to action, may relate to some exercise behaviours (e.g., Slenker et al. 1984), the model as a whole has been relatively unsuccessful in predicting the adoption and/or maintenance of physical exercise. Indeed, it could be argued that there is greater support for beliefs from the HBM predicting *non-participation* in exercise (e.g., Biddle and Ashford 1988; Lindsay-Reid and Osborn 1980). The exercise and HBM studies are summarised in Table 3.1.

There is little doubt about the general heuristic appeal of the HBM. However, a number of points can be made in criticism of the model and associated research (see Sonstroem 1988; Wallston and Wallston 1985).

First, one must question the holistic nature of the model. Is it one model or merely a collection of individual variables? Indeed some workers have argued that because the list of potential variables is so large, the model is untestable (Wallston and Wallston 1985). Similarly, what relationships

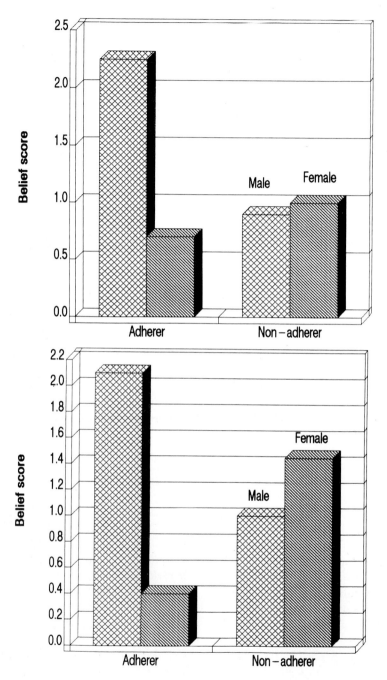

Figure 3.5.a–c Interaction effects between gender and adherence for perceptions of, **a**, heart problems, **b**, lung problems and, **c**, obesity problems. (Adapted from Olson and Zanna 1982.)

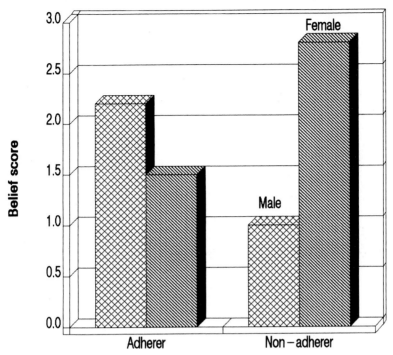

Figure 3.5.c

exist between the variables and how should the model variables be tested? Some research studies test the variables in linear combination while others test multiplicative interactions.

Second, there has been a lack of consistency in the operationalising of variables and the measuring tools used. Although Janz and Becker (1984) point out that the results obtained from a diversity of measuring instruments add to the validity of the model, such diversity does not make for easy comparison across studies. Although recent psychometric developments have been made in the measurement of exercise benefits, outcomes and barriers (Sechrist et al. 1987; Steinhardt and Dishman 1989), these instruments were not developed as tools for the direct assessment of the HBM.

Another criticism is that many of the studies measure health beliefs retrospectively, although some prospective studies do exist in health (King 1982) and exercise (Lindsay-Reid and Osborn 1980). Inevitably, the retrospective studies fail to resolve the temporal patterning of beliefs and behaviour: do beliefs cause the behaviour or does the behaviour produce the beliefs?

In terms of exercise research, one of the major problems associated with the HBM is that it was developed to predict an isolated illness-avoidance behaviour, such as attendance at a clinic. Exercise is a complex behaviour

Table 3.1. Summary of Research on Exercise and the Health Belief Model

Study	Sample	Measures	Study purpose(s) and design	Results	Comments
Lindsay-Reid and Osborn (1980)	124 sedentary male fire-fighters	3 major health belief indices and adherence to exercise programme	Prospective study of the relationship between HBM variables and exercise adherence	Exercise adherers reported low perceptions of risk of heart disease and illness probability. Beliefs in the benefits of health action were significant predictors of exercise adoption	Susceptibility beliefs predicted in contrary direction to HBM
Tirrell and Hart (1980)	32 men and women who had recently undergone coronary bypass surgery	Health beliefs, knowledge, exercise adherence	Relationship between health beliefs and knowledge and adherence to a walking programme	Adherence associated with perceptions of few barriers, exercise knowledge and perceived efficacy for exercise	Composite HBM measure unrelated to adherence
Olson and Zanna (1982)	60 new members of four fitness clubs (24 male; 36 female)	A multitude of social, psychological, and biological factors, including health beliefs	3-month prospective study of predictors of exercise adherence	Regular attenders had lower perceptions of susceptibility to heart, blood pressure and respiratory problems. However, this pattern was mainly due to	Consistent interaction on beliefs between adherence and gender. Requires further study

Study	Sample	Variables	Aim	Results	Comments
Slenker et al. (1984)	124 joggers, 96 non-exercisers	HBM variables, knowledge, motivation, health locus of control	(a) development of a valid questionnaire based on the HBM (b) test questionnaire as predictor of jogging behaviour	Barriers to jogging major predictor. Other HBM variables contributing smaller amounts of variance ... females with males showing the opposite trend	
O'Connell et al. (1985)	69 obese and 100 non-obese adolescents	HBM variables, knowledge, and weight locus of control	To test the HBM in predicting dietary and exercise behaviours in obese and non-obese adolescents	Exercise behaviour for obese adolescents predicted by cues to exercise (poor muscle tone, peer pressure, poor health). None of the HBM variables predicted exercise behaviour of non-obese adolescents	Only study located on HBM, exercise and children
Biddle and Ashford (1988)	433 men and women (Study 1). 468 men and women (Study 2).	HBM variables, knowledge, attributions	Retrospective street surveys of aerobic exercisers and non-exercisers	Both studies show exercisers and non-exercisers to differ, but mainly contrary to HBM predictions on vulnerability	

and, at least where adherence is concerned, is a *process* more than a single behaviour (Dishman 1987; Sonstroem 1988). For example, exercise is likely to involve stages of adoption, maintenance, relapse and re-adoption in many cases. Similarly, motives for adopting and maintaining exercise can be diverse, and may not include health enhancement or illness avoidance. The evidence presented here suggests that the illness-avoidance orientation of the model is not appropriate for the explanation or prediction of exercise behaviours.

Parts of the HBM, or at least beliefs themselves, may remain within a wider model of exercise behaviour (see Dishman 1990, Dishman and Dunn 1988). Although the HBM may not be wholly appropriate for the prediction of exercise, its historical significance should not be underestimated. However, there appears to be a strong case for modifying the existing HBM for the prediction of exercise behaviours.

The Exercise Behaviour Model

From the review of the literature so far it has been suggested that the HBM is incomplete for the study of exercise. Noland and Feldman (1984, 1985), however, attempted to answer this criticism with their Exercise Behaviour Model (EBM). This is illustrated in Fig. 3.6.

Essentially, Noland and Feldman (1984, 1985) proposed that there are four major predispositions in influencing exercise. These are perceived control over exercise behaviour (exercise locus of control; see Chap. 4), attitudes toward physical activity, self-concept, and values related to exercise. As with the HBM, the EBM specifies a number of "modifying" factors, such as demographics, cues to action, as well as perceived benefits and barriers. According to Noland and Feldman (1984, p. 33), "the Exercise Behaviour Model is intended as a comprehensive, theoretical model which attempts to outline and relate factors that are most likely to interact to produce an individual's decision to engage in regular, vigorous exercise".

Regrettably, as outlined in Chap. 4, where locus of control is discussed, parts of the model have no reported psychometric validity. As yet the EBM remains exploratory, although the creation of an exercise-specific model is to be applauded. Nevertheless, preliminary analyses of the model show that attitude and locus of control are related to exercise behaviour in only weak and inconsistent ways. Also, contemporary views of motivation and social cognition suggest that their measures of attitudes and values need reappraising (see Dzewaltowski 1989).

Attitudes

It is often seen to be a statement of the obvious that attitudes are about feelings and behaviour. However, the study of attitudes in social psychology

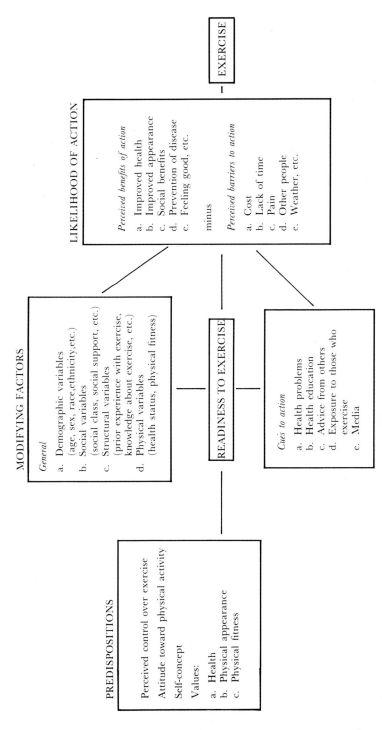

Figure 3.6. The Exercise Behaviour Model (Noland and Feldman 1984, 1985). Reprinted with permission from *Health Education*, March/April 1984, p. 35. *Health Education* is a publication of the American Alliance for Health, Physical Education, Recreation and Dance, 1900 Association Drive, Reston, VA 22091, USA.)

has a long, yet controversial, history, particularly when attempting to predict behaviour from stated attitudes. Indeed, it is common to find attitude change as a clearly stated goal in situations such as health care and education, presumably because of the belief that attitude change will lead to behaviour change. Of course, things are not quite as simple as that and it is necessary to explore the theoretical research in the social psychology of attitudes in order to develop a clearer understanding.

So far, this chapter has concentrated on the beliefs people may hold about health and exercise and whether these have any influence on subsequent behaviours. A three-component model of attitude (Hovland and Rosenberg 1960), however, suggests that this is an incomplete view of the attitude process. In addition to attitudes having a belief (cognitive) component, they also have affective (emotional) and behavioural components (Ajzen 1988; Eiser 1986, 1987; Stahlberg and Frey 1988) (see Fig. 3.7).

Attitude, like personality, motivation and some other psychological constructs, is hypothetical and not open to direct observation. The responses often used to infer attitudes can be either verbal or non-verbal in each of the cognitive, affective and behavioural categories of the three-component model. These are illustrated in Table 3.2, with examples from physical exercise.

Attitudes toward Physical Activity: A Descriptive Approach

The study of attitudes has interested sport and exercise scientists for quite a long time although the initial research efforts were primarily descriptive. For example, Kenyon (1968), in his widely cited research, developed the Attitude Toward Physical Activity (ATPA) inventory in which he identified six sub-domains. These domains reflected Kenyon's belief that physical activity could be reduced to more specific components based on their "perceived instrumentality". Kenyon's model, therefore, suggested that

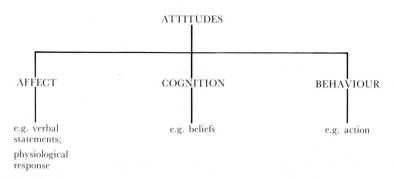

Figure 3.7. Simplified diagram of the three-component view of attitudes. (Adapted from Hovland and Rosenberg (1960).)

Table 3.2. Responses Used in Inferring Attitudes Toward Exercise (Adapted from Ajzen 1988)

Response mode	Response category		
	Cognitive	Affective	Behavioural
Verbal	Expressions of belief about exercise	Expressions of feelings towards exercise	Expressions of intention to exercise
Non-verbal	Perceptual reactions to exercise	Physiological reactions (independent of effort) to exercise	Exercise approach or avoidance behaviours.

physical activity was perceived as (a) a social experience, (b) health and fitness, (c) the pursuit of vertigo (thrill and adventure-seeking activities), (d) an aesthetic experience, (e) catharsis, and (f) an ascetic experience. Numerous studies have used the ATPA scale, and a modified version has been developed for children (Schutz et al. 1985).

While the description of attitudes about physical activity may have some use in research and be of some heuristic value (Miller Lite 1983), such expressions of attitudes have been found to be poor predictors of actual behaviour. For example, Sidney et al. (1983) found differential attitude profiles on the ATPA among over-60-year-olds in an endurance exercise programme. But these attitudes were unrelated to reported participation patterns, daily records of activity, and measures of physical fitness. Similarly, Biddle and Bailey (1985) found significant attitude differences, using Kenyon's scale, between male and female participants in fitness classes, but found no relationship between these attitudes and stated reasons for participation.

Kenyon (1968) states that the area of social attitudes has been plagued by problems of definition and measurement. However, Kenyon (1968, p. 567) defines attitude as: "a latent or nonobservable, complex, but relatively stable behavioural disposition reflecting both direction and intensity of feeling *toward a particular object* ..." (our emphasis). This definition, therefore, means that the ATPA scale will assess a generalised attitude toward physical activity rather than attitude toward a specific behaviour, such as jogging or recreational walking. It is not surprising, therefore, that behaviours are not strongly predicted from such a measure.

Attitude-behaviour Models

The descriptive approach to attitude measurement inevitably led researchers to question whether attitudes actually did predict behaviours at all – the "attitude-behaviour discrepancy". Indeed, Eiser (1986, p. 60) states that this discrepancy is "essentially an artefact of the haphazard selection of specific behavioural indices which researchers have tried to relate to general verbal measures of attitudes", but goes on to say that "if we are as selective in our choice of behavioural indices as we are at present in our choice of verbal indices, the 'attitude-behaviour discrepancy' may disappear as a substantive problem".

Such a critique is consistent with a more contemporary view of the role of attitudes in predicting behaviour. In social psychology in general, as well as exercise psychology research in particular, the Theory of Reasoned Action (TRA) model has been used extensively in the belief that specific measures of attitude, in conjunction with social influences, will predict behavioural intention and subsequent behaviour.

The Theory of Reasoned Action

Proposed by Ajzen and Fishbein (Ajzen and Fishbein 1980; Fishbein and Ajzen 1975), the TRA is concerned with "the causal antecedents of volitional behaviour" (Ajzen 1988, p. 117). It is based on the assumption that intention is an immediate determinant of behaviour, and that intention, in turn, is predicted from attitude and social (subjective) normative factors. The TRA is illustrated in Fig. 3.8.

Ajzen and Fishbein suggest that the attitude component of the model is a function of the beliefs held about the specific behaviour, as well as the evaluation (value) of the likely outcomes. The measurement of such

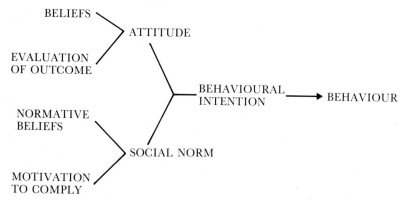

Figure 3.8. Theory of Reasoned Action. (Adapted from Ajzen 1988.)

variables, they suggest, should be highly specific to the behaviour in question. Specifically, four factors should be considered:

1. action: attitude and behaviour need to be assessed in relation to a *specific* action, such as taking part in an aerobic dance class rather than a general attitude object such as physical activity
2. target: reference should be made to specific target groups, such as aerobic exercisers
3. context: reference should be made to the context in which the behaviour takes place (e.g. private vs. public)
4. time: specificity of time should be considered

The social norm component of the TRA ("normative component") is comprised of the beliefs of significant others and the extent that one wishes or is motivated to comply with these beliefs. The relative importance of the attitudinal and normative components will depend on the situation under investigation. For example, one might hypothesise that adolescent health behaviours, in some contexts, will be more strongly influenced by the normative component than the attitudinal component, but that this trend may be reversed with adults.

TRA and Exercise Research. The TRA has received a great deal of attention in social psychology (see Ajzen 1988; Eiser 1986) and has also been used as a model for the investigation of a number of health behaviours (see Eiser 1986; McCaul et al. 1988). Although not without its critics, particularly in respect of the causal structure of the model (see Liska 1984), it has also been recommended and used in exercise research (Godin and Shephard 1990; Smith and Biddle 1990a; Sonstroem 1982b, 1988).

Riddle (1980) tested the TRA in predicting jogging behaviour in adult women and men. Specifically, she found that the intention to jog was significantly predicted from both the attitudinal and normative components of the model, although the attitudinal component was stronger. The beliefs held about the consequences of jogging were the factors most clearly distinguishing joggers from non-exercisers with, as expected, joggers having the more positive beliefs. Similarly, Pender and Pender (1986) found that both attitudinal and normative components of the TRA predicted intention to exercise in a community sample, although only attitude predicted intentions to attain or maintain recommended body weight and avoid highly stressful situations.

The work of Godin and co-workers has been the most extensive test of the TRA in exercise settings (Godin et al. 1986a,b,c; Godin et al. 1987a, b; Godin and Shephard 1984, 1986a,b, 1990; Godin et al. 1989; Valois et al. 1988). Godin and Shephard (1986a) tested the predictive utility of the Kenyon model against the TRA. In terms of predicting intention to be physically active the TRA attitude component was superior to the sub-domains of Kenyon's model, thus supporting earlier statements about the need to measure specific attitudinal factors in predicting behaviour.

In a further test of the theory, Godin and Shephard (1986b) studied 698 Canadian children aged 12–14 years. They found that boys were more active than girls and that boys had a greater intention to exercise, and higher scores on the attitudinal and normative components of the TRA, although these declined in both boys and girls across the three cohorts studied. Overall, the TRA was only partially supported in its ability to predict exercise intentions. The attitude component was found to be a better predictor of intention than the normative component.

Those children with a strong intention to exercise were found to have significantly different beliefs about exercise and the consequences of exercise from those with weak intentions, although even those with weak intentions held reasonably positive beliefs about exercise. These differences are illustrated in Figs 3.9 and 3.10.

Godin and Shephard (1986b) also analysed data on 192 children where parental information was also available. Although, when testing the full TRA, the normative component was less predictive of intentions than the attitudinal component, nevertheless the researchers did find that strength

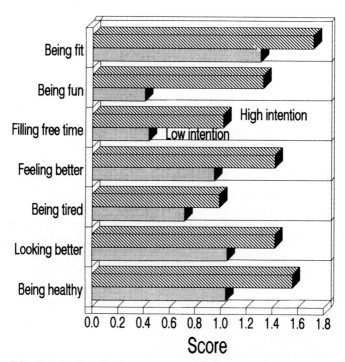

Figure 3.9. Exercise beliefs of children. Possible range is −2 to +2. (Adapted from Godin and Shephard 1986b.)

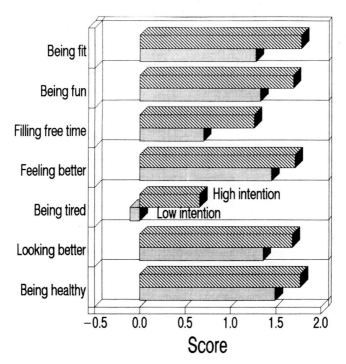

Figure 3.10. Evaluation of consequences of exercise outcomes by children. Possible range is −2 to +2. (Godin and Shephard 1986b.)

of the children's intention to exercise was related to the mother's intention to exercise, the father's current physical activity levels, and the family's socio-economic status, thus confirming the importance of some family influence variables. However, this requires further investigation since Godin et al. (1986a) found little relationship between the activity levels of parents, as perceived by the children, and the children's own activity levels. However, given the problems children have in accurately assessing their own levels of physical activity (Saris 1986), the validity of their reports of levels of parental activity must be questioned.

In a study of 62 lower-limb-disabled adults, Godin et al. (1986c) revealed that intention was a significant predictor of exercise, but the two TRA components did not predict intention, thus leading the researchers to conclude that the TRA had failed with this particular sample.

Greenockle et al. (1990), however, found that the amount of exercise taken by 14-year-old students in a physical education class was mediated by intention and the normative component of the TRA was a stronger predictor of intention than attitude.

Smith and Biddle (1990b) were not able to discriminate between adherers and non-adherers to an exercise programme in a commercial health club in terms of either attitudes towards the exercise programme or social norm beliefs. However, they found that the attributions given for adherence/non-adherence clearly discriminated between the two groups. The main attributions for adherence were ease of the task and personal effort, and the main attribution for non-adherence was luck. Future studies may wish to investigate the role of attributions in modifying the attitude-behaviour relationship, particularly in situations of ongoing behaviour such as exercise adherence.

TRA: Conclusion and Critique. The TRA has received some support in exercise contexts, although by no means have the results been clear-cut. Based on the evidence presented, the TRA attitudinal component appears to be influential in predicting intentions to exercise (Godin and Shephard 1986b). From a practical standpoint this suggests that interventions that attempt to alter beliefs and affective perceptions of the outcomes of exercise may be useful. More is needed to be known about the physical sensations and senses of satisfaction and enjoyment attached to beginning exercise routines before definitive statements can be made here (see Chap. 2). However, it appears that the physically demanding routines associated with rigorous training regimes would be quite unsuitable for the majority of people wishing to start and maintain a health-related exercise programme. Educational interventions in terms of both the cognitive and affective components of exercise attitudes appear warranted.

Although the normative component of the TRA has not been a strong predictor of exercise intentions, it has sometimes contributed in a small way. Interventions that are possible include public health campaigns (e.g. Biddle and Armstrong 1990a) that persuade the public that exercise is normal and not just for the young, fit and "sporty". The concept of persuading people through "fear appeals" will be dealt with later in the chapter.

The TRA has not been without its critics, and, as already demonstrated, it has only been partially successful in predicting exercise intentions, let alone actual behaviour. Eiser (1986) high-lights a number of limitations of the TRA:

1. the TRA is a unidirectional model and fails to offer the possibility that variables in the model can act in a reciprocal manner
2. the TRA predicts behaviour from measures of behavioural intention taken at one point in time. Similar attitudinal models of behaviour (e.g. Triandis 1977; Bentler and Speckart 1981) take into account prior behaviour or "habit". In the exercise context, habitual physical activity is often the goal of public health initiatives and therefore research may usefully investigate the role of habit in addition to other TRA variables. As it stands, the TRA may only predict new behaviours rather than habitual ones

3. the TRA was developed to account for behaviours that are under volitional control (Ajzen 1988). Consequently, the theory may not predict behaviours where other factors may be influential. In the case of exercise, there may be a number of behavioural barriers preventing the behaviour being totally volitional (e.g. responsibilities to others, job etc)

A revised TRA, the "Theory of Planned Behaviour" (TPB; see later in this chapter), is an attempt to account for behaviour under "incomplete" volitional control.

In addition, insufficient attention has been paid to the measurement of behaviour within the TRA (Smith and Biddle 1990a). Without an accurate measure of the behaviour under investigation, the principle of correspondence cannot be applied. This casts some doubt on several of the studies cited here, such as Riddle (1980) and Godin and Shephard (1986b). Riddle's research used self-report of jogging behaviour whereas Godin and Shephard measured only intentions rather than exercise behaviour. The definition of the behaviour and its measurement present particular problems for the study of exercise adherence within the TRA (Smith and Biddle 1990a).

Alternative Attitude Models

In addition to the widely cited TRA, other models of attitude have been proposed, and some have been used in exercise research. The models reviewed here will be: Triandis' Theory of Social Behaviour, Ajzen's Theory of Planned Behaviour, and Rogers' Protection Motivation Theory.

Triandis' Theory of Social Behaviour. Triandis (1977) proposed an attitude model that has some similarities with the TRA (see Wallston and Wallston 1985; Valois et al. 1988). The model specifies that the likelihood of acting out a particular behaviour will be dependent upon: (i) prior behaviour ("habit"); (ii) behavioural intention, and (iii) facilitating conditions. In contrast to the TRA, the Triandis model suggests that as the strength of habit increases, so the level of volition decreases, and hence proposes that in addition to intention researchers must also assess habit and facilitating conditions.

Valois et al. (1988) compared the Triandis model with that of the TRA in predicting both exercise behaviour and intention. Using 166 adults aged 22–65 years of age, Valois et al. (1988) found that the two models were equally effective in predicting actual exercise behaviour (with each model predicting about one-third of the variance in exercise), but they also found that whereas the Triandis model accounted for 25% of the variation on exercise *intentions*, the TRA accounted for only 9%. This suggests a difference between intentions, in the form of "decision making" and actual behaviour or "decision implementation" (Kendzierski 1990). This is discussed more fully later.

In a similar study by Godin et al. (1987b), measures were taken of past exercise behaviour (habit), attitude, social norm, and both proximal (after 3 weeks) and distal (after 2 months) exercise participation. The results showed that intention was directly influenced by both attitude and habit, proximal behaviour was the result of habit *only*, and distal behaviour was influenced by a combination of intention and proximal behaviour. These researchers concluded that their results had two clear practical implications. First, if the target group is sedentary adults, intervention should take place through the attitude component as this, and not subjective norm, influences intention. However, for children the intervention should be in the form of developing the exercise habit and positive attitudes since this group is unlikely to have developed these adequately at this age.

Theory of Planned Behaviour. The TRA has provided a model that has been partially successful in predicting behaviour and intentions for actions that are primarily *volitional* and *controllable*, which include a large number of every-day behaviours. However, in the case of physical exercise, and other health-related behaviours such as smoking and weight control, volitional control is likely to be "incomplete" (Ajzen 1988). As outlined in Chap. 4, perceptions of behavioural control have a potentially important role in many health-related behaviours.

Ajzen's theorising and research (Ajzen 1988; Ajzen and Madden 1986; Ajzen and Timko 1986; Schifter and Ajzen 1985) suggest that the TRA is insufficient for behaviours where volitional control is incomplete. Consequently, Ajzen has proposed an extension of the TRA for such behaviours and has called this the Theory of Planned Behaviour (TPB). The TPB is the same as the TRA but with the additional variable of perceived behavioural control, as illustrated in Fig. 3.11.

Perceived behavioural control is defined by Ajzen (1988, p. 132) as "the perceived ease or difficulty of performing the behaviour"; he goes on to say that it is assumed "to reflect past experience as well as anticipated impediments and obstacles". Fig. 3.11 links perceived control with both intentions and behaviour. This suggests that the variable is proposed to have a motivational effect on intentions, such that individuals wishing to exercise, for example, but with little or no chance of doing so (because of largely insurmountable behavioural barriers at the time) are unlikely to exercise regardless of their attitudes towards exercise or the social factors operating. Similarly, Ajzen (1988) argues that perceived behavioural control will accurately predict behaviour under circumstances when *perceived* control closely approximates *actual* control. For example, whereas some people may have a strong perception of control over their body weight, the reality might be different since there are biological factors likely to affect weight gain and loss which are beyond personal control. In such situations one would not expect perceived control to be a strong predictor of weight

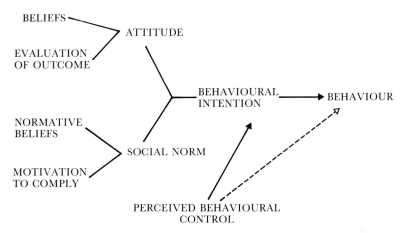

Figure 3.11. Theory of Planned Behaviour. (Adapted from Ajzen 1988.)

change, although it is possible for it to predict to a lesser degree. Similarly, one would expect better predictions of exercise *behaviour* (e.g., frequency of exercise) from perceived control compared with exercise *performance* (e.g., a fitness test score) since the latter is less controllable, because of factors such as heredity and the test environment.

Evidence from the Theory of Planned Behaviour. The TPB has interesting potential for use in the study of exercise, particularly as exercise is a behaviour that has many participation barriers, thus making it a behaviour that is only partly under volitional control. Consequently, the use of TPB is appropriate in exercise settings and should extend the results reported using the TRA. However, to date the testing of the TPB has been modest, although has included health behaviours which may be similar to exercise, such as weight loss. One must remember, though, that weight loss is a health outcome whereas exercise might be described as a health behaviour or process. Nevertheless, this research gives some insight into the TPB in a health context.

Schifter and Ajzen (1985) studied 83 American female college students who included overweight and normal weight subjects, although overweight students were encouraged to participate. The study tested the TPB for weight loss and subjects were weighed at the beginning and end of a 6-week period and, at the same time, asked to complete questionnaires testing the TPB. The adherence rate over the 6 weeks was 91%. Subjects were assessed at the beginning of the study on their attitudes, subjective (social) norms, perceived control and intentions for weight loss, and other variables assessed included Health Locus of Control, ego-strength, and self-knowledge. After 6 weeks the subjects were assessed on control and competence scales.

Schifter and Ajzen (1985) analysed their results in terms of the relationship between the three model variables of attitude, norm and control with both intention to lose weight and actual weight loss. All three variables were found to correlate significantly with the intention to lose weight, but only perceived control correlated significantly with actual weight loss. These correlations are illustrated in Fig. 3.12.

The bivariate correlations illustrated in Fig. 3.12, however, do not test the model adequately. Consequently, Schifter and Ajzen (1985) used multiple regression analysis in predicting intention and found that attitude, norm and perceived control all made significant and independent contributions to intention (multiple R = 0.74). Further analyses showed that the greatest weight loss was experienced by those with a high perception of control and strong intentions to lose weight. At low levels of perceived control, however, no effect for weight loss was found.

These results suggest that actual weight loss was much more a function of *perceived control* over weight loss than the intention to lose weight. This is consistent with Ajzen's (1988) argument that the TRA is insufficient when the behaviour in question is not totally under volitional control.

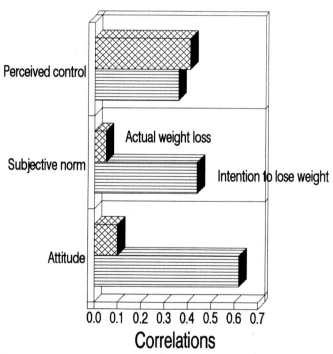

Figure 3.12. A test of the Theory of Planned Behaviour (TPB), showing weight loss intentions, actual weight loss, and TPB variables. (Adapted from Schifter and Ajzen 1985.)

Gatch and Kendzierski (1990) tested the TPB in predicting the intentions of 100 female American students in attending an aerobic exercise class. They found that perceived behavioural control significantly increased the prediction of intention over and above that accounted for by attitude and subjective norms. No measure of actual exercise behaviour was taken in this study.

Protection Motivation Theory. Earlier in this chapter the Health Belief Model was discussed at some length. A model that has some similarities with the HBM, as well as with the TRA/TPB, is that of Rogers' Protection Motivation Theory (PMT; Rogers 1983). This, too, is a cognitive model based on expectancy-value principles. It was originally developed as an explanation for the effects of "fear appeals" in health behaviour change, although "health threats" might be a better term as the model is really one of health decision-making (Wurtele and Maddux 1987).

Health behaviour intentions ("protection motivation") are predicted from the cognitive appraisal mechanisms shown in Fig. 3.13. The "threat appraisal" is in turn determined by perceptions of vulnerability and the possible severity of the health outcome. Similarly, the "coping appraisal" is predicted by perceptions of efficacy and the costs of undertaking the action.

Support has been found for the model (Rippetoe and Rogers 1987). Similarly, Prentice-Dunn and Rogers (1986) contrast the PMT with the HBM and suggest that the PMT has some distinct advantages. They say that the PMT has more of an organisational framework and is not open to the criticism of merely being a catalogue of variables. Second, the division of cognitive appraisals into threat and coping categories helps to clarify how people think about health decision-making. Third, PMT includes self-efficacy, a variable found to be a powerful mediator of behaviour change in other studies (see Chap. 5). Also, PMT accounts for the role of emotion in health behaviours.

To date, only one study has tested PMT in an exercise context. Wurtele and Maddux (1987) made 160 sedentary undergraduate women read persuasive appeals for increasing their exercise. The appeals were varied along the four dimensions of severity, vulnerability, response efficacy and self-efficacy. (Consistent with Bandura's (1977a, b) theory of self-efficacy, PMT includes two types of efficacy. "Response efficacy" refers to the belief that a response will produce the desired outcome whereas "self-efficacy" refers to the belief in one's own ability to initiate and maintain the desired behaviour; see Prentice-Dunn and Rogers (1986)).

Wurtele and Maddux (1987) found that only vulnerability and self-efficacy predicted intentions to exercise, which in turn were predictive of self-reported exercise. These researchers also found that subjects with high self-efficacy also had strong intentions to exercise even though they were not exposed to the vulnerability-enhancing or response efficacy-

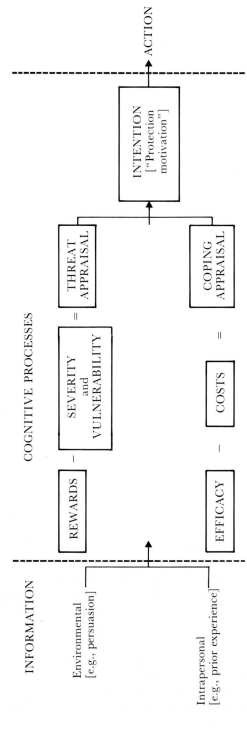

Figure 3.13. Adapted version of the Protection Motivation Theory Model. (Adapted from Prentice-Dunn and Rogers 1986.)

enhancing conditions in the study. This confirms the important role of self-efficacy in behaviour change. Wurtele and Maddux (1987) also found that the threat appeals were ineffective in changing exercise intentions.

Decision-making Theories

Kendzierski (1990) and Kendzierski and LaMastro (1988) have studied the role of attitudes and exercise from the perspective of decision-making theories. In particular they high-light Edwards' (1954) Subjective Expected Utility (SEU) theory and Kuhl's (1985) Action Control (AC) perspective.

SEU theory suggests that decisions about exercise are made on the basis of the individual's belief in the worth or value of exercise, or more specifically of the outcome from exercise, and the probability that this outcome will occur should participation take place. Whether exercise takes place, or the type of exercise participated in, will be determined by the behavioural alternative with the most favourable value and probability. Interestingly, SEU theory considers alternative courses of action, and thus when used in exercise research will shed light on the individual's beliefs about *not* exercising as well as about participation itself. This approach has rarely been used in exercise research.

Kendzierski and LaMastro (1988) found that SEU theory predicted interest in exercise (weight training) but not actual adherence. They concluded that SEU theory may be more useful in situations involving simple choices, whereas they argue that exercise adherence is a complex behavioural process.

Kendzierski (1990) conducted further research along these lines. Specifically, she investigated SEU theory and Kuhl's (1985) AC theory in predicting intentions, adoption of and adherence to aerobic exercise. Subjects were assessed on Kuhl's "action control scale" which categorises subjects into action-oriented or state-oriented individuals. Action-oriented are those who tend to focus on and plan for future actions, whereas state-oriented individuals are those who do not plan for the future and focus on the present or past.

Kendzierski (1990) found that SEU theory predicted exercise intentions but not adherence, leading her to suggest that it was important to make the distinction between decision *making* and decision *implementation*. The correlation between intention and behaviour was slightly stronger for action-oriented individuals, giving some support to Kuhl's AC theory. This theoretical perspective may be useful in investigating perceptions of control (see Chap. 4), and the use of planning strategies in exercise. Some authors have suggested (e.g. Dishman 1990; Dishman and Dunn 1988) that self-regulatory planning skills may be important in the exercise adherence process. Similarly, SEU theory requires further study in exercise research, including the investigation of attitudes towards *not* exercising (Kendzierski and LaMastro 1988; Smith and Biddle 1990a).

Concluding Remarks

Despite these theoretical models, little is still known about the nature of attitude change in the domain of exercise (see Godin and Shephard 1990). McGuire's (1985) process model of persuasion might usefully be tested in exercise contexts. This model suggests five stages are required for the successful change in behaviour from a message. The five stages are: attention, comprehension, yielding, retention, and behaviour (see Stroebe and Jonas 1988).

The early research into attitudes and physical activity was largely descriptive and failed to provide consistent data on attitude–behaviour links. The subsequent adoption of attitude and belief models, some of which have been reviewed here, and the commonalities and differences evident in structure and research results, suggests that no one model is going to be sufficiently predictive that other models can be dismissed. Nevertheless, in exercise psychology there are still a number of theoretical models that have yet to be tested, and still others that require testing against each other to assess their relative effectiveness. The social psychological emphasis may also have to be broadened to account for psychobiological factors, such as emotions and physical sensations, that will accompany the exercise experience.

4

Perceptions of Control

The literature about health and fitness is consistent in its message that changes in exercise and health behaviours are associated with the need to "take control" or "take charge" of personal lifestyles. The information that many of the modern diseases linked with premature mortality are "lifestyle-related" (Powell 1988) has the implicit message that we, as individuals, are at least partly responsible, thus implying the need for personal control and change.

Corbin et al. (1987a) have outlined a "stairway to health-related fitness" as a working model of objectives for the teaching of fitness and health to school students. In this model they suggest that students need to progress to a state of relative "fitness independence" in which they have achieved the knowledge and skills to enable them to have a measure of control and expertise to change or maintain levels of fitness and exercise independent of advice from teachers or other people. Similarly, Biddle (1987a), in an outline of practical aspects of motivation and lifestyle change in exercise, says that behaviour change is something that can be brought about through perceptions of increased control. This can also be found in the literature about weight control (Mahoney and Mahoney 1976). In describing their "wellness" approach to exercise and fitness, Patton et al. (1986, p. 26) state that "wellness-oriented health/fitness programmes have a philosophical base similar to that of humanistic psychology and humanistic education, which recognise self-responsibility as being integral to genuine self-growth".

It should also be recognised, however, that there are potential problems with health messages that consistently encourage personal control as the *only* way of changing behaviour. Feelings of guilt can develop when problems arise that are out of the individual's control (e.g., disease related to environmental pollution) but which might cause other people to blame the victim for a lack of motivation or moral behaviour (see Biddle 1989a; Sparkes 1989). Similarly, positive changes in behaviour can be achieved by allowing some control to be exerted by others, such as doctors.

This chapter, therefore, will discuss the psychological issues associated with perceptions of behavioural control in the context of health and exercise (see Lau 1988). A number of psychological orientations focus on this issue, including locus of control of reinforcements, attribution theory, and intrinsic motivation.

Locus of Control of Reinforcements

Theoretical Origins

Locus of control of reinforcements refers to the extent that people perceive that reinforcements are within their own control, are controlled by others, or are due to chance factors.

The locus of control (LOC) construct stems from an approach to personality known as social learning theory (Rotter 1954) where general beliefs are thought to develop from expectations based on prior reinforcements and the value attached to such reinforcements. This is an expectancy-value approach to motivation (see Weiner 1980). In his seminal monograph on LOC, Rotter (1966, p. 2) says that "it seems likely that, depending on the individual's history of reinforcement, individuals would differ in the degree to which they attributed reinforcements to their own actions". This led Rotter to formalise the construct of LOC and suggest that a generalised belief existed for internal versus external control of reinforcement. Rotter (1966, p. 1) defined "internals" and "externals" as follows:

> If the person perceives that the event [the reinforcement] is contingent upon his/her own behaviour or his/her own relatively permanent characteristics, we have termed this a belief in *internal control*.
>
> When a reinforcement is perceived . . . as following some action of his/her own but not being entirely contingent upon his/her action, then . . . it is typically perceived as the result of luck, chance, fate, as under the control of powerful others, or as unpredictable . . . When the event is interpreted in this way, . . . we have labelled this a belief in *external control*.

In the same monograph Rotter presented psychometric evidence for the measurement of LOC with his internal–external (I–E) scale. This was (Rotter 1966, pp. 1–2) a measure of "individual differences in a generalised belief for internal or external control of reinforcement". The 29-item scale yields one score of LOC (high score indicating high externality) thus suggesting that LOC is a unidimensional construct. This has been challenged by a number of researchers. It should be noted, however, that Rotter stated that his I–E scale was a measure of *generalised* expectancy and, therefore, was likely to have a relatively low behavioural prediction but would apply across a wide variety of situations. It was also likely to have greater predictive powers in novel or ambiguous situations since in specific well-known contexts more specific expectancies will be used (see section on Self-Efficacy Theory in Chap. 5).

Two developments in LOC research that have a bearing on exercise involvement are the multidimensional nature of LOC and the behavioural specificity of measuring instruments.

Multidimensional LOC

In terms of multidimensionality, a number of researchers have suggested that the unidimensional I–E split is insufficient (Cherlin and Bourque 1974; Collins 1974; Duffy et al. 1977; Levenson 1981; Palenzuela 1988; Reid and Ware 1973), although they do not all agree on the exact nature of the multidimensionality. Nevertheless, there is some agreement that at least the external pole of LOC should be divided into "chance" and "powerful others" since those believing that their life is "unordered" (chance "control") would be different from those believing in events being controlled by powerful others (Levenson 1981; Whitehead and Corbin 1988; see Fig. 4.1). This distinction could have important implications for exercise and health research, as discussed later.

Specificity of Measurement

Since Rotter's I–E scale was developed as a generalised measure, it was inevitable that researchers would predict that more situation-specific measures of LOC would allow for better prediction of specific behaviours. One of the most widely used of such measures is the Multidimensional Health Locus of Control Scale (MHLC; Wallston et al. 1978) which yields scores on internal, chance and powerful others subscales and is a

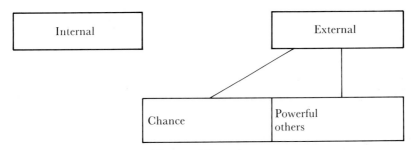

Figure 4.1. Multidimensional Locus of Control.

development from the unidimensional version (Wallston et al. 1976). The MHLC, however, has had mixed success in predicting health behaviours, largely because of the wide range of possible behaviours it encompasses. It is also orientated towards illness and, therefore, may have little relationship with more overt health-enhancing behaviours such as exercise (Whitehead and Corbin 1988). Nevertheless, early reviews of the literature (Strickland 1978, 1979; Wallston and Wallston 1978, 1981) concluded that there was evidence for a link between health LOC and specific health behaviours.

Other health-specific scales have been developed, such as Saltzer's (1982) Weight Locus of Control scale (WLOC). This 4-item inventory has been shown to possess validity such that WLOC internals were more likely to complete a weight-control programme than externals, and of those who did complete the programme, internals with a high value for physical appearance or health were more successful in achieving their initial weight-loss goals compared with externals who also valued health and appearance (Saltzer 1982).

Exercise Research and LOC

Research into the link between perceived control, as measured by LOC scales, and participation in exercise has taken three routes. First, some researchers have tried to identify links between generalised LOC and exercise, some have used health LOC, and, more recently, exercise- and fitness-specific measures have been developed and tested. These studies are summarised in Table 4.1.

General and Health LOC Measures

Sonstroem and Walker (1973) studied the relationship between LOC and both physical fitness and activity levels. They administered the Rotter I–E scale, Kenyon's (1968) Attitude Toward Physical Activity (ATPA) scale (a general measure of activity attitudes with domains of social experience, health/fitness, catharsis, ascetic, aesthetic, and vertigo (thrill/risk); see Chap. 3), and a questionnaire to assess the extent of voluntary participation in physical activity to 102 final year American university students. In addition, a 600-yard run was administered as an index of cardiovascular fitness. However, current thinking suggests that such a test is a poor indicator of this component of fitness (AAHPERD 1984). The same test had been administered to these students in their first year at the university.

The results were analysed by means of a one-way analysis of covariance, with first-year fitness (run) scores as the covariate in an effort to control for initial fitness levels. The students were placed in one of four groups on the basis of an *a priori* decision of a median split on the I–E scale and at the 45th and 55th percentile ranks on the ATPA. It was found that internals with a positive attitude score ran significantly faster than all other groups. A one-way analysis of variance (ANOVA) on the activity levels produced the same result. However, when 2 (internal/external) by 4 (ATPA quartiles for full sample) ANOVAs were performed on activity level, only a main effect for attitude (value) was found. No post-hoc analyses were reported but the raw data provided by Sonstroem and Walker (1973) suggest that activity levels were higher for those with more positive attitudes, and particularly so for those in the top quartile. A trend could be observed such that internals had higher activity levels within each quartile.

Such results suggest that LOC may have a small influence on activity and fitness scores. However, the fitness results are questionable on grounds of test validity.

Sonstroem and Kampper (1980) also used a generalised measure of LOC in a study of pre-adolescent boys. This investigation attempted to predict participation and adherence to school sports from measures on Sonstroem's (1978) Physical Estimation and Attraction Scales (PEAS) and Bialer's (1961) LOC scale for children. Participation in sports was predicted by scores on both estimation and attraction, but not by LOC. Adherence to a cross-country running programme was not predicted by any of the study variables.

A more popular approach in exercise LOC studies has been to administer the MHLC scale and then try to discriminate between groups of exercisers and non-exercisers. O'Connell and Price (1982) compared those who adhered to a 10-week exercise programme delivered on-site to employees of an American insurance company with those who dropped out and a control group of non-participants. The results showed small, but significant, differences such that the adherers were more internal than the drop-outs who, in turn, were more internal than controls. No differences were found for the chance or powerful others subscales.

Similar results were found by Slenker et al. (1985) in an analysis of joggers and non-exercisers. Joggers were more internal, but not different on chance and powerful other scales, compared with non-exercisers, although age may have been a confounding variable since it was found that the joggers were significantly younger.

Carter et al. (1987) studied 110 women who had enrolled on a 15-week college aerobic exercise programme. The MHLC was administered alongside a questionnaire eliciting reasons for joining the class. Subjects were classified as "internal" if they scored above the median on the internal scale *and* below the median on the chance scale. Subjects were considered to have a high "value" for fitness if they rated physical fitness as their prime reason for attending the class. A 12-min run test was given to the subjects in which they had to run or walk as far as possible in 12 minutes. Although it is generally recognised that this is a better measure of cardiovascular

Table 4.1. Tabular Summary of Studies of Locus of Control and Exercise and Fitness

Study	Sample	LOC Measure	Study Purpose(s)	LOC Results	Remarks
A. Generalised LOC Measures					
Sonstroem and Walker (1973)	American male senior undergraduates (n = 102)	Rotter's I–E scale	Investigated the relationship of LOC and health/fitness value to fitness and activity	Internals with high fitness value had faster run times and greater activity levels	Fitness measure (600 yd run) lacks validity
Duke et al. (1977)	74 boys and 35 girls aged 6–14 years	Nowicki-Strickland Internal–external control scale	Investigated changes in LOC over 8-week sports camp	Shift to more internal LOC and improvement in physical fitness scores	No control group. Numerous explanations possible for LOC shift
Sonstroem and Kampper (1980)	393 boys aged 12–13 years	Bialer's LOC scale	Prediction of school sport participation and adherence from psychometric scales of physical estimation and attraction, and LOC	LOC not predictive of either participation or adherence	
B. Health LOC Measures					
Dishman and Gettman (1980)	Adult male participants in supervised exercise programme (n = 66)	Health LOC (HLOC)	Prospective study of psychobiological predictors of adherence/drop-out	Health LOC at programme entry not a significant discriminator between adherers and drop-outs. Externals with low fitness value were more likely to drop out.	

Study	Sample	Measure	Aim	Findings
Blair et al. (1980)	504 company employees	HLOC	Investigated leisure-time physical activity as intervening variable with HLOC and social support in health behaviours	Vigorous exercisers with internal HLOC had better scores on a medical examination and the Cornell Medical Index
O'Connell and Price (1982)	Male and female adult participants in a corporate fitness programme (n = 89)	Multi-dimensional health LOC (MHLC) scale	MHLC differences between adherers and drop-outs	Adherers slightly more internal than drop-outs
Olson and Zanna (1982)	24 male and 36 female Canadian adults in community fitness clubs	MHLC	Social psychological predictors of adherence	Male drop-outs characterised by high scores on powerful others
Laffrey and Isenberg (1983)	Women from adult education classes (n = 70)	MHLC	Interrelationships of MHLC, health value, exercise importance, and physical activity in leisure time	No relationship between internal health LOC and activity
Slenker et al. (1984)	124 adult joggers and 96 non-exercisers	MHLC	a) Development of a questionnaire based on the Health Belief Model (HBM); b) Utility of questionnaires in predicting jogging/non-exercising	MHLC did not significantly add to HBM variables in predicting jogging

Table 4.1. Continued

Study	Sample	LOC Measure	Study Purpose(s)	LOC Results	Remarks
Slenker et al. (1985)	132 adult joggers and 93 non-exercisers	MHLC	Differences between joggers and non-exercisers on MHLC	Joggers more internal. No differences on chance and powerful others	Joggers were also younger
Carter et al. (1987)	110 women on 15-week college aerobic exercise programme	MHLC	Association of LOC and fitness value with fitness, success expectancies and effort ratings	LOC unrelated to fitness. Internals with high fitness value reported that they were willing to exert more effort than others	
C. Exercise/Fitness LOC Measures					
Noland and Feldman (1984)	Adult women (n = 64)	Exercise locus of control (EXLOC) measure	Relationship between aspects of the exercise behaviour model, including EXLOC, and exercise participation	External (environment) subscale of EXLOC inversely related to participation	Psychometric properties of EXLOC unknown
Noland and Feldman (1985)	Adult women (n = 215)	EXLOC	As for 1984 study	No relationship between EXLOC and participation for 25–45-yr olds.	As above

McCready and Long (1985)	Adult women in community fitness programme (n = 61)	Exercise objectives LOC scale (EOLOC)	Relationship between exercise adherence, physical activity value, and LOC	Greater amounts of exercise related to higher internal and lower chance and powerful others scores on EXLOC for 46-65-yr olds	Factorial validity of powerful others dimension of EOLOC unclear
Long and Haney (1986)	Sedentary women (n = 68)	EOLOC	a) To assess impact of counselling on initiating a more active lifestyle. b) To assess EOLOC and related variables in the context of a)	EOLOC unrelated to adherence. Levenson's LOC external scales weakly related. Weak relationship between EOLOC (with value) and activity increases	
Whitehead and Corbin (1988)	3 groups of American undergraduates (total n = 377)	Physical fitness LOC (FITLOC)	Psychometric construction of FITLOC	Preliminary evidence for validity and reliability of FITLOC with college sample. Weaker concurrent validity with activity measure	Requires testing with other samples and with value measures

fitness than the 600-yard run test mentioned earlier, it is still highly dependent on pacing skills and motivation and is only moderately correlated with $\dot{V}O_{2max}$ (Safrit et al. 1988).

Carter et al. (1987) found by means of an ANOVA that those with a high value placed on fitness scored better on the run test regardless of LOC scores. However, when asked how much effort they would be willing to put in to the run, the highest effort scores were recorded by both the internal and high value groups.

Laffrey and Isenberg (1983) studied 70 American women aged 24–65 years on the following variables: (a) leisure time physical activity (LTPA; assessed through a modified version of the Minnesota Leisure Time Activity Questionnaire), (b) the internal scale of the MHLC scale, (c) a measure of "health value" based on Rokeach's scale of terminal values, and (d) a measure of "perceived importance of physical exercise" on a 9-point Likert scale.

The results showed no relationship between LTPA and internal health LOC or health value. Activity and perceived importance (value) of exercise were significantly correlated ($r = 0.53$, $p < 0.001$). A step-wise multiple regression analysis predicting LTPA from the three other variables showed that 21% of the variance in LTPA was explained by perceived importance/value of exercise. Health value and internal health LOC added a minimal amount to the prediction.

In a study of joggers and non-exercisers, Slenker et al. (1984) tested out items related to the Health Belief Model (HBM) but also included a measure of health LOC (MHLC). In a multiple regression analysis using all HBM variables and MHLC, 61% of the variance in jogging behaviour was explained by eight of these variables. However, health LOC did not contribute significantly to the prediction.

Finally, Dishman and Gettman (1980) used the unidimensional health LOC measure developed by Wallston et al. (1976) as part of a battery of measures in attempting to predict exercise adherence and drop-out in a 20-week prospective study of adult men (see Chap. 2). Health LOC did not significantly add to the discrimination between adherers and drop-outs in a discriminant analysis even though adherers had higher internal scores than drop-outs. Similarly, in attempting to predict days of exercise participation, a step-wise multiple regression analysis showed that only the variables of self-motivation, body fat and body weight enhanced the prediction equation, accounting for 45% of the variance. Health LOC entered as the fifth variable but did not add to the prediction. Nevertheless, it was found that subjects with an external health LOC and low value score on Kenyon's ATPA health/fitness scale were less likely to adhere to the programme than subjects with an internal health LOC and high health/fitness attitude score.

Dishman and Gettman's (1980) data provide, at best, moderate support for the concept of health LOC in predicting participation in a supervised exercise programme. Given their use of multivariate statistics in researching variables that discriminate between adherers and drop-outs, it is possible to conclude that LOC is a relatively weak influence when placed in the context of other factors.

These results collectively provide rather weak support for LOC in predicting fitness and exercise behaviours, although the extent that this could be a reflection of the inadequacies of the fitness or LOC measures remains to be seen. At best these studies suggest that some group differences may exist between exercisers and non-exercisers at a cross-sectional level on LOC. However, one cannot ascertain whether such differences developed as a result of involvement or whether they influenced the initial decisions to become active. The conclusion from these studies, therefore, appears to be that health LOC does not strongly predict, or relate to, exercise behaviour although some association has been found in some studies.

Such an equivocal conclusion has prompted researchers to ask why such is the case. Three main possibilities exist. First, the theory could be wrong or not applicable to exercise; second, the measuring tools are not sensitive or appropriate enough to demonstrate a relationship between LOC and exercise participation, and third, fitness/exercise "externals" are rare people, thus making it difficult from a research perspective to demonstrate relationships or discriminate between groups. Given the theoretical predictions of LOC research, and the extensive testing of the theoretical constructs involved, one could still propose that a relationship should exist. Most of the studies where no relationship has been found suggest that the LOC measures have not been specific enough to exercise and fitness behaviours, and this includes health LOC. Dishman and Gettman (1980) conclude by saying that not all people will perceive exercise as a health-promoting behaviour anyway. Calls for greater specificity in measurement have been met, with several recent studies that have addressed this issue in exercise and physical fitness.

Measurement of Exercise and Fitness LOC

Several researchers have attempted to develop exercise or fitness LOC scales (McCready and Long 1985; Noland and Feldman 1984; Whitehead and Corbin 1988). In a study of female participants in a university health education evening class programme, Noland and Feldman (1984) tested parts of their proposed Exercise Behaviour Model (EBM), as outlined in Chap. 3. They assessed exercise with a shortened version of the Minnesota Leisure Time Physical Activity Questionnaire and also administered questionnaire items on physical activity attitudes and values. LOC was assessed with their own Exercise Locus of Control scale (EXLOC). This scale was purported to measure internal, chance, powerful others, and environment subscales of LOC. Noland and Feldman (1984, p. 34), in terms of the internal scale, said that "it deals with the belief that the individual controls his/her own exercise behaviour". This is conceptually different, of course, from locus of control beliefs of *reinforcement* as postulated by Rotter (McCready and Long 1985; Palenzuela 1988; Rotter 1966, 1975).

Significant relationships between attitude and exercise ($r = 0.315$, $p < 0.05$) and the environment subscale of the EXLOC and exercise ($r = -0.332$, $p < 0.01$) were found. This suggests that exercise is related to positive attitude and inversely related to beliefs that the environment (e.g., weather, exercise equipment) has some control over participation in exercise. A multiple regression analysis of all variables on exercise showed that attitude, value and the four EXLOC scales in combination accounted for 20% of the variance in exercise behaviour, although no single variable was significant.

In a follow-up study of 215 women, Noland and Feldman (1985) assessed the variables of exercise, attitude values and EXLOC once again. In addition, they assessed the extent to which the women perceived 15 barriers to exercise, including costs and lack of time. Analyses were performed separately for those between 25 and 45 years of age and for those between 46 and 65 years. For the younger group, no relationship was found between any of the EXLOC scales and exercise. For the older group, it was found that greater amounts of exercise were related to higher scores of internal control and lower scores on the chance and powerful others scales. The four EXLOC scales, in combination with attitude, fitness value, and perceived barriers accounted for only 17% of the variance in exercise for the younger group. For the older group, however, attitude plus chance (negatively) significantly predicted exercise, with the addition of the other EXLOC scales, fitness value and barriers. Interestingly, whereas the environment scale was the best EXLOC predictor in the Noland and Feldman (1984) study, it was the weakest of the EXLOC scales in the 1985 report.

The Noland and Feldman (1984, 1985) studies were the first to report an exercise-specific LOC scale. However, their research reporting leaves many unanswered questions. First, no psychometric validation procedures for EXLOC are reported, although Noland and Feldman (1985, p. 31) say they "found that the chance, powerful others and internal scales of the EXLOC had positive relationships with each of the respective scales of Levenson's (1974) general, multidimensional locus of control measure". However, these correlations are not reported, nor are any details given as to how such data were collected. The size of the correlations is important as very strong relationships would be indicative of EXLOC measuring almost the same as "general" LOC instead of the intended exercise LOC. No factorial validity is reported, either, for the addition of the environment subscale. Their research leaves open the question: is the weak link between exercise LOC and participation in exercise a result of poor instrumentation or the existence of a genuinely weak relationship? Further research on the *measurement* of exercise-related LOC appears warranted.

McCready and Long (1985) also reported the use of an exercise-specific LOC scale. They studied 61 women aged between 15 and 57 years who were participating in an 8-to-12-week aerobic exercise programme but had exercised regularly (2 to 3 times/week) during the past year. The study investigated the influence of LOC and attitudes on adherence to the programme. Four measures were used: (a) Levenson's LOC scale, (b) a revised version of the Children's Attitude Toward Physical Activity scale (CATPA; Schutz et al. 1985), (c) shortened version of Crowne and Marlowe's (1960) social desirability scale, and (d) the "Exercise Objectives Locus of Control" scale (EOLOC). Preliminary evidence for its validity and reliability is presented by McCready and Long (1985). EOLOC is based on Levenson's multidimensional model of LOC and assesses internal, chance and powerful others scales through an 18-item inventory. The factor structure of EOLOC, however, is still in need of clarification since McCready and Long (1985) report two factor analyses producing 5 factors, although with an increase in the number of subjects in their second factor analysis they could eliminate one of these factors after rotation. However, this still leaves four factors, with internal and chance looking fairly pure. The powerful others items loaded on two factors although it is not clear why this should be. The only detectable difference in the questions is that the three statements loading on factor 3 refer to "exercise objectives" whereas the three statements loading on factor 4 refer to "exercise goals". Further work is required to clarify this.

Analyses revealed that subjects classified into low-, moderate- and high-attendance groups did not differ from each other on the EOLOC scales or CATPA scores. A step-wise multiple regression analysis was used to predict attendance. The results showed that three attitude scores and the two external scales of Levenson's inventory were weak predictors of attendance. EOLOC did not predict attendance at all. This led McCready and Long (1985, p. 352) to conclude that:

> individuals with higher percent attendance tended at the beginning of the fitness programme to have less positive attitudes toward physical activity as a means of continuing social relations and achieving health and fitness, and more positive attitudes toward physical activity for release of tension. They also held weaker beliefs that their reinforcements are controlled by powerful others and a stronger belief that chance elements affect their lives.

These results might seriously question the EOLOC as a measure of exercise-specific LOC, particularly when Levenson's general scale was more predictive. However, the results reported by McCready and Long (1985) show that their subjects had a very narrow range of scores on the internal scale. From a maximum possible score of 30, 72% of subjects scored 29 or 30 (group mean = 27)! Such a biased sample and lack of variability are bound to weaken any statistical analysis relating adherence to internal EOLOC. This supports the contention that it is unlikely many exercise/fitness externals will be found.

Long and Haney (1986) also used the EOLOC and CATPA scales in a study of sedentary women. They investigated the effects of counselling on the initiation of a physical activity programme. Three groups were studied: counselling plus information (about programmes and services in the community), counselling with no information, and a control group on a waiting list. Counselling included the identification of facilitators and barriers to activity, and clarification of any misunderstandings about exercise. All subjects were followed-up after 1 month.

The two counselling groups increased their activity levels significantly over the 1-month period compared with the control group. However, in attempting to predict the increase in exercise from a combination of EOLOC and CATPA scores only weak support was found for these variables. In the control group, it was found that subjects who scored less on EOLOC powerful others and who did not view exercise as a means of risk taking and hard training were more likely to increase their activity levels. However, no such trend emerged for the counselling groups. Regardless of group, however, internal EOLOC, combined with positive attitudes towards activity as a means of improving body shape, enhancing health and reducing tension, were related to an increase in activity. This relationship, however, was statistically weak and accounted for only 5% of the variance.

The consensus has to be that EOLOC has, to date, failed to provide evidence that a LOC measure specific to exercise is a better predictor than other LOC measures. Indeed, one could safely argue that it does not predict exercise behaviours at all well.

One of the problems with the exercise-specific measures of LOC so far reported is that the psychometric properties of the scales (i.e., EXLOC and EOLOC) are still unclear. A more recent and rigorous attempt to develop a LOC scale for physical fitness behaviours has been reported by Whitehead and Corbin (1988). They present preliminary evidence for the validity and reliability of FITLOC – multidimensional scales for the measurement of locus of control of reinforcement for physical fitness behaviours – with American college students. Items were written to reflect the three dimensions of internal, chance and powerful others, and "physical fitness behaviours" were defined (Whitehead and Corbin 1988, p. 110) as "any behaviours which would be likely to result in a change in a subject's organic physical fitness status". Items were then administered to four experts in exercise psychology to test for face validity. This produced 18 items which were then reduced to 11 through a variety of procedures, including factor analysis, alpha reliability and item discrimination analyses.

The 11 items of FITLOC contained three for internal control (IFit), and four each for chance (CFit) and powerful others (PFit). Further analyses with a new sample supported the factorial validity of the scale, and concurrent validity was demonstrated by predicted relationships with Levenson's subscales, although this was more strongly supported for the CFit and PFit scales rather than IFit. Concurrent validity was only marginally demonstrated with correlations between the FITLOC scales and a measure of physical activity recall (see Fig. 4.2). The correlation coefficients, while in the expected directions, were unconvincing in their strength. Whitehead and Corbin (1988) suggested that future research needs to include measures of value if concurrent validity is to be adequately demonstrated. Their own analysis had to assume that value scores were equal across subjects.

The FITLOC requires further testing, particularly with more hetero-geneous samples. As Whitehead and Corbin (1988) themselves point out, further work needs to include measures of value as well as expectancy, including the nature of social relationships people might have with powerful others.

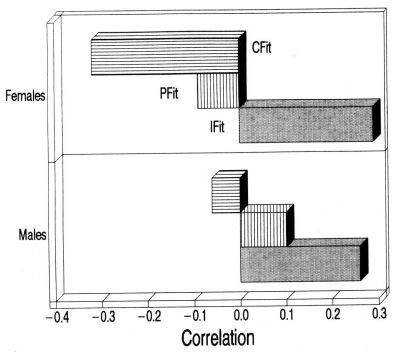

Figure 4.2. Correlations between physical activity estimations and FITLOC subscales for males and females. (Adapted from Whitehead and Corbin 1988.)

A Critique of Locus of Control

The research on LOC so far reported has originated from the construct as outlined by Rotter (1966). Subsequent developments have included the use of multidimensional and situation-specific instruments. However, the overall conclusion one can reach about the relationship of LOC (however measured) and participation in exercise or fitness activities is largely weak or inconclusive. Current interest in the use of meta-analytic reviews in psychology (Hunter et al. 1982) suggests that a meta-analysis of the LOC literature might help resolve the inconclusive nature of the narrative review presented here. Alternatively, a critical look at the LOC construct itself, or at least the way it has sometimes been used in research, may also shed further light on the problem (see also Mineka and Hendersen 1985; Palenzuela 1988; Rotter 1975).

Rotter (1975) has outlined three main problems and misconceptions about the I–E LOC construct. First, he suggests that the most consistent problem in LOC research is the avoidance of measuring reinforcement value, a point echoed by Whitehead and Corbin (1988). It would be an over-simplification to suggest that internals will act in a certain way simply because of their control beliefs. Differences in their interests and values associated with the behaviour could easily override any internal or external orientation. In terms of exercise behaviour this could account for some of the equivocal results reported, although some of the studies have attempted measures of value (or attitude). For example, the current interest in some forms of exercise (e.g., mass jogging, aerobic exercise-to-music classes) might suggest that one important factor operating here is social compliance to a "fashion". Research suggests that externals may be more compliant than internals. If some externals valued health and physical fitness and wanted to comply with the current fashion of mass jogging, one would predict higher levels of involvement for *externals* rather than internals.

A second problem outlined by Rotter (1975) is that of specificity-generality. He suggests that the ambiguity of the situation may also be important in determining whether LOC has an effect on behaviour. In novel and ambiguous situations people have little or no information to draw on, and hence are more likely to be influenced by generalised beliefs in LOC. However, for more familiar situations, LOC beliefs are likely to be less important since beliefs specifically related to the behaviours in question may acquire greater salience. Again, this may account for the weak relationships between LOC and participation reported in the sport and exercise literature. It could be hypothesised that people already possess beliefs about their physical abilities, competence and so on. They are more likely, therefore, to draw on these specific beliefs than more generalised LOC beliefs.

The third problem Rotter (1975) outlined was referred to as the "good guy–bad guy" dichotomy. By this he meant that researchers had often erroneously assumed that it was "good" to be internal and "bad" to be external. Although it may be an advantage to hold internal LOC beliefs at times, it could also be argued that such beliefs can be maladaptive. Palenzuela (1988) has argued this in his cogent analysis of the LOC construct. He suggests that an interactionist perspective is required such that the "advantage" of internal or external beliefs will depend on the situation. Guilt and frustration may be created in children who have always been led to believe that their propensity for being overfat was "their fault" (high internality) whereas it may be more a function of their parents' influence on the childrens' lifestyles; a case of genuine lack of control. Palenzuela (1988) suggests that an interactionist perspective may help resolve the good guy–bad guy dichotomy.

Another problem with the LOC construct is that of multidimensionality. Many of the health and exercise research studies have utilised scales consisting of internal, chance and powerful others subscales. However, it has already been suggested that these three dimensions are by no means clear cut (see McCready and Long 1985). Palenzuela (1988, p. 613) suggests that the dimensionality of the LOC construct should be determined by the "nature and definition of the construct and then confirmed at an empirical level, not the opposite way round". This supports Rotter's (1975) argument that simply factor analysing his own I–E scale and finding several factors does not, in itself, demonstrate the multidimensionality of LOC. The results of the factor analysis are likely to be dependent on the sample and "only reveal the kinds of similarities perceived by a particular group of subjects for a particular selection of items".

However, Rotter (1975, p. 63) is not arguing against the use of factor analysis *per se*, rather he says that: "they may be useful if it can be demonstrated that reliable and logical predictions can be made from the subscales to specific behaviours and that a particular subscale score produces a *significantly higher relationship than that of the score of the total test.*"

Similarly, the distinction between positive and negative outcomes is often ignored in LOC research in exercise. Brewin and Shapiro (1984) have argued that it is illogical to speak of internally controlled negative events since one could assume that the negative outcome was unintended. They found that Rotter's I–E scale correlated only with responsibility for positive outcomes. They also provided psychometric evidence for separate scales for the measurement of responsibility for positive and negative outcomes. This distinction is also supported by Gregory (1978). However, in the exercise and health field, it is difficult to know when an individual is trying to avoid a negative outcome (e.g., obesity) or trying to attain a positive one (e.g., a desirable body shape).

Several authors have questioned the concepts of locus of control of *reinforcement* and locus of causality of *behaviour* (Ajzen 1988; Palenzuela 1988). For example, Ajzen's Theory of Planned Behaviour (outlined in Chap. 3) includes the variable "perceived behavioural control" rather than generalised beliefs in LOC of reinforcement. Ajzen (1988) has argued that such generalised beliefs are likely to be unrelated to specific behavioural tendencies when target, action and context factors are considered. Ajzen (1988, p. 104), therefore, concludes that generalised LOC beliefs cannot "be expected to permit accurate prediction". He goes on to say (p. 105) that: "in terms of conceptualising control beliefs that are compatible with a particular behaviour of interest, one need not stop at the level of perceived achievement responsibility or health locus of control. Instead, one can consider perceived control over a given behaviour or behavioural goal".

Ajzen (1988) suggests that Bandura's (1977b) Theory of Self-Efficacy (see Chap. 5) is an appropriate framework here. However, self-efficacy and LOC are conceptually different. Self-efficacy beliefs refer to the beliefs that an individual is *capable* of a particular action whereas LOC beliefs are those associated with the belief in control over *reinforcements*. Indeed, Bandura's distinction between efficacy and outcome expectations is important here since outcome expectancies are more closely related to LOC beliefs than efficacy expectancies, although Palenzuela (1988) has argued that even these concepts are different.

In conclusion, the often-stated belief that "control" over behaviour is necessary for individuals to lead active or healthy lives has not been supported by the LOC literature. This is probably due to a combination of weak methodology, inadequate instrumentation and the likelihood that LOC is, in any case, only a small part of the explanation of exercise behaviours. Future work needs to consider its place in a wider research model and, by implication, its relationship with related constructs.

There is little doubt, however, that a number of theoretical concepts in psychology have a potential relationship with LOC or more specific beliefs in behavioural control, such as attributions, intrinsic motivation, extrinsic rewards, self-efficacy, learned helplessness, and attitudes. Consequently, although the way some of these concepts were originally conceptualised may make them appear independent, it is important to use composite research models to test for similarities and to explain greater amounts of variance in exercise behaviour.

The remaining sections of this chapter will deal with some of these related concepts, including attributions and intrinsic motivation.

Attributions and Exercise

Theoretical Origins

It is not the intention here to provide a comprehensive review of attribution theory *per se* as this can be found elsewhere (see Eiser 1986; Hewstone 1983, 1989; Hewstone and Antaki 1988; Weiner 1986). However, the role attributions may play in perceived control of exercise behaviours is potentially important (Knapp 1988) although, as yet, research focussing specifically on exercise (as opposed to competitive sport) is sparse.

Attributions are the perceived causes and reasons people give for an occurrence and, because the focus is often on the perceived causality of behaviour, the term "causal attributions" is often used. For example, a child may state "I failed the class test because I didn't revise enough". Similarly, a person may attribute a rejected offer of a dinner-date to a personal perception of not being "good looking". These examples illustrate that attributions may be made in both achievement and affiliative domains of behaviour. However, it is in the former that a great deal of research has been accumulated, particularly concerning academic achievement (see Weiner 1980, 1986), but also in sport (see Brawley and Roberts 1984; Rejeski and Brawley 1983). However, to date very little has been written about the role of attributions in health-related exercise contexts, although studies of other health areas have used an attributional approach.

Early Perspectives

Heider (1944, 1958) is seen as the most influential figure on early attribution work with his writings on interpersonal perception and the psychology of "everyday actions". Heider (1958) proposed that:

1. an adequate understanding of individual behaviour is dependent on knowing how people perceive their social environment
2. people seek a predictable and stable environment and consequently indulge in frequent causal thinking
3. people look towards dispositional properties of the person (themselves or others) in accounting for actions, as well as assessing environmental influences

He suggested that an outcome was dependent on "personal force" (motivation and ability) as well as "environmental force" (task difficulty). Subsequent developments in attribution theory (AT) still subscribe to similar views (Weiner 1986) and will be discussed later.

Jones and Davis (1965) produced an influential paper on attributions of other peoples' actions, rather than self-perception. They argued that prior to attributing a cause to another's behaviour, two types of information are processed. First, information related to the social desirability of the behaviour is assessed. For example, more is revealed about someone who acts in an unusual way, such as jogging at 5 a.m.! One could assume more about that person's motivation to jog from this than if the run was with four friends at midday. The second type of information processed is associated with choice. Again, more information about the person is revealed when the behaviour in question has relatively "unique effects". The effects which are relatively unique to exercise are likely to yield important information about why people participate. For example, if people choose to attend an exercise class rather than go to the pub, the motive of affiliation is common to both and, therefore, gives little information about why exercise is chosen. Only unique effects will yield such information, such as the need for exercise and the desire to control body weight, neither of which are likely to be satisfied at the pub! In other words, this analysis allows for a better judgement of why one action was taken in preference to another. Such a perspective, which has yet to be tested in exercise psychology, could provide some insight on participant–leader interaction in exercise settings (Biddle 1986a).

Another perspective adopted in AT is that of Kelley (1967). He used the ANOVA statistical model as an analogy to explain how people arrive at attributions. He suggested that people process information about relationships (covariation) between responses and outcomes in arriving at decisions and attributions. If running is only enjoyed in the summer when the weather is fine, for example, attributions related to running enjoyment become clearer. He has suggested that information pertaining to distinctiveness of the behaviour (whether other people also behave in that way), consistency (whether you have behaved like this before), and consensus (how other people behave in such a situation) interact in the process of making attributions. Again, this has largely gone untested in exercise research (see Biddle 1986a; Biddle and Ashford 1988), although it does feature in other health contexts, such as predicting attendance at clinics where blood pressure levels are screened (King 1983).

Attributions and Perceptions of Control

One of the most widely known approaches to attributions is that proposed by Weiner (1980, 1986). Although Weiner originally worked in the field of educational achievement, his theory of achievement motivation and emotion has application to a broader range of issues (Weiner 1986).

The main attribution elements used in Weiner's research were ability, effort, task difficulty and luck. Table 4.2 summarises some of the cues used in making such attributions. Fig. 4.3 shows the classification model for categorising such elements into the dimensions of locus of control (later renamed locus of *causality*) and stability. The locus of causality dimension classifies attributions as they relate to the individual (internal) or reside outside the individual (external). The stability dimension refers to the classification of attributions in relation to their temporal stability, with some attributions being transient (unstable) and others relatively permanent (stable) over time.

Weiner (1979) later modified this model to include a "controllability" dimension. The locus of control dimension then became locus of causality to reflect better the distinction between this and the "new" dimension. The controllability dimension classifies attributions in terms of whether they

Table 4.2. Antecedents of the Main Attribution Elements. (Adapted from Weiner 1980)

Attribution Element	Antecedents
Ability	Percentage, number and pattern of success; level of difficulty of the task; ego-involved goals
Effort	Relationship between performance and value of the task/goal; perceived physical effort; mastery goals; persistence
Task difficulty	Social norms and comparison; characteristics of the task
Luck	Uniqueness of the outcome; independence, randomness of outcome

are controllable or uncontrollable. For example, effort is often seen to be internal yet unstable whereas ability (at least in the "natural ability" sense) is internal but stable. One could argue, therefore, that effort is controllable whereas ability is not. This kind of argument led to the creation of the extra dimension, as illustrated in Fig. 4.4. The nature and measurement of the controllability dimension, however, remains a point of debate in the literature (Biddle 1988b; Russell 1982).

Weiner has argued that the attribution dimensions are related to the consequences that attributions may have for motivation, cognition and emotion. For example, making attributions to stable factors is likely to lead to expectations that similar results will recur in the future, whereas unstable attributions provide less clear-cut information about expectations. Similarly, attributions to internal factors are thought to heighten emotional feelings

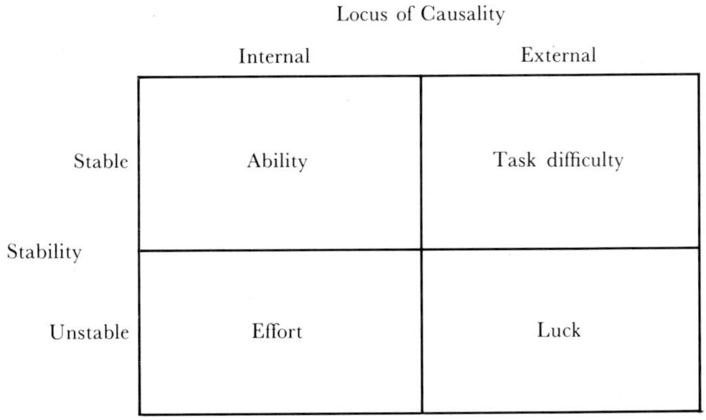

Locus of Causality

		Internal	External
	Stable	Ability	Task difficulty
Stability	Unstable	Effort	Luck

Figure 4.3. Weiner's original 2 × 2 (locus × stability) attribution classification model.

Locus of causality

Internal attribution.   External attribution

	Stable	Unstable	Stable	Unstable
Controllable	Stable effort	Unstable effort	Stable effort (other's)	Unstable effort (other's)
Uncontrollable	Ability	Mood	Task difficulty	Luck

Controllability

Figure 4.4. Weiner's reconceptualised $2 \times 2 \times 2$ (locus × stability × controllability) attribution classification model.

whereas external attributions may be related to a lowering of emotion. This has subsequently been refined such that locus of causality is thought to be related to feelings of self-esteem and pride whereas the controllability dimension is thought to be related to social emotions, such as guilt and pity. For example, attributing the completion of a half-marathon to well-planned training (internal) could increase the feeling of pride associated with the run. If, however, the run was not completed due to a lack of personal effort (controllable), guilt may ensue, or , in the case of someone trying hard but failing due to a perceived lack of ability (uncontrollable), others may feel pity for the individual (see Weiner 1986). Attribution-emotion relationships have been demonstrated in competitive sport (Biddle and Hill 1988; Vallerand 1987) but not in health-related exercise contexts.

One area of attribution research that may be important in the study of exercise is that of learned helplessness. Again, the relationship with exercise is speculative due to a lack of research, although evidence in educational and clinical psychology does exist (see Abramson et al. 1978; Dweck and Leggett 1988; Forsterling 1988; Peterson and Seligman 1984). Apart from a position paper by Dweck (1980), surprisingly little research has been generated in sport or motor-performance contexts (see Johnson and Biddle 1989; Prapavessis and Carron 1988).

Essentially, early work with animals who were found to give up after exposure to uncontrollable failure, even when the situation became potentially controllable, was extended to humans and, later, to include an attributional perspective. In short, Abramson et al. (1978) suggested that uncontrollable failure, when attributed to personal inadequacy (internal, stable attributions), and generalised to other situations ("global" attribution), would generate feelings of helplessness. As a result of such proposals, attribution "retraining" methods were suggested in an effort to change maladaptive attributions for failure (Forsterling 1985, 1988).

Learned helplessness hypotheses retain a great deal of intuitive appeal, although there is much disagreement as to the exact mechanisms underpinning such phenomena (Alloy et al. 1988; Brewin 1988). Research based on this hypothesis might be a fruitful avenue for investigating those who drop out from, or do not initiate, an exercise programme. For example, studies could look at the cognitions of adults quitting, or failing to initiate, activity programmes, and compare them with their more active counterparts. However, this would only suggest cross-sectional differences. Developments should, therefore, include investigations of attributions at the point of drop-out, or over time for those who never participate. Longitudinal studies are required which investigate the development of cognitions in childhood and their relationships, if any, with participation patterns in adulthood.

Attribution Research in Health

The general notion of perceived control in health has a long history. However, it is only relatively recently that formal AT paradigms have been applied. Several researchers have investigated the causal beliefs attached to chronic illness (Gotay 1985; Lowery and Jacobsen 1985). However, in a study of cancer patients, Gotay (1985) did not find extensive attributional thinking (use of the "why me?" question). Chance was the most frequently cited attribution for cancer. Gotay (1985) suggested that avoiding making attributions could be one form of coping strategy. However, Lowery and Jacobsen (1985) did find partial support for Weiner's AT predictions with patients who were chronically ill.

The patients studied by Lowery and Jacobsen (1985) were interviewed and asked to respond to a question about how well they were doing with their illness. A 4-point scale was collapsed into "success" and "failure" categories and the patients were asked why they thought things were going well or not so well. In addition, ten possible causes for the disease were listed and patients rated the importance of each factor. These were based on Weiner's (1979) locus, stability and controllability attribution dimensions.

Patients who attributed their illness to external, unstable or uncontrollable factors tended to perceive themselves as having been unsuccessful in their illness outcome. However, only 66% of the "failure" patients offered an attribution. For the "success" patients, attributions were offered by 79% and tended to be internal and somewhat controllable (mainly effort-based). No evidence was found for a link between stable/unstable attributions and expectations of future success. The sample studied by Lowery and Jacobsen (1985) was strongly optimistic and, therefore, did not expect failure in the long term. Overall, the results partially supported AT predictions for patients who were chronically ill, but further work is required before a clearer understanding of a theory developed in achievement environments has validity in the illness contexts studied here (see Lau and Hartman 1983; Pill and Stott 1985; Rodin 1978; Sechrist 1983; Stoeckle and Barsky 1980).

Bar-On and Cristal (1987) studied 89 male post-myocardial infarction (MI) patients who were admitted to an intensive coronary care unit after their first MI. Two main questions were posed: "why did the MI happen?" and "what will help you cope with it?". Subjects selected their answer from 20 alternatives for each question. These responses were then factor analysed and five main factors appeared: "Fate and luck", "denial", "control of future" (no causes; just internal control for coping), "limits and strengths" (personal strengths and weaknesses), and "the physical model of man" (heredity, poor lifestyle, medication will help etc).

Two rehabilitation measures were assessed: a subjective assessment of ability to function physically, sexually and at work, rated in comparison with their pre-MI perceptions, and a more objective measure, including the number of times they were readmitted to hospital and the number of subsequent MIs.

The results supported an attributional perspective on cardiac rehabilitation. Patients who attributed their MI and its outcomes after hospital treatment to the luck/fate factor returned to work more slowly and were lower on the functioning score compared with patients who attributed the MI to "limits and strengths". This was largely independent of the severity of the MI, level of education, and depression. However, whether this reflects a more stable "attributional style" or perceptions developed in treatment has yet to be determined. Nevertheless, partial support for an attributional perspective in medical settings was provided by this study.

Haisch et al. (1985) investigated the effects of attribution retraining in weight loss and found positive effects. Subjects who were taught to reattribute weight problems to internal and unstable (controllable) factors were more successful in weight control after a 23-week intervention programme than subjects not participating in attribution retraining. This was also shown to be successful after a 10-month follow-up. Again, this suggests that attributions may be important variables in health behaviours, and, in this case, in relation to perceptions of control. This is supported by work by Eiser and co-workers on smoking behaviours (Eiser 1982; Eiser et al. 1978; see also Eiser 1986; Eiser and van der Pligt 1988).

Attribution Research in Exercise

As already stated, attribution research in the domain of physical activity has been almost exclusively on competitive sport. This has tended to be focussed on the attributional patterns of winners and losers, sex differences, and, to a lesser extent, emotional correlates of attributions after competition. Knapp (1988) suggests that attributional factors may be important in behavioural change strategies in exercise but provides a cautionary note on the excessive use of extrinsic rewards. This will be discussed in more detail later in the chapter.

Biddle and Ashford (1988) conducted a cross-sectional retrospective survey of beliefs, including attributions, of exercisers and non-exercisers. In their first study, 433 adults were interviewed, in a street survey, on beliefs about cardiac and general health. It was found that aerobic exercisers (defined as those who participated in aerobic exercise at least twice per week) differed from non-exercisers (those who participated in aerobic exercise "occasionally" or "never") on numerous variables. Of interest to this discussion is that exercisers had significantly higher perceptions of control over their cardiovascular health than non-exercisers. However, this study assessed the three attributional variables of locus of causality, stability and controllability of cardiac health. Therefore, in a second study (n = 468) Biddle and Ashford (1988) also assessed the attributional variables proposed by Kelley (1967), those of "consensus", "distinctiveness" and "consistency". Also, all attributions were made in relation to exercise behaviours rather than cardiac health.

Again, exercisers and non-exercisers were different in their attributions. Exercisers reported higher scores on internality (locus) and controllability over exercise, as well as higher scores on consensus and consistency attribution information (see Fig. 4.5). This suggests that exercisers were more likely to have been active in the past (consistency) and were more likely to have modified other health habits (consensus). However, with cross-sectional surveys of this type causality or direction of influence are unknown. However, the trends are sufficiently important to continue research along these lines but using prospective designs.

In a study of adherence to exercise in a commercial health and fitness club, Smith and Biddle (1990b) found clear differences in attributions for adherence between adherers and non-adherers. These are shown in Fig. 4.6. Adherers reported that their attendance was due to their own effort and ease of the task, whereas non-adherers reported that their lack of attendance was due mainly to luck, but not due to the difficulty of the task, or their own lack of ability or effort.

The research methods proposed by George Kelly may also provide a useful insight into these cognitive processes (Bannister and Fransella 1971; Kelly 1955, 1963). Kelly's "personal construct" theory of personality, while posing logistical difficulties for researchers with the use of individualised repertory grids, is a humanistic phenomenological approach which looks at how individuals organise and perceive their own world. Such an approach may be an interesting route within the attributional framework outlined here (Weiner 1980).

This chapter, so far, has discussed the psychological constructs of locus of control and attributions in relation to exercise, although with attributions the limited amount of exercise research has meant that related fields had

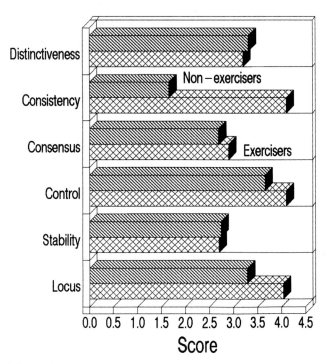

Figure 4.5. Attributions for aerobic exercise involvement reported by aerobic exercisers and non-exercisers. (Adapted from Biddle and Ashford 1988, study II; maximum score possible = 5.)

to be considered. Finally, this chapter will consider the notion of control in the context of intrinsic motivation, which is a motivational construct frequently mentioned as being at the core of exercise adoption and adherence.

Intrinsic Motivation, Perceived Control and Exercise

Motivational issues *per se* have been considered in Chap. 2, yet a discussion on intrinsic motivation in the context of self-determination and perceived control is appropriate at this point.

Intrinsic and extrinsic motivation are well-known constructs in psychology and, although often under different names, in every-day situations too. Intrinsic motivation is motivation to do something for its own sake in the absence of external (extrinsic) rewards. Often this involves fun, enjoyment and satisfaction, such as recreational activities and hobbies. The enjoyment is in the activity itself rather than any extrinsic reward such as money, prizes or prestige from others. Such intrinsically pursued activities are

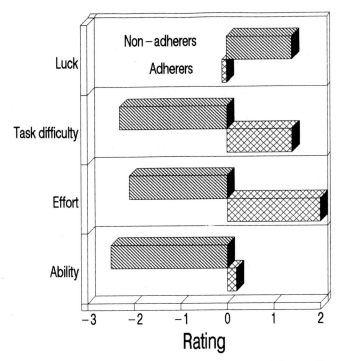

Figure 4.6. Ratings of attributions for exercise adherence and non-adherence in a commercial health club (Smith and Biddle 1990b).

referred to as "autotelic" (self directing) by Csikszentmihalyi (1975). Such a notion is useful for the present discussion since it suggests that intrinsically motivated behaviour is linked to feelings of self-control or self-determination (Deci and Ryan 1985).

Extrinsic motivation, on the other hand, refers to motivation directed by rewards, money, and other external factors (e.g., grades in school). This suggests that if these rewards were removed, motivation would decline in the absence of any intrinsic interest.

The relationship between intrinsic and extrinsic motivation was, at one time, thought to be quite simple in that "more" motivation would result from adding extrinsic to existing intrinsic motivation. This appeared logical given the evidence from behaviourists who have demonstrated that reinforcements (i.e., extrinsic rewards) will increase the probability of the rewarded behaviour reoccurring. However, a number of studies and observations, mainly with children, started to question whether intrinsic motivation was actually *undermined* by the use of extrinsic rewards.

Rewards and Cognitive Evaluation Theory

Cognitive Evaluation Theory (CET) developed from the study of the effects of rewards on intrinsic motivation and is an attempt to explain the possible undermining effects of reward systems on subsequent motivation.

Lepper et al. (1973) tested the relationship between intrinsic motivation and extrinsic rewards with pre-school children (aged 3–5 years). Baseline data on intrinsic interest were collected. Intrinsic motivation was operationally defined as the amount of time spent playing with brightly coloured "magic marker" highlighting pens during a break in the school day. The children were then assigned randomly to one of three groups:

1. "expected reward condition": the children agreed to play with the pens and expected a reward for doing so (a certificate with seal and ribbon)
2. "unexpected reward condition": the children agreed to play with the pens but were not told anything about receiving a reward (although they did receive one afterwards)
3. "no reward condition": these children neither expected nor received a reward for playing with the pens.

The children then participated in the experimental manipulation and were tested individually in a separate room in one of the three conditions. They were observed unobtrusively, on a later occasion, by the use of a one-way mirror. The pens were available in a classroom alongside a variety of other play equipment. The amount of intrinsic interest (involvement) was recorded. Fig. 4.7 shows the amount of time, expressed as a percentage of free-choice time, spent playing with the pens for each of the three groups. The expected reward group played for a significantly smaller amount of time than the other two groups.

A similar experiment was conducted by Lepper and Greene (1975) with children of the same age as in the previous study. This time they used interest in playing with attractive puzzles as the operational definition of intrinsic motivation, and offered the reward of being able to play with a collection of toys. Two reward conditions were created: expected reward and unexpected reward, as before. In addition, the researchers had three surveillance conditions. Some children were told that while they were playing with the puzzles their performance would be monitored by a video camera most of the time (high surveillance), occasionally (low surveillance) or not at all (no surveillance). Three weeks after the experimental manipulation, the children were unobtrusively observed playing with the puzzles in the classroom.

The results showed no difference between the high and low surveillance conditions and so the data were collapsed across these two conditions. Fig. 4.8 shows the percentage of subjects playing with the puzzles in the classroom. These results show that intrinsic motivation was lower under

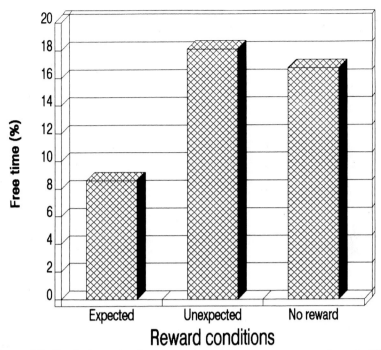

Figure 4.7. Intrinsic motivation, as expressed by time spent on task, and different reward conditions. (Adapted from Lepper et al. 1973.)

surveillance and expected reward conditions, although the two independent variables did not interact.

These two studies supported earlier work by Deci (see Deci and Ryan 1985) who found that people paid to work on intrinsically motivating tasks spent less time on the tasks when given an opportunity in free time. Collectively, the results of these studies suggest what has been termed an "overjustification effect". By rewarding people for participating in an intrinsically interesting task, subsequent involvement in the task when the reward is no longer available is reduced. Various researchers (Deci and Ryan 1985; Kassin and Lepper 1984) explain this in terms of "cognitive evaluation theory" and aspects of attribution and self-perception theories (Bem 1972; Kelley 1967).

The overjustification effect is based on the premise that the behaviour would have occurred anyway, without the need for extrinsic rewards. However, with the use of expected rewards a shift in perceptions occurs from intrinsic to extrinsic. The task is pursued for reasons of obtaining the reward rather than for intrinsic value. Therefore, the reward "overjustifies" the behaviour and, in the event of the reward no longer being offered, the individual shows a reduced intrinsic motivation (for an extended discussion

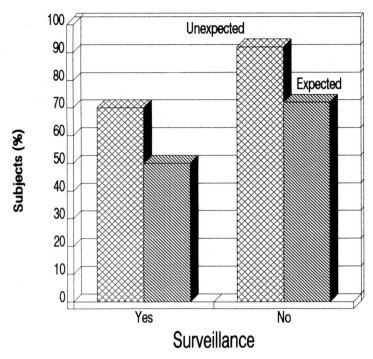

Figure 4.8. Intrinsic motivation, surveillance and reward conditions. (Adapted from Lepper and Greene 1975.)

of explanations for this effect with young children, see Kassin and Lepper 1984).

However, the studies by Lepper and his co-workers demonstrated that it was not the rewards *per se* that were the problem, but whether the rewards were *expected* or not. This suggests, therefore, that rewards need not be detrimental to intrinsic motivation in all situations. This led to the formulation of "cognitive evaluation theory" (Deci and Ryan 1985; Lepper and Greene 1975; Lepper et al. 1973). This theory stated that rewards were likely to serve two main functions: information and control. If the reward provides information about the individual's *competence* then it is quite likely that intrinsic motivation can be enhanced with appropriate rewards. However, if the rewards are seen to be controlling behaviour (i.e., the goal is to obtain the reward rather than participate for intrinsic reasons), then withdrawal of the reward is likely to lead to subsequent deterioration in intrinsic motivation. Attribution theory provides the framework for this analysis since the controlling function of rewards suggests that attributions for participation will be externally focussed. This will be likely to reduce positive emotions under conditions of success and lead to perceptions of lack of control in situations of failure. While the informational function of rewards can be positive due to the recognition of competence, this will, of course, only be true for those succeeding. Regular use of rewards for successful outcomes to individuals in groups (e.g. at school) could equally de-motivate unsuccessful people as they have their incompetence reinforced. This is referred to by Deci and Ryan (1985) as the "amotivating" function and is conceptually related to the concept of helplessness alluded to earlier in this chapter. Fig. 4.9 summarises these possibilities.

In summarising cognitive evaluation theory, Deci and Ryan (1985) present three propositions.

Proposition 1. (Deci and Ryan 1985, p. 61). "*External events relevant to the initiation and regulation of behaviour will affect a person's intrinsic motivation to the extent that they influence the perceived locus of causality for that behaviour. Events that promote a more external locus of causality will undermine intrinsic motivation, whereas those that promote a more internal perceived locus of causality will enhance intrinsic motivation*".

Deci and Ryan (1985) say that events that lead to an external locus of causality undermine intrinsic motivation because they deny people "self-determination", that is they control people's behaviour. On the other hand, internal locus of causality may enhance intrinsic motivation by facilitating feelings of self-determination, thus creating greater autonomy.

Proposition 2. (Deci and Ryan 1985, p. 63). "*External events will affect a person's intrinsic motivation for an optimally challenging activity to the extent that they influence the person's perceived competence, within the context of some self-determination. Events that promote greater perceived competence will enhance intrinsic motivation, whereas those that diminish perceived competence will decrease intrinsic motivation*".

As proposition 2 suggests, intrinsic motivation is not just about feelings of control but also about perceived competence, Again, the suggestions made earlier about helplessness and negative affect in exercise have relevance here. The two right-hand routes in Fig. 4.9 relate to competence perceptions.

Proposition 3. (Deci and Ryan 1985, p. 64) "*Events relevant to the initiation and regulation of behaviour have three potential aspects, each with a functional significance. The informational aspect facilitates an internal perceived locus of causality and perceived competence, thus enhancing intrinsic motivation. The controlling aspect facilitates an external perceived locus of causality, thus undermining intrinsic motivation and promoting extrinsic compliance or defiance. The amotivating aspect facilitates perceived incompetence, thus undermining intrinsic motivation and promoting amotivation. The relative salience of these three aspects to a person determines the functional significance of the event.*"

Deci and Ryan conclude that, generally speaking, choice and positive feedback are perceived as informational, while rewards, deadlines and surveillance tend to be controlling. Negative feedback is seen to undermine motivation and is, therefore, referred to as "amotivating".

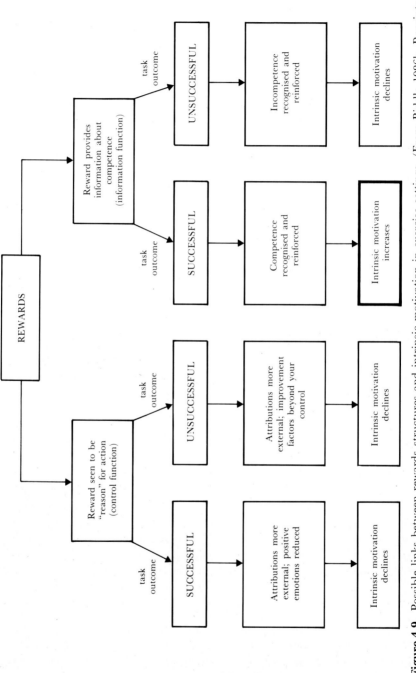

Figure 4.9. Possible links between rewards structures and intrinsic motivation in exercise settings. (From Biddle 1986b. Reprinted with permission.)

   Since exercise, like some other aspects of human behaviour, often requires persistence, effort, time management, self-regulatory skills and many other things related to motivation, it is relevant to consider the role of intrinsic motivation and self-determination in exercise psychology. Regrettably, research in the physical domain has almost solely focussed on competitive sport, although some studies are related to general intrinsic motivation processes and physical fitness (see Vallerand et al. 1987). Whitehead and Corbin (1989) test part of the CET in the context of fitness-testing with children. This study is discussed more fully in the section on youth fitness incentive schemes later in this chapter.

   Thompson and Wankel (1980) have provided some evidence for the role of perceived choice and control in exercise. Their study investigated the influence of activity choice on adherence and future exercise intentions. Adult women (n = 36) who had recently enrolled at a health club were the subjects and they were asked to list their activity preferences. Subjects were then matched on the basis of these preferences and then randomly assigned to either a "choice" or "no choice" group. The choice group were told that their exercise programme was based solely on the choices they had made, whereas the no choice group were told that their programme was based on a standard format for exercise rather than their own preferences. In reality both groups received activities they had initially selected. The experimental manipulation was in terms of *perceived* choice only. Subjects were monitored over a 6-week period. The results are shown in Fig. 4.10 and show that the choice group had a significantly better attendance record towards the end of the 6-week period, suggesting that perceived choice is an important factor in exercise motivation and is consistent with an intrinsic motivation perspective.

Measurement of Intrinsic Motivation

The discussion so far has considered intrinsic motivation as a unidimensional construct. However, Ryan (1982) has proposed that the higher-order construct of intrinsic motivation is underpinned by four factors: interest-enjoyment, competence, effort, and tension-pressure. These are measured with his Intrinsic Motivation Inventory (IMI). The structure of the IMI has been confirmed in exercise and sport settings with adults of college age (McAuley et al. 1989a,b; McAuley and Tammen 1989) and children (Whitehead and Corbin 1989). Similarly, Harter and her co-workers have proposed that children hold at least five different motivational orientations which have intrinsic–extrinsic parameters (Harter 1981; Harter and Connell 1984) and this has been used in sport and physical education contexts (Biddle and Armstrong 1990b; Weiss et al. 1985). This was discussed in chapter 2 in the context of exercise adherence.

   The work of Ryan (1982) does suggest that more needs to be known

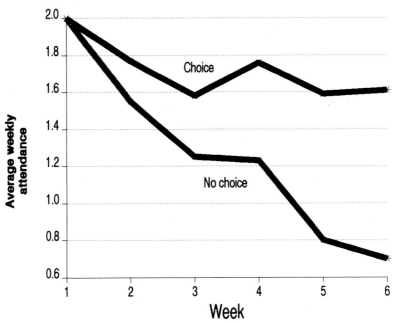

Figure 4.10. Adherence to exercise and perceived choice of exercise programmes. (Adapted from Thompson and Wankel 1980.)

about the antecedents of different intrinsic motivational subscales, as well as the possibility of different subscales of intrinsic motivation having different consequences for behaviour.

Implications for Exercise Participation

It is generally accepted that intrinsic motivation is a desirable quality for continued involvement in physical activities. However, the complex interrelationship between intrinsic motivation, perceptions of control and competence, and extrinsic rewards remains to be fully tested in exercise settings. Summary evidence on adherence (Dishman et al. 1985) suggests that adults will adopt exercise for reasons of health yet are more likely to continue participation because of feelings of well-being and enjoyment and, possibly, other intrinsic reasons. The Canada Fitness Survey (1983a) reports ten major reasons given for being active. While it is not easy to distinguish intrinsic from extrinsic reasons, the dominant reason (to feel better) is intrinsic. This is also true for "activity-limited" and disabled Canadians (Canada Fitness Survey 1986), as shown in Fig. 4.11.

Figure 4.11 shows that the intrinsic reason of "feeling better" is important to both active and inactive people, although, as expected, to varying degrees. This suggests that adults have an intrinsic orientation to exercise, whether they exercise or not. No doubt the more extrinsic influences of wanting to look "good" in front of others (e.g., body shape), or participating to please others, will also be important factors for some people. Exercise leaders and health promoters should be aware, however, of the interrelationship between rewards and intrinsic motivation. For example, the use of reward systems ("token economies") in health clubs has been a common strategy (Franklin 1988), though no systematic evaluation of their effectiveness has been reported. While the short-term influence on adherence may be positive, the research reported in this chapter suggests that those wishing to promote greater participation in exercise must be cautious in their use of extrinsic rewards, particularly for those already high in intrinsic motivation. Rewarding competence may be appropriate, and it may also be better to reward and reinforce exercise *behaviours* rather than performance. In other words, encourage the *process* of activity by reinforcing frequency and participation, rather than solely reinforcing the *product* of exercise through rewarding high fitness scores or the use of comparative reward

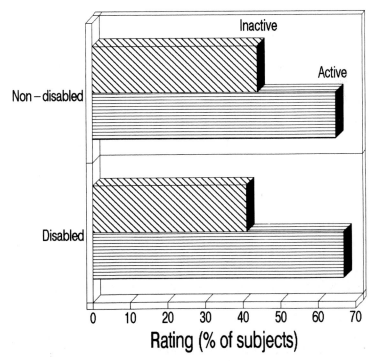

Figure 4.11. Percentage rating "Being active to feel better" as "very important". (Adapted from Canada Fitness Survey 1983a, 1986.)

structures. The rewarding of participation is more likely to lead to feelings of control and self-determination.

Youth Fitness Incentive Schemes

The issue of motivating children to become and remain physically active has attracted the attention of physical and health educators, yet little systematic evidence on the motivation of children and youth has been collected (Biddle and Armstrong 1990b; Dishman 1989; Dishman and Dunn 1988). Despite this, it is commonplace in schools and within some national agencies to operate extrinsic reward systems for the promotion of children's sporting and fitness behaviours. British examples include the "five-star" award scheme for (track and field) athletics, an award scheme for gymnastics, and a plethora of badges available through various swimming and life-saving activities. Similar schemes exist elsewhere, and in the USA there has been much debate about the type of award scheme to implement for physical fitness (Corbin et al. 1988; Whitehead et al. 1990). Ironically, the award scheme implemented by the President's Council for Physical Fitness and Sports (PCPFS) requires participants to achieve very high goals before they are rewarded (reaching the 85th percentile on five test items), yet they state that one of their goals is to "motivate boys and girls to develop and maintain a high level of physical fitness" (AAHPER 1965, cited in Corbin et al. 1988). Such standards seem more likely to demotivate, given that so few are likely to achieve them. Positive goal-setting should include goals that are challenging yet realistic.

Vallerand et al. (1987) suggest that future research on intrinsic motivation and sport should also look at exercise and fitness environments (as distinct from sporting environments) since the motivational factors may not be the same in each. Similarly, youth award schemes, if they are established to promote activity for health, must take note of both the psychological and physiological evidence currently available. The American Alliance for Health, Physical Education, Recreation and Dance (AAHPERD) have developed the "Physical Best" fitness award scheme (see AAHPERD 1988; McSwegin et al. 1989). This scheme promotes three types of awards ("recognition system") as shown in Table 4.3.

In explaining their three awards, McSwegin et al. (1989, p. 25) state that "extrinsic rewards . . . may not always motivate children and youth to strive to develop activity habits beneficial to lifelong fitness. How a student views an award inflences that student's behaviour, prompting that student to be more involved or less involved in the activity". Clearly, McSwegin et al. (1989) are aware of the potential problems of extrinsic rewards and the overjustification hypothesis. This makes a pleasant contrast to the belief, which is often stated in discussions of physical education, that awards are motivational, regardless of the circumstances.

Some physical educators have suggested that children should be rewarded

Table 4.3. The "Physical Best" "Recognition System" (AAHPERD 1988; McSwegin et al. 1989)

Award	Behaviour
Fitness Activity Award	Recognition of the student's participation in physical activities outside school physical education. Student keeps an "activity log/diary" and sets personal goals and activities in consultation with the teacher
Fitness Goals Award	Recognition for obtaining individual fitness and exercise goals, set in consultation with the teacher. Goals can be set in cognitive, psychomotor and affective learning domains
Health Fitness Award	Recognises the attainment of fitness levels associated with minimal risk or risks of health problems. Students have to attain the standards for all six items (distance run, skin-fold measures, body mass index, sit and reach flexibility, sit-up, and pull-up)

for *participation* in exercise (what Corbin et al. (1988) call "process awards"), rather than superior performance against others. Not only could the latter approach produce spurious results in terms of implications for health ("I'm fitter than X therefore I don't need to exercise"), but it is also likely to lead to a more external perceived locus of causality. Of course, rewarding exercise behaviour is also open to the negative aspects of rewards as much as are "performance awards" but, as with all reward schemes, the key must lie in their use as *information on competence by providing positive feedback*. As Corbin et al. (1988, p. 213) conclude, "in the absence of research to document various award schemes designed to motivate fitness and regular exercise among youth, we would be wise to apply the best theoretical evidence available". Similar cautionary comments have been made in the British physical education literature (Biddle 1984, 1986b).

One of the few studies on the psychological effects of fitness testing with children was reported by Whitehead and Corbin (1989). They studied 105 American children aged 12–13 years on an agility running test. Specifically, they tested Deci and Ryan's (1985) proposition 2 from CET that external events which increase or decrease perceived competence will increase or decrease intrinsic motivation. Intrinsic motivation was measured by the IMI (Ryan 1982), thus producing scores on interest-enjoyment, competence, effort, and pressure-tension. The children ran the agility course and were given feedback that they were either in the top 20 per cent for their age group, or were in the bottom 20 per cent. A further group received no feedback and acted as a control group.

The results provided clear support for CET such that those receiving the negative feedback (low percentile) showed a reduction in intrinsic motivation, and those receiving positive feedback (high percentile) increased in intrinsic motivation. Path analyses revealed that the changes in the subscales of the IMI were almost exclusively mediated by changes in perceived competence.

Conclusion

As stated at the beginning of this chapter, the popular literature on health and physical fitness constantly makes reference to the concept of "control" over lifestyle, fitness and health. The evidence presented here has been accumulated from three main sources: locus of control and causality, attribution theories, and intrinsic motivation. One could conclude that there is, observable throughout, a "thread" that suggests perceptions of control are moderately important mediators of exercise behaviours. However, such a conclusion is based largely on research that has been conducted outside the exercise setting, although the LOC literature does contain a number of studies specifically on exercise and physical fitness. Even so, the integration between the theoretical perspectives chosen in this chapter does point towards the utility of exercise psychology research being conducted in these fields, and preferably in an integrated way.

5

Self-confidence and Exercise

One psychological construct that appears to have clear intuitive logic and forms part of our every-day language is that of self-confidence. The term is used regularly in achievement contexts, such as education and sport, and can be identified in many other spheres of life, such as social interaction. In terms of exercise it is likely to be implicated in many of the mechanisms discussed in this book. For example, the adoption and maintenance of an exercise programme (see Chap. 2) may well depend, in part, on having the confidence to initiate and then sustain exercise (Desharnais et al. 1986), and the potential benefits to mental health discussed in Section C, may be influenced by the development of feelings of confidence and mastery. Similarly, the constructs associated with perceptions of control (Chap. 4) would appear to act as mechanisms for changing confidence. Indeed, Bandura (1986) refers to his own theory of self-efficacy as being associated with people's sense of control over events in their lives.

The need to study the theories and mechanisms of confidence should, therefore, be self-evident. However, there are a number of issues that need addressing. It is not known whether there are different types of confidence in exercise, such as the confidence to initiate exercise in the first place or the confidence that exercise will bring about desired results, such as loss of weight or gains in fitness. The role of state versus trait factors is not known, although contemporary approaches to the study of self-confidence (e.g., Bandura 1977a, b, 1986) suggest that situational cues will dominate over and above any personality disposition towards confidence as a trait. Also, the permanence of confidence in particular situations, or across different groups (e.g., age, gender, class, race) is rarely studied. This all suggests that self-confidence, despite recent interest in this area of psychological research, and the intuitive logic and appeal of the topic, requires further study before application can be made in some fields.

Approaches to the Study of Confidence

The shift from reliance on stable personality traits as predictors of behaviour to a more social-cognitive approach (Bandura 1986) has led to the development of a number of theoretical perspectives on self-confidence. These approaches range from efficacy expectations (Bandura 1977a, b, 1986) to performance expectations (Corbin 1984), specific situational influences (Lenney 1977), perceptions of competence (Harter 1978, 1983), and cognition-emotion relationships with likely behavioural consequences (e.g. learned helplessness; Abramson et al. 1978).

This diversity of approaches has been mirrored in the literature on sport and physical activity, with studies on self-efficacy theory, performance expectancies, trait and state sport confidence, and movement confidence (see Feltz 1988a). While a number of these approaches will be considered, Bandura's self-efficacy construct will form the central theme of the chapter. This theoretical perspective has received considerable research interest in recent years and provides a heuristic device by which the study of self-confidence in exercise can be undertaken.

Self-Efficacy Theory

Perhaps the most widely tested of theories associated with confidence is that of Self-Efficacy Theory (SET; Bandura 1977a, b, 1986, 1990). Not only has SET been applied in clinical settings (Bandura and Adams 1977) but it has subsequently been tested in a variety of physical activity and health contexts, such as sport (Feltz 1982; Feltz and Mugno 1983), weight loss (Weinberg et al. 1984), exercise compliance (Desharnais et al. 1986; Kaplan et al. 1984), and with other health-related behaviours (see O'Leary 1985; Strecher et al. 1986). Bandura (1986, p. 391) defines perceived self-efficacy as: "people's judgements of their capabilities to organise and execute courses of action required to attain designated types of performances. It is concerned not with the skills one has but with judgements of what one can do with whatever skills one possesses".

The key phrase here is "capabilities to organise and execute courses of action" since Bandura has always differentiated between *efficacy* expectations and *outcome* expectations. By this it is meant that beliefs related to the ability to carry out a particular behaviour are efficacy expectations whereas beliefs as to whether the behaviour will produce a particular result are outcome expectations. For example, efficacy expectations might be the belief that one can successfully adhere to a prescribed exercise programme of jogging three times each week for 20 minutes each run. However, outcome expectations might refer to whether one believes that such a programme will produce the weight loss that was desired at the beginning of the programme. The differentiation between these two types of expectations is illustrated in Fig. 5.1.

Although Bandura's SET refers to the two expectancies as being different, they are both part of the self-confidence concept in exercise. People are likely to be concerned about *both* types of expectancy and both require study in research on the psychology of exercise (see Desharnais et al. 1986). For example, it is important to know whether efficacy expectations are influential in the adoption of exercise programmes, yet it is also likely that outcome expectations will affect the maintenance of such programmes and the reinforcement necessary for continued involvement. Studies apparently testing SET, however, do not always make it clear whether they are investigating efficacy or outcome judgements.

Sources of Efficacy Information

Four main sources of information for self-efficacy beliefs have been identified by Bandura (1986). These are: performance attainment, imitation and modelling, verbal and social persuasion, and judgements of physiological states.

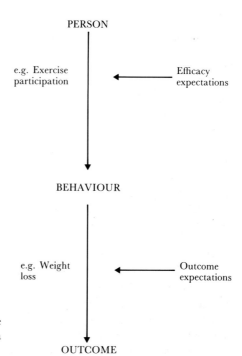

Figure 5.1. Efficacy and outcome expectations. (Adapted from Bandura 1977a.)

Performance Attainment. This is thought to be the most powerful of efficacy sources since it is based on personal experience of success and failure. However, as alluded to in the previous chapter, the appraisal of such events (i.e. attributions) is likely to influence expectations of future success. Bandura (1986, p. 399) states that "successes raise efficacy appraisals; repeated failures lower them, especially if the failures occur early in the course of events and do not reflect a lack of effort or adverse external circumstances". Attribution theory (Weiner 1986) predicts that internal and stable causes of failure, such as lack of ability, are more likely to lead to debilitating and demotivating cognitions and negative emotions than factors which appear more changeable, such as lack of effort or poor strategy, and research has shown that attributions can influence efficacy perceptions (Schunk 1981, 1982, 1983, 1984). However, the role of attributional variables in perceptions of self-efficacy in exercise contexts has not been studied in any depth.

The extent that efficacy expectations gained in one context generalise to other contexts is not known, although Bandura (1986) does suggest that some generalisation is likely. Clearly, the generalisation is predicted to be strongest in similar events to the original source of efficacy judgements. Again, attributional factors are likely to be important here. For example, research into learned helplessness has suggested that the nature of the attributions given in response to failure may influence the extent to which negative perceptions generalise beyond the event itself. "Global" attributions for failure are those which generalise beyond the situation in which failure occurred. For example, if an individual believes that inability to play a competent game of tennis is due to lack of co-ordination, this will probably generalise to other sports situations. However, a "specific" attribution for failure will not generalise and is regarded as a more positive way to think about such situations as it is more likely to protect self-esteem (Abramson et al. 1978).

Imitation and Modelling. Self-efficacy can also be developed through the vicarious experiences of imitation and modelling. Observing others succeed or fail could affect subsequent perceptions of personal capabilities, particularly if the model is perceived to be similar to oneself. This casts some doubt on the use of elite sports models in the promotion of exercise for the recreational participant, at least from the point of view of self-efficacy.

Bandura (1986) suggests that imitative learning is more likely to be influential when the individual has little or no actual experience of the task since the information from the model is more salient in such situations.

Bandura (1986) also suggests that the social comparison element of vicarious experience is important since in some situations it is not always possible to gauge your success without some kind of reference point, such as another person's score. He says (Bandura 1986, p. 400) "Because most performances are evaluated in terms of social criteria, social comparative information figures prominently in self-efficacy appraisals". However, it is doubtful whether this is always the case with health-related exercise. While exercise through competitive sport requires, by necessity at times, social comparison, success in recreational exercise, such as aerobic conditioning, could easily be judged by enhanced feelings of well-being or personal self-improvement (mastery). Indeed, some have argued that this is likely to be a more positive way of encouraging participation in preference to comparisons with others (Fox and Biddle 1988), although the matter requires further testing.

Verbal and Social Persuasion. Depending on the source of such efficacy information, persuasion from others is likely to influence perceptions of self-efficacy. However, it is thought to be a relatively weak source in comparison to the two already mentioned. The success of such initiatives is also dependent on the realistic nature of the persuasion, and hence is similar to goal-setting. Given the potential for regular contact between exerciser and instructor in supervised programmes, verbal persuasion is likely to be a source of self-efficacy worthy of note.

Judgements of Physiological States. The original theorising on SET was based on experiences in clinical settings, and in particular the modification of reactions to aversive events, such as phobias (Bandura 1977b). In such situations it was found that self-efficacy was related to how one appraised internal physiological states such as heart rate. Bandura (1986, p. 401) says that "treatments that eliminate emotional arousal to subjective threats heighten perceived self-efficacy with corresponding improvements in performance". The use of such somatic feedback can be a positive influence on self-efficacy and will be elaborated on when specific exercise studies are reviewed subsequently. It is also the case that accurate monitoring of physical effort, such as that required in some exercise programmes, is not easy and hence commonly prescribed intensities (e.g. 60% of maximum heart rate for aerobic programmes) produce markedly differing results within groups (Dishman 1988b). Teaching people how to monitor physiological signs, therefore, may not only be safer but provide for the possibility of enhancing efficacy perceptions. The role of perceived (or preferred) exertion scales is something to be investigated here (Borg 1973; Dishman 1988b; Dishman et al. 1987) (see Chap. 2).

Self-efficacy, therefore, is believed to have four main sources, as outlined. Ewart (1989, p. 684) summarises the application of these in the context promoting exercise in a rehabilitation situation:

the most effective way to encourage patients to adopt exercise activities for which they lack self-efficacy is to expose them to the recommended activity in gradually increasing doses (performance), arrange for them to see others similar to themselves performing the activity (modeling);

have respected health care providers offer encouragement by providing reassurance and emphasizing the patient's accomplishments (persuasion), and arrange the setting of the activity so as to induce a relaxed but 'upbeat' mood (arousal; *physiological state*) [*words in italics added*]

The hypothesised relationship among the four sources of self-efficacy information outlined and the consequences of such information is shown in Fig. 5.2.

In addition, self-efficacy will vary along the dimensions of magnitude, strength, and generality (Bandura 1977a). Magnitude of SE refers to the ordering of tasks by difficulty, such as feeling that one is capable of sustaining a walking programme but not one for running half marathons. The strength of SE refers to the assessment of an individual's capabilities for performing a particular task. For example, people are able subjectively to rate their likelihood of maintaining a jogging programme of 3 miles every other day. Finally, the generality of SE refers to the extent to which efficacy expectations from one situation generalise to other situations, such as efficacy gained through a walking programme generalising to the lifting of weights in a body-conditioning programme (see Ewart et al. 1983). Each of these measures of SE should, if conforming to Bandura's theory, be taken. Rarely is this actually the case (see Table 5.1).

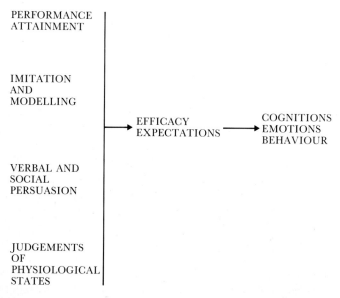

Figure 5.2. Sources of self-efficacy and behavioural predictions. (Adapted from Feltz 1988a.)

Self-efficacy in Exercise and Health: Research Findings

There are relatively few studies that have investigated SE and health-related exercise, although several studies on sports psychology have been completed. However, these tend to be focussed on performance and anxiety rather than health behaviour change (Feltz 1988a; Wurtele 1986). Studies of exercise and SE are summarised in Table 5.1.

Research with Patients

Ewart and co-workers have conducted a number of studies on SE and exercise (Ewart 1989). Ewart et al. (1983) studied SE in patients who had suffered a myocardial infarction (MI) and later started exercising on a treadmill. Before and after treadmill exercise SE was assessed on walking, running, stair climbing, sexual intercourse, lifting and general exertion. The improvements in SE are illustrated in Fig. 5.3.

Fig. 5.3 shows that positive changes in SE took place following treadmill exercise, and that this was greatest for running, suggesting that SE effects do generalise but appear to have stronger effects on similar exercise modes (see also Brody et al. 1988). When counselling also took place it was found that SE perceptions for sexual intercourse, lifting, and general exertion significantly increased above the level attained after treadmill running. This was not true for the other activities, indicating that generalisability of SE is enhanced for dissimilar activities when additional intervention is given.

Ewart et al. (1983) also found that SE, after treadmill running and counselling, significantly correlated with self-reported activity at home. This is an important finding in the quest for ways of enhancing activity levels away from supervised environments.

Ewart et al. (1986a) investigated the specificity of SE perceptions with 40 men with documented coronary heart disease (CHD). The exercise of circuit weight training was used. SE ratings taken prior to a variety of tests of physical fitness were shown to correlate more strongly with results of tests for activities specific to the SE judgements. For example, SE ratings for the performance of lifting activities was significantly correlated with the arm strength test but not with the aerobic endurance treadmill test. Conversely, SE ratings of jogging were significantly correlated with the aerobic endurance tests but not with tests of arm, grip or leg strength. The correlations between performance on tests of arm strength and aerobic endurance and measures of self-efficacy in five different physical activities are illustrated in Fig. 5.4.

Kaplan et al. (1984) studied patients with chronic obstructive pulmonary disease (COPD) and tested whether generalised expectancies (i.e. health locus of control) would differ from specific expectancies (self-efficacy) in changes of exercise behaviour. The results showed superior effects for SE

Table 5.1. A Summary of Studies on Self-Efficacy (SE) and Exercise

Study	Subjects and design	Behaviours	SE Measure Strength	Generalisation	Magnitude	Results
Ewart et al. (1983)	40 men (mean age = 52) tested 3 weeks after MI. Treadmill run test. SE assessed before and after	SE for various physical activities	∨	∨	∨	SE increases for activities similar to treadmill exercise were greatest after treadmill running; increases for dissimilar activities were greatest after counselling. SE after treadmill run correlated with home based activity
Kaplan et al. (1984)	60 COPD men and women (mean age = 65); walking exercise prescription given after treadmill testing	SE for various physical activities. Health LOC	∨	∨	∨	SE increased with intervention (cognitive-behavioural, cognitive and behavioural) but not with attention control after 3 months follow-up. Efficacy expectations changed in activities as a function of their similarity to walking. HLOC not

Study	Description	SE measure				Results
Ewart et al. (1986a)	40 men with CHD. Strength tests on arms and legs and test of aerobic endurance followed by either walk-jog and circuit weight training or walk-jog and volleyball	SE for performing arm and leg activities	√	√	√	SE related to specificity of task. SE and type of training independently contributed to performance gains
Ewart et al. (1986b)	40 men with CHD. Pre-jog SE assessed. Subjects' heart rate then monitored during jog	Jog-SE	√	x	√	Adherence to target HR related to jog-SE. Those with high jog-SE over-estimated training heart rate and those low in jog-SE under-estimated

clearly associated with walking behaviours but efficacy-behaviour relationships greater for internals

Table 5.1. Continued

Study	Subjects and design	Behaviours	SE Measure Strength	Generalisation	Magnitude	Results
Davis et al. (1984)	854 male and female workers surveyed on 6 areas of health including exercise	Various, including exercise efficacy and intent to change	√	x	x	Perceptions of low efficacy predictive of intent to change and dissatisfaction with current activity levels
Taylor et al. (1985)	30 post-MI men and their wives. 10 wives observed husbands on treadmill test, 10 did not, 10 participated themselves. Counselling also given about patients' capacities	Wives' efficacy ratings of husbands' cardiac capabilities. Husbands also rated SE	√ √	x x	x x	Patients' SE in cardiac capabilities improved significantly after exercise and counselling. Wives who participated in treadmill exercise showed significant increase in judgments of husbands' cardiac and physical efficacy
Sallis et al. (1986)	1411 men and women surveyed	Activity habits and SE	√	x	(√)	SE predictive of: a) adoption of vigorous

Study	Sample	Variables				Findings
			✓	x	x	activity (men and women) b) maintenance of vigorous activity (women only) c) adoption and maintenance of moderate activity (women only)
Desharnais et al. (1986)	98 young men and women assessed at entry to fitness programme	Outcome and efficacy expectations for fitness programme adherence	✓	x	x	Efficacy expectation discriminated between adherers and drop-outs, although both efficacy and outcome expectancies were significant mediators of adherence
Dzewaltowski (1989)	136 male and 192 female students attending required physical education classes	Exercise frequency, variables from Social Cognitive Theory (Bandura, 1986), including SE, and from the Theory of Reasoned Action	✓	x	x	Social Cognitive Theory predicted exercise better than the Theory of Reasoned Action. SE was the best predictor

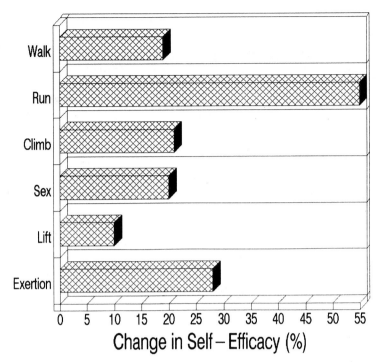

Figure 5.3. Increases in self-efficacy after treadmill running. (Data from Ewart et al. 1983.)

as a mediator of changes in walking behaviour. Experimental subjects showed significant gains over control subjects in "walking SE". This generalised to similar activities such as stair climbing. Interestingly, an interaction between SE and health locus of control was found such that correlations between SE perceptions and physical activities were only significant for those with an internal health locus of control. This is consistent with an expectancy-value approach in psychology (see Weiner 1980).

Ewart et al. (1986b) investigated the role of SE in subjects' ability accurately to gauge intensity of exercise. Through the use of devices which monitored ambulatory heart rate, they found that subjects, who were known to have CHD, were generally inaccurate in estimating their heart rate (HR) training prescriptions (i.e., 70%–85% maximal treadmill heart rate; see American College of Sports Medicine 1986). SE scores were shown to be related to over- or under-estimation of HR such that those with high jogging SE tended to over-estimate HR whereas those who under-estimated had lower jogging SE. These results may be important for future studies in which psychological variables in exercise prescription are investigated; these studies are usually dominated by physiological guidelines only (Rejeski

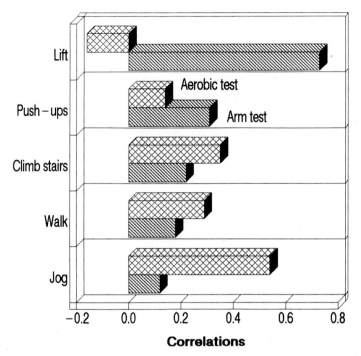

Figure 5.4. Correlation between performance on arm strength and aerobic endurance tests and self-efficacy ratings for selected physical activities. (Data from Ewart et al. 1986a.)

and Kenney 1988). However, the problems associated with HR monitoring as a means of exercise prescription require further research and discussion (see Dishman 1988b).

One of the sources of SE information, according to Bandura (1977a, b, 1986) is through vicarious processes. Taylor et al. (1985) investigated the influence of spouse involvement in the SE beliefs and rehabilitation of post-MI men. The patients performed a symptom-limited treadmill test under one of three conditions of spouse involvement. For one group the spouse was uninvolved, for another group she was an observer for the treadmill exercise. The third group had their wives both observe the treadmill task and participate in the same test later on.

Results showed that there was no difference in spousal judgements of their husband's cardiac or general physical capabilities in the "uninvolved" or "observation only" groups. However, for the group where the spouse participated in the treadmill test there was a significant rise in spousal judgements of efficacy related to their husband's cardiac capability. Given prior research in cardiac rehabilitation through exercise, where spouse support has been found to be an important influence on exercise adherence

(Oldridge 1988), these results are potentially significant. Strategies which involve spouses more directly in the rehabilitation process, therefore, may yield more positive results.

The studies discusssed so far have focussed on subjects with known medical symptoms, such as documented CHD. The extent that such studies can be generalised to other people remains problematic. Given that SE is a social-cognitive variable open to environmental and perceptual inter-vention, it might be unwise to generalise from these studies. For example, Ewart (1989) suggests that post-coronary patients are often limited more by fear of exertion than by their actual medical condition. This is quite different from the situation in individuals free from disease symptoms.

Research with Subjects Free of Known Disease

Davis et al. (1984) investigated psychosocial and risk factors in the prediction of participation in health programmes at American worksites. A low perception of "personal efficacy" was predictive of individuals' *intent* to change their exercise habits and their dissatisfaction with current activity levels. Unfortunately, it appears that the measure of "personal efficacy" used in this study does not closely approximate the concept of self-efficacy as suggested by Bandura (1986). Davis et al. (1984, p. 369) report that three items were used to assess personal efficacy for exercise. These were "when I am exercising or playing sports, I feel self-conscious about the way I look"; "I am the kind of person who does not get enough exercise"; "it's hard for me to find time in a day to get some exercise". These items appear to be assessing a wider notion of confidence than the individual's perception of ability (efficacy) to carry out exercise.

Desharnais et al. (1986) studied 98 young adults at the beginning of an 11-week fitness programme at a Canadian university. All participants were assessed on their "expectation of outcome" which represented their perceptions of the potential benefits and value of the fitness programme and, hence, is the same as Bandura's "outcome expectancy". They were also assessed on efficacy expectations in terms of whether they expected to be capable of attending the fitness programme until its completion.

The results showed that adherers and drop-outs from the programme were significantly different on both outcome and efficacy expectancies, with self-efficacy being the stronger discriminator.

Finally, Sallis et al. (1986) studied potential predictors of changes in people's levels of community activity. Three measures of physical activity were examined over one year with 1411 Californian adults. The main results can be summarised as follows:

1. SE was predictive of the adoption of vigorous activity for both sexes
2. SE was predictive of the maintenance of vigorous activity for women only

3 SE was predictive of the adoption and maintenance of moderate exercise for women only

Such gender differences are not easy to explain but are certainly worthy of further study. Lenney (1977) and, subsequently, Corbin (1984) highlight possible gender differences in achievement behaviours and physical activities. Socialisation effects may account for differences in SE between males and females, particularly in activities strongly sex-typed. They will be discussed in more detail later in the chapter.

Self-efficacy appears to be a concept worthy of continued investigation in exercise research. Collectively, the results reported here suggest that SE may be an effective mechanism for behaviour change in exercise settings. This supports Dishman's (1986b) comment that, although sparse, the study of self-efficacy in health-related exercise and activity is encouraging. However, until recently, no research had been conducted that compared SET with other social psychological models in predicting exercise. Dzewaltowski (1989) compared Bandura's (1986) Social Cognitive Theory (SCT), the central part being self-efficacy, with Fishbein and Ajzen's Theory of Reasoned Action (TRA; see Chap. 3). Specifically, three measures associated with SCT were assessed. These were self-efficacy related to participation in an 8-week exercise programme, outcome expectancies, and self-evaluated dissatisfaction/satisfaction with the outcomes of exercise. All subjects were students attending compulsory classes in physical education, although the measure of exercise behaviour included activity both inside and outside the class.

The results showed that SCT predicted exercise better than the TRA, and that SE was the strongest predictor of the three SCT variables. However, while this might suggest that SCT should be used instead of the TRA, the measure of behavioural intention, central to the TRA in linking attitudes and social norms to behaviour, was very high in nearly all subjects, and hence had a very restricted range. This reduced the possibility of intention predicting behaviour. Similarly, the study suffers from a crude measure of exercise. Only the number of days on which exercise took place was assessed, and this was elicited via unvalidated self-report rather than known measures of activity recall (Blair 1984). However, perhaps of greater concern is the fact that all subjects were recruited from compulsory classes in physical education. The extent of their activity is almost certain to be affected by being in such a situation. Had the classes had some element of voluntary attendance about them, such as in commercial fitness clubs, then the theories would have been tested in a more useful context.

Despite these criticisms, Dzewaltowski (1989) has provided an important step in comparing two well-known psychological perspectives in predicting exercise. A more realistic situation is required for future research of this kind before competing models can be adequately compared.

Self-Efficacy: Methods and Measurement

SET has not been without criticism (Kazdin 1978; Smedslund 1978). However, some of the comments were written soon after the theory was articulated (Bandura 1977a, b) and before a large body of research had been accumulated. Nevertheless, there are methodological issues concerning SET in exercise that require attention.

Bandura proposes at least three types of SE measure (strength, magnitude and generality), but studies have not usually assessed all three. In the literature on sports psychology it has been usual to measure the strength of SE for one particular task (see Feltz 1988a). In health-related exercise research it is important that measures of magnitude and generality are also taken as these factors are potentially influential in guiding interventions (Ewart et al. 1983; Strecher et al. 1986).

Bandura has recommended that SE be measured at a micro, task-specific, level. Some researchers, however, believe that the global assessment of self-efficacy in physical settings may be useful. Consequently, Ryckman et al. (1982) developed the Physical Self-Efficacy Scale (PSE) and identified two subscales: Physical Self-Presentation Confidence scale (PSPC) and Perceived Physical Ability scale (PPA). However, when tested by McAuley and Gill (1983) in gymnastics, it was found that event-specific efficacy perceptions were more highly correlated with performance than were scores on the PPA scale. This supports Bandura's (1986) recommendation for the measurement of SE at the level of high behavioural specificity. Fig. 5.5 illustrates the relationships found by McAuley and Gill (1983).

Sherer et al. (1982) report the development of what they call The Self-Efficacy Scale. However, inspection of the test items and rationale for test construction suggests that their inventory is more akin to a general self-motivation scale and does not approximate Bandura's conceptualisation of self-efficacy.

In addition to the reliance on self-report measures of SE, a full test of Bandura's theory should involve measures of physiological function. However, when such measures were collected in a sports psychology research programme (Feltz 1982; Feltz and Mugno 1983), physiological arousal (as measured by heart rate) was not a significant predictor of SE, but perceived arousal was. Feltz (1988b) also found gender differences such that heart rate prior to performing a back dive did predict initial performance but only for females. Autonomic perception predicted self-efficacy prior to the first trial in both males and females.

Finally, it is important in the context of exercise and health that research identifies the underlying mechanisms of SE in behaviour change and actual health outcomes. For example, Bandura and his co-workers have also suggested that SE may act as a coping mechanism in reducing the potential ill-effects of stress. He provides evidence showing that when perceived coping efficacy is high, exposure to stressors has no adverse physiological

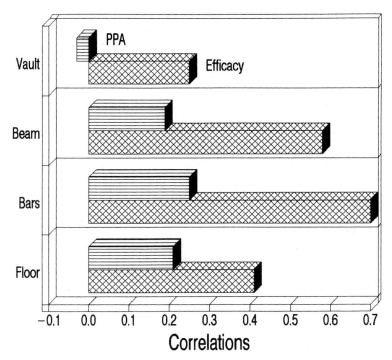

Figure 5.5. Correlation coefficients between event-specific efficacy expectations, Perceived Physical Ability Scale (PPA), and gymnastics performance. (Data from McAuley and Gill 1983.)

effect; physiological effects such as heightened autonomic arousal and activation of stress-related hormones are observed when the same stressors are in evidence in the absence of perceived coping efficacy (Bandura 1989; Bandura et al. 1985, 1988). Bandura (1989, p. 490) summarises by saying that "the types of biochemical reactions that have been shown to accompany a weak sense of coping efficacy are involved in the regulation of immune systems".

This area of research links to that of aerobic fitness and psychosocial stress reactivity, discussed in Chap. 6, and has important implications for research on exercise and immune function (see Chap. 1). It further strengthens the need for continued investigation of SE in health and exercise contexts.

The construct of self-efficacy is part of a broader conceptualisation of human thought and action proposed within Bandura's (1986) Social Cognitive Theory. Future studies, such as that reported by Dzewaltowski (1989), should assess other aspects of SCT, including the role of SE.

Further issues for consideration in SE and exercise might include:

1. the influence of SE in diverse settings; for example, a comparison should at least include "free-living" versus supervised exercise settings where social influences are likely to be different

2. the similarity in relationships between SE for subjects with a known pathological symptom and those classified as asymptomatic. As reported, the majority of exercise, as opposed to sports, studies use subjects in clinical settings, such as CHD rehabilitation

3. the role of attributional variables in SE and exercise has yet to be systematically explored. For example, the utility of learned helplessness models and exercise non-participation requires investigation (see Chap. 4)

4. gender differences in SE also need further research. Feltz (1988b) reports gender differences in the analysis of causal elements of SE in the performance of a high avoidance sport task (backwards dive into a swimming pool). Such research needs extending into health/exercise settings

5. SE theory has rarely been tested in exercise contexts where the prolonged influence of SE is studied, although the work of Sallis et al. (1986) is an exception. For example, Ewart et al. (1983) predicted home-based activity from SE measures but this cannot be called a study of exercise maintenance since no analysis took place over time. This is now required alongside research into the role of SE in relapse behaviour in exercise. Many exercisers have temporary fluctuations in their activity patterns and, therefore, research into SE should be broadened to account for such behaviours (Knapp 1988; Marlatt 1985)

6. the longevity of SE is not known. Given the situational specificity of SE it may not be appropriate to look towards confidence "traits". Nevertheless, it might be appropriate to investigate the influence of SE in particular activities in childhood and see whether such cognitive factors influence adult activity patterns. The "behavioural carry-over" into adulthood is something which is concerning researchers into public health and physical education at present (Blair et al. 1989a; Dishman and Dunn 1988; Simons-Morton et al. 1987, 1988b)

7. Dishman and Dunn (1988) have put forward a multidimensional model of exercise behaviour suggesting that the major "guiding models" for the study of exercise adherence through the life-span are psychological, biobehavioural (e.g., perceived exertion), and social-environmental (see Fig. 2.11). With self-efficacy featuring as one of many theories in the psychological category it is obvious that research must look towards an integration not only of psychological models, but also of models and theories from different disciplines (e.g., physiology). This is not unique to SE, of course (see Dzewaltowski 1989).

Other Approaches to the Study of Confidence and Exercise

Performance Estimation

Bandura's SET and SCT clearly differentiate between efficacy and outcome expectations. However, at the beginning of the chapter it was stated that both types of expectancy are likely to be important in physical activity settings. Using a similar construct to outcome expectations, Corbin and his co-workers have investigated the issue of self-confidence in exercise from the view point of performance estimations (Corbin 1981, 1984; Corbin et al. 1981, 1983; Corbin and Nix 1979). This research programme was based around theorising by Lenney (1977) in the area of women and achievement behaviour. She suggested that while evidence pointed to under-achievement by females in some achievement contexts, this was not invariably so. Lenney pointed out that female self-confidence was dependent on "situational vulnerability" which was determined by three main factors:

1. the sex-typed nature of the task: confidence is likely to be low in situations where the task is perceived as "inappropriate". That is to say, a role conflict may be apparent such as in performing tasks sex-typed as "masculine". An example would be women in the context of a weight-training class where some, although by no means all, might lack self-confidence

2. social evaluation: Lenney (1977) has suggested that females will under-estimate their ability when they are being evaluated or compared, such as in competition

3. feedback: it has been proposed that females achieve better levels of performance when given objective and accurate feedback. However, this was not found to be the case by Corbin et al. (1981) when Lenney's first two factors were held constant

These factors point to important variables in the exercise environment and, while originated from the study of women in achievement contexts, could also apply to men in some situations, such as activities sex-typed "feminine" (e.g., dance; exercise-to-music). However, given the predominantly masculine stereotyping of many physical activities, particularly sports, the emphasis has been placed on research into female self-confidence (Corbin 1984). Although this research has focussed on sport, the implications would appear to be evident for participation in health-related exercise.

Corbin and Nix (1979) studied the self-confidence of young boys and girls (aged 8–10 years) before and after cross-sex competition. It was found that activities sex-typed "male" (i.e., those involving strength, power and speed) created significantly lower expectations of success for girls compared to boys. However, this was not the case for activities sex-typed "male–female". After girls experienced as much success as boys, they had confidence levels equal to the boys.

In a subsequent study, Corbin (1981) used a sex-typed "neutral" activity but manipulated the perceived ability of the subject's opponent. All subjects competed against a confederate and lost 4 out of 5 games. Post-performance confidence of females was equal to that of males after competing against opponents perceived to be low in ability. However, they were significantly less confident after competing against subjects perceived to be high in ability. Corbin (1981) suggested that competing against someone perceived to be good created vulnerability in the females but not in the males, possibly supporting Lenney's (1977) assumption that females are more situationally dependent on external information for performance estimations.

Corbin et al. (1983) tested whether the gender differences in self-confidence were the result of genuine low confidence in females or boastfulness on the part of males since they reported that boasting may be seen as "unfeminine". Using a leg endurance task perceived to be "male" by both boys and girls (aged 15–17 years), performance estimates and performance scores were elicited under one of two conditions. Subjects in one group were attached to a "polygraph" whereby their physiological responses to stress were assessed. The other group was not involved with this apparatus. The polygraph condition was an attempt to elicit truthful performance estimates since subjects were told that untruthful responses would be detected.

The results are illustrated in Fig. 5.6 and show that males made significantly higher performance estimates than females, although the actual performance scores, while favouring males, showed a difference that was not statistically significant. The main effects for the conditions (polygraph versus no polygraph) was also not significant suggesting that the gender differences in performance estimates are not necessarily due to male boastfulness. Corbin et al. (1983, pp. 409–410) concluded that "the significant difference in performance estimates between the sexes and the lack of a significant sex by treatment interaction might be used to support Lenney's (1977) contention that females lack self-confidence in certain situations such as those present in this investigation".

The mechanisms of self-confidence in physical exercise are far from clear. So far, this chapter has reviewed two lines of research that suggest that efficacy expectations can be manipulated through four sources of information, while performance estimates, for females at least, may be the result of situational vulnerability through perceptions of task sex-typing, social evaluation, and feedback.

Both theoretical perspectives draw on prior work on perceptions of "mastery" or "competence". For example, Corbin (1984) states that in order for self-confidence to be increased, participants in physical activity should be rewarded for mastery attempts.

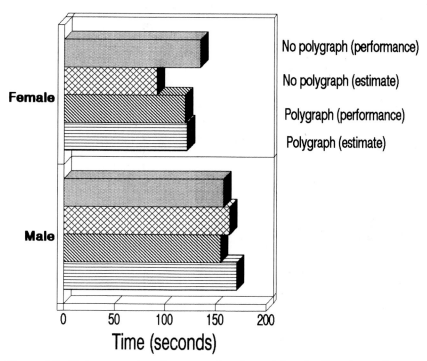

Figure 5.6. Estimates and performance of males and females for a leg endurance task under conditions of polygraph and no-polygraph. (Data from Corbin et al. 1983.)

Perceptions of Competence and Mastery

The link between self-efficacy, performance estimates and perceptions of mastery or competence should now be self-evident. However, there has been considerable interest recently in theories associated with mastery and competence (Harter 1983; Nicholls 1984), and this has been extended into the literature of sports psychology (Duda 1987; Roberts 1984). Some of these approaches, including Cognitive Evaluation Theory and Personal Investment Theory, were discussed in Chaps 4 and 2, so little more will be added here. However, from the point of view of exercise confidence, it should be noted that the theories proposed by Harter and Nicholls, when tested in physical activity settings, have almost exclusively involved young people in sports environments. There is a need not only to test these theories with older people in health-related exercise and fitness activities, but also to test them alongside other confidence-based theories, such as SET. Bandura (1986, pp. 410–411) states that at present "extensive theoretical comparisons" between SET and effectance motivation (a competence/mastery perspective on motivation) are not possible as the theory of effectance motivation "has not been formulated in sufficient detail". However, it would now be possible to compare the effectiveness of SCT and SE in predicting exercise against related theoretical perspectives such as Personal Investment Theory (Maehr and Braskamp 1986; see Chap. 2).

Sport Confidence

Vealey (1986a) developed a sport-specific, interactional model of self-confidence in which she constructed scales for the measurement of state and trait sport self-confidence. A scale measuring perceptions of competitive orientation was also developed. This is analogous to Nicholls' (1984) ego-oriented and mastery-oriented goals in achievement motivation. Vealey's (1986a) rationale for using such a conceptual framework was that it allowed for individual differences in defining the meaning of success in sport.

Vealey (1986a, p. 222) defined "sport-confidence" as "the belief or degree of certainty individuals possess about their ability to be successful in sport". However, the focus of this book is more aligned to recreational involvement in physical activity from the point of view of health rather than sports performance. Vealey's model, therefore, will not be discussed further except to say that the instruments developed to measure sports confidence could provide useful guidelines for research into confidence in health-related exercise contexts. Similarly, the Competitive State Anxiety Inventory (CSAI-2; Martens et al. 1990) has a self-confidence subscale alongside scales for somatic and cognitive anxiety. However, Feltz (1988a) argues that, although self-confidence has been conceptualised as being opposite to cognitive anxiety, its identification through factor analytic procedures does not mean that self-confidence is part of anxiety or vice versa.

Movement Confidence

Griffin, Keogh and co-workers have proposed a model of movement confidence for children that they claim is different from other conceptualisations of self-confidence (Griffin and Keogh 1982; Griffin et al. 1984; Keogh et al. 1981). Griffin and Keogh (1982, p. 213) state that "we are viewing movement confidence as an individual feeling of adequacy in a movement situation". However, although they recognise the similarities between their model and other conceptualisations of competence and motivation, Griffin and Keogh (1982, p. 215) say that they are "proposing an important additional consideration for movement situations in terms of the sensory experiences which are directly related to moving". Hence, their "movement involvement cycle" depicts movement confidence being a product of an interaction between movement competence (i.e. perceptions of personal skill within the confines of a particular task), and movement sense ("personal expectations of sensory experiences related to moving") (Griffin and Keogh

(1982, p. 214). The model is shown in Fig. 5.7. The uniqueness of the components of the model have been questioned by Feltz (1988a) who says that the movement confidence model can be explained in terms of self-efficacy theory. The "unique" addition of movement sense to the model is, according to Feltz, already part of SET since one source of efficacy information is autonomic perception. While the search for the nature and make-up of confidence appears appropriate (Griffin et al. 1984), the research programme based around the movement confidence model has failed to support initial propositions that confidence is more than just competence. For example, Griffin et al. (1984) found that the major contributor to movement confidence was the perception of competence. Although some variations on this theme were found, the evidence was not convincing. Indeed, analysis of the "Movement Confidence Inventory" (which purports to assess movement competence, personal preference to enjoy the expected moving sensations, and perceived potential for physical harm), has failed to verify that movement confidence is anything more than global perceptions of movement confidence rather than the subcomponents suggested, although Griffin & Crawford (1989) have provided more convincing data recently. Self-efficacy may, however, be an adequate substitute term for movement confidence applied to exercise settings.

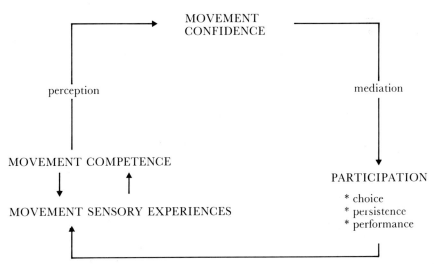

Figure 5.7. Movement Confidence Model. (From "A model for movement confidence" by N.S. Griffin and J.F. Keogh (1982) in J.A.S. Kelso and J.E. Clark (eds) *The Development of Movement Control and Co-ordination*, p. 214. Reprinted by permission of John Wiley & Sons, Ltd.)

Implications of the Study of Self-confidence

The theories and perspectives on self-confidence and physical exercise are becoming increasingly diverse. While the amount of activity in studying this phenomenon might at first appear a positive thing, one could argue that such disparate research efforts are not likely to lead to reliable practical applications. For this reason the implications for practice will be drawn primarily from self-efficacy theory and the work presented on performance estimates. The other perspectives are either too narrowly specified (e.g., sport; children) or too recent to lead to definitive conclusions (e.g., movement confidence; sport-confidence).

A rationale for increasing activity levels in the population at large for reasons of health promotion and disease prevention has been outlined in Chap. 1. However, the extent to which current low levels of activity are associated with low levels of self-confidence in exercise is not known. Practical implications, therefore, can only be drawn from research with small samples in relatively narrow contexts, such as the studies with post-MI men by Ewart and co-workers (Ewart 1989; Ewart et al. 1983, 1986a, b).

SET gives clear intervention possibilities through each of its four sources of efficacy information (Bandura 1986). For promoting health-related activity, the following guidelines based on these sources are offered:

1. *Performance attainment.* In recreational activity it is less important to participants whether they succeed in an objective way (i.e. win the game). However, efficacy expectations for the *adoption* of exercise are likely to be enhanced by prior experience in similar situations. Regrettably many people's experience of physical activity stems from a narrow range of competitive games at school, although recent trends in physical education may provide a better balance for more recent school leavers. Nevertheless, White and Coakley (1986) provided evidence from an English study that showed that negative perceptions of school physical education (PE) could be related to post-school participation. In their study of young people in south-east England they attempted to identify the factors on which young people based their decisions about participation in leisure-time sport and recreation. They found that involvement in sport reflected factors beyond those associated with competitive sport itself, suggesting that sport is just one form of physical activity for recreation. One factor deemed important by these people was the experience they had had in school PE and sport. Lack of participation was seen to be related to negative memories of PE, with boredom, lack of choice, negative evaluation from peers, and feelings of stupidity and incompetence being the most commonly cited factors. Girls were more likely to associate physical education experiences with discomfort and embarrassment and this seemed to affect their orientation to leisure time (White and Coakley 1986). Such experiences, according to SET, are

likely to alter efficacy expectations in those activities experienced in school PE which may then generalise, to differing degrees depending on the activities, to other exercise modes.

A similar analysis is possible for school leavers who have experienced courses in health and fitness activities. Their SE for initiating their own activity programme is likely to be influenced by their experience at school. The traditional images of "sergeant-major"-led drill and "exercise as punishment" have almost certainly been negative influences on activity patterns in leisure time. Interventions, therefore, must come in the form of enjoyable reinforcing physical activity where individual perceptions of mastery and intrinsic motivation are enhanced (see Chap. 9).

2. *Vicarious experience.* Related to the discussion above it could be argued that people's early experience in exercise, and the success of those around them, will influence SE expectations and, hence, exercise patterns. Seeing people of similar build and physical ability "succeed" in exercise is likely to have positive effects. However, such effects have a greater probability of occurrence when "success" is perceived in individualistic mastery-oriented terms (i.e., self-improvement). Constant comparison with others (an ego-involved orientation) is more likely to lead to disappointment and potential drop-out (Dweck and Leggett 1988; Roberts 1984).

3. *Social and verbal persuasion.* Although this usually refers to persuasion from others, self-talk has sometimes been found to be an effective strategy for enhancing SE (Wilkes and Summers 1984) although the results have been mixed (Feltz 1988a). In terms of exercise, it is likely that self-talk and personal perceptions of the costs and benefits of exercise will play a role in adopting or maintaining exercise. Research in strategies for controlling body weight (Mahoney and Mahoney 1976) has shown that "positive self-talk" can influence behaviour. This is also likely in exercise.

4. *Physiological arousal.* This is probably more important in avoidance behaviours and SE perceptions, although a relaxed approach to exercise has been advocated to enhance the mental health benefits (Glasser 1976; Steptoe and Bolton 1988). A greater awareness of physiological symptoms of effort and pain could also be beneficial in maintaining an exercise programme at an appropriate level.

Corbin (1984), although restricting his research in self-confidence to estimations of *performance* rather than *efficacy*, gives a variety of practical guidelines for enhancing self-confidence that are based on both his research and SET itself. With reference to ensuring successful behaviours, Corbin recommends the following:

a. establishment of realistic goals

b. establishment of progressively difficult tasks, although this is more likely to appeal to those exercisers who wish to be challenged

c. physically aid the performance of progressive tasks through "participant modelling" techniques (Feltz et al. 1979)

d. avoidance of situational vulnerability until some confidence has been built. An educational programme is also needed here to reduce the "negative" stereotyping of some physical activities for certain groups

e. proper use of feedback such that females in particular receive immediate and objective feedback

In terms of using positive reinforcement and role models, Corbin (1984) suggests: reward mastery attempts, be a positive role model, expose females to appropriate and respected role models who do not communicate disapproval of involvement in physical activities. Finally, he encourages good use of communication techniques, such as positive self-talk and praise, as well as techniques for anxiety reduction.

In summary, self-confidence has been found to have heuristic appeal and, despite the varied attempts at theoretical explanations of the construct, a general agreement on the possibilities of intervention to enhance exercise confidence is beginning to emerge. However, self-confidence must be seen in the context of related psychological constructs outlined in this book rather than in isolation.

PSYCHOLOGICAL OUTCOMES OF EXERCISE

6

Psychological Effects of Exercise for the Normal Population

The association of a healthy mind with a healthy body has long been recognised, but only recently have scientists begun to investigate this association in a systematic way. An unhealthy mind may be manifested in psychological problems; personally, or by association, such problems will affect the lives of a large number of people in contemporary society. Official reports (Mental Disorder Programme Planning Group 1985) suggest that 20% of the population will have to cope with some form of mental illness. Depression, one of the most common psychological problems, is estimated to affect one in four Americans and Europeans (American Psychiatric Association 1980). With a potential for such a high proportion of the population becoming mentally ill, it is obvious that cost-effective and efficient treatments must be found. It is possible that for some of these psychological problems regular involvement in physical activity can have a therapeutic effect. It is also possible that exercise can have a positive effect on psychological states that do not normally require treatment, such as mental fatigue, feelings of tension, and loss of self-confidence. The relationship of mind and body for these normal every-day states has not been investigated until recently. In this section the psychological effects of exercise will be discussed for both normal and clinical populations. In addition, a chapter will be devoted to reviewing the possible mechanisms which underlie the psychological effects which have been observed. In general, reference will be made to people who exercise for recreation rather than at a high competitive level.

Descriptive Studies

In this section studies which have described the perceived effects of exercise will be reviewed.

An important publication on the interrelationship between exercise and mental health considered four large population surveys in the United States and Canada (Stephens 1988). Stephens examined data from the National Health and Nutrition Examination Survey I which spanned the early to mid-1970s, the Canada Health Survey completed at the end of the 1970s, the National Survey of Personal Health Practices and Consequences from 1979, and the Canada Fitness Survey of 1981. In these surveys, approximately 56 000 people were investigated and Stephens specifically analysed the data on physical activity and mental health indices. Six different measures of mental health were used across the surveys.

Stephens (1988) conducted 32 analyses – eight mental health measures (two were used in two surveys and analysed separately) for each sex and two age groups split at 40 years. Twenty-five of these analyses demonstrated a positive association between physical activity and mental health, with the remaining seven showing no association. Stephens (1988, pp. 41–42) concluded as follows:

> The inescapable conclusion of this study is that the level of physical activity is positively associated with good mental health in the household population of the United States and Canada, when mental health is defined as positive mood, general well-being, and relatively infrequent symptoms of anxiety and depression. This relationship is independent of the effects of education and physical health status, and is stronger for women and those age 40 years and over than for men and those under age 40. The robustness of this conclusion derives from the varied sources of evidence: four population samples in two countries over a ten year period, four different methods of operationalising physical activity and six different mental health scales.

The question remains, of course, whether good mental health precedes or is a consequence of physical activity. Stephens (1988) suggests that while good mental health may be a necessary condition for activity, it is not a sufficient condition in itself. However, poor mental health in the form of low self-esteem and depression may well predict low levels of activity. More will be said of this later.

Several large surveys have noted that very high percentages (60%–92%) of non-elite runners feel that running provides psychological benefits (Callen 1983; Carmack and Martens 1979; Jorgenson and Jorgenson 1979; Mutrie and Knill-Jones 1985). These benefits include reports of "feeling better" (Carmack and Martens 1979), an increased sense of well-being (Jorgenson and Jorgenson 1979), anxiety and tension reduction (Callen 1983; Mutrie and Knill-Jones 1985), and increased self-image and self-confidence (Callen

1983). Few sex differences have been noted for these effects although Callen (1983) did note two interesting differences between the sexes in his survey of American runners. Firstly, more women (72%) than men (62%) felt that running improved their mood, and secondly, more women (69%) than men (52%) reported that running relieved feelings of depression. This latter finding has been supported by Mutrie and Knill-Jones (1985) who also found that more women (50.6%) than men (37%), in a sample of Scottish non-elite marathon runners, reported that running relieved feelings of depression.

The opposite of a "feel better" effect has been noted when exercisers miss their regular workout. Glasser (1976) has described symptoms of withdrawal from exercise, which include increased irritability, guilt, and tension. Carmack and Martens (1979) and Summers et al. (1982) have also reported that when runners missed their regular exercise they experienced bad moods, guilt, irritability, depression, and sluggishness. Similar findings have been reported by Robbins and Joseph (1985), but they noted that distress from missing a run was more common in the women in their study.

An added dimension to descriptive studies is an examination of the mood states of people involved in different intensities of exercise. Tooman et al. (1985) found that competitive runners (13 men and 7 women, with an average running speed in training of 6.13 min/mile), had more positive mood states than recreational runners (14 men and 6 women, with an average running speed of 8.31 min/mile). The mood states were measured by the Profile of Mood States (POMS, McNair et al. 1971) which is a questionnaire comprised of six subscales. The subscales are named as tension, depression, anger, vigour, fatigue and confusion and these six scales can also be totalled to give a global mood score. Wilson et al. (1980) compared the POMS scores of a group of marathon runners, a group of joggers, and a group of non-exercisers. They found that both the marathon runners (weekly mileage = 36–100 miles) and the joggers (weekly mileage = 3–10 miles) had lower depression, anger, and confusion scores and higher vigour scores than the non-exercisers. They also found that the marathon runners had more positive mood profiles than the joggers. However, only men were included in this study.

The suggestion that different intensities of exercise may be associated with different mood profiles developed from the idea that athletes may differ from non-athletes. Morgan and Pollock (1977) suggested that athletes have more positive mood profiles (as measured by POMS) than the normal population. The athletes' mood profiles were characterised by lower than normal levels of tension, depression, anger, fatigue and confusion, and higher than normal levels of vigour. Morgan (1980b) has described this configuration as the "iceberg profile". A hypothetical iceberg profile is shown in Fig. 6.1. Morgan's work was conducted on male athletes only and very little evidence exists for a similar "iceberg profile" amongst women exercisers. However, Gondola and Tuckman (1982) and Berger and Owen

(1983) found that both male and female recreational exercisers (runners and swimmers) did display an "iceberg profile" in comparison to non-exercising controls.

Descriptions, of course, do not provide evidence that exercise causes psychological benefits. There are many alternative reasons which could be offered to explain the differences in mood profiles that have been described. For example, it could be argued that people who generally experience positive moods are more likely to exercise than those who do not. The relationship between exercise and affect, as described by these studies, remains associative rather than causal. Descriptive studies, despite their limitations, are nevertheless valuable because they provide hypotheses which can be tested in experimental situations.

Experimental and Quasi-experimental Studies

True experimental studies, which employ random assignment of subjects to experimental and control conditions, are hard to find in the literature examining the psychological effects of exercise. Folkins and Sime (1981) have suggested that as few as 15% of studies in this area qualify as true experiments, and most of them have examined clinical populations. Hughes (1984) comments that even when studies in this area are experimentally designed there are flaws, such as demand characteristics associated with the experimenter or expectations of the subject, which are not controlled for. Most of the designs are at best quasi-experimental in which a group receiving exercise is compared with a non-equivalent group in a control condition. Alternative explanations of effects, such as local history or selection bias, remain plausible with this type of design. Other designs do

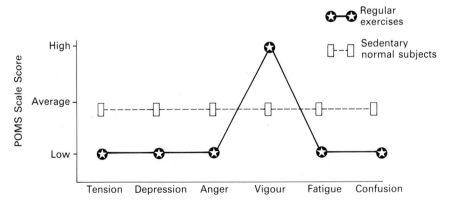

Figure 6.1. A hypothetical set of POMS scores for regular exercisers and sedentary normal subjects. The configuration for the regular exercisers is known as the "iceberg profile".

not incorporate control conditions at all. Cook and Campbell (1979) warn that there are several factors which threaten validity in this kind of design, namely local history, statistical regression, and testing effects. In other words, this type of design does not allow causal inference regarding the treatment effects. Only when subjects are randomly assigned to treatments can reasonable causal inference be made. The effect of exercise could be more clearly identified in future studies by using placebo control groups in which all variables, except the one under investigation, remain constant. With these caveats in mind, and with the hope that current research will spawn future work which is more appropriately designed, the experimental and quasi-experimental literature will now be reviewed.

The Effect of Acute Exercise Involvement

Several studies have measured the effect of a single exercise session on mood. Nowlis and Greenberg (1979) measured the effects of a 12.5-mile run on mood in 18 experienced runners (13 men and 5 women). They found that the runners reported increased "pleasantness" after the run, and that this effect was reported by both men and women.

Berger and Owen (1983) measured the mood profiles of novice (n = 25) and intermediate swimmers (n = 33) before and after one swimming lesson. They found that, compared to a control group who had been to a lecture class (n = 42), the swimmers reported greater decreases in levels of tension, depression, anger, and confusion, and greater increases in vigour after one swimming lesson. These effects were found for both men and women. Berger and Owen (1983, p. 429) concluded that "swimmers really do report 'feeling better'", but this should, however, be accepted with caution. The swimming in this study was performed as part of a lesson. It is not clear from this design whether the swimming itself or some other aspects of the teaching/learning interaction was responsible for the mood elevation. A similar problem arose in a study by Reiter (1981) in which the effects of one general exercise session were measured on a group of elderly women. Reiter (1981) found that this kind of exercise had a positive effect on the group's reported sense of well-being, while control groups in arts and crafts classes did not report a change in sense of well-being. Again, it is not clear if it was the exercise itself, or some other aspect of the exercise environment, such as the charisma of the exercise leader, which was responsible for the mood elevation.

Bahrke and Morgan (1978) compared the effects of walking on a treadmill (at 70% of maximum heart rate), meditating, and resting in a comfortable chair, on measures of state anxiety. The finding, that all three groups decreased state anxiety scores after treatment, was interpreted as evidence for exercise as a diversion from normal activities. Bahrke and Morgan (1978), therefore, suggested that one mechanism of the psychological benefits of exercise may be that it provides a distraction for the participant. However, these results can be interpreted in another way: it could be that all groups were more anxious before the experiment, because they did not know exactly what to expect. Thus, a fall in state anxiety would be predicted after the experiment was over. When the changes in the control group are in the same direction as those in the treatment groups it is unusual to claim that there has been a treatment effect which can be associated with the treatment itself, rather than with extraneous variables (such as the Hawthorne effect), for which the control group provides comparisons.

Schwartz et al. (1978) conducted a study which offered another explanation to the findings of Bahrke and Morgan (1978). Schwartz et al. (1978) suggested that anxiety has both somatic and cognitive components, and that a global measure of anxiety, such as the Spielberger State Trait Anxiety Inventory (Spielberger et al. 1970), which was used by Bahrke and Morgan (1978), does not reveal the true effects of exercise on anxiety. Schwartz et al. (1978) found that both meditation and participation in an exercise class reduced anxiety scores. However, the exercise reduced somatic anxiety while meditation reduced cognitive anxiety. This suggested that Bahrke and Morgan (1978) might have found differences between the three treatment groups in their experiment, if they had used a different scale.

Berger and Owen (1988) studied the acute effects of four different forms of activity – swimming, physical conditioning, hatha yoga, and fencing – on mental health (specifically mood states) and suggested that in addition to the type (mode) of exercise, other factors to consider in the relationship between exercise and mood might include the absence or inclusion of competition, the predictability of the activities, and the degree of repetitive or rhythmical action involved (see Table 6.1). Berger and Owen (1988) studied students before and after physical education classes.

The results were based on changes in anxiety and mood states before and after the activity class. Little change took place in swimming, with the

Table 6.1. Exercise Mode Requirements in Four Physical Activities. (Adapted from Berger and Owen 1988)

Activity	Mode requirements			
	Aerobic	Competition	Predictable	Repetitive rhythmical
Swimming	Yes	No	Yes	Yes
Conditioning	1/2[a]	No	Yes	Yes
Yoga	No	No	Yes	Yes
Fencing	No	Yes	No	No

[a] The conditioning class was half aerobic and half anaerobic.

group having a highly positive mood profile before the class. For the physical conditioning class, the students reported greater fatigue after the class than before. No other mood benefits were observed for this class; in fact 12 of the 28 class members dropped out of the course suggesting that high levels of exercise intensity can be counter-productive to adherence. Overall, the yoga participants showed significant positive changes in mood, while the fencing group reported greater vigour after the class than before.

The study by Berger and Owen (1988), therefore, shows that positive mood changes are possible after different exercise modalities, but that high intensity exercise may be detrimental from the point of view of positive affect and adherence.

At the present time the literature on the acute effects of exercise is not sufficiently well developed to allow unequivocal conclusions to be drawn; it does point the way, however, for future study in this area.

The Effect of Chronic Exercise Involvement

Several studies have investigated the effects on mental health of a programme of exercise. These programmes typically last between 8 and 10 weeks with two to four exercise sessions each week. For example, after a 10-week jogging class, Folkins et al. (1972) found that fitness improvements were positively correlated with measures of psychological well-being for a group of college students (n = 44). It was noted that this effect was stronger for the women than for the men. Brown et al. (1978) studied the effects of various types of exercise on 71 male and 96 female college and high school students. They found decreased depression scores (although scores were below clinical levels) in those who performed 30 minutes of exercise (tennis, wrestling, or jogging), three times per week for 10 weeks, but not in a non-exercising control group and a team of softball players. No differences were noted between the sexes in this study, but the selection bias involved in using intact groups may have confounded the results. In a more controlled study, Blumenthal et al. (1982) compared mood profiles of 16 exercisers (11 women and 5 men) and 16 sedentary, matched control subjects.

The comparisons were made before and after the experimental subjects engaged in a 10-week exercise programme. By the end of the exercise programme reduced levels of trait and state anxiety were reported by the experimental group and they had more positive mood profiles than the control group. Blumenthal et al. (1982) acknowledge that selection bias may provide an alternative to exercise as an explanation of the results.

Taken together, these results provide some support for the idea that chronic involvement in exercise leads to psychological benefits, but they also highlight flaws in the research. The complete picture will not be available until designs which incorporate random assignment to treatment groups replicate the findings. To date only one such study has been completed. Moses et al. (1989) randomly assigned 94 volunteers to either a high intensity (70%–75% of maximum heart rate) aerobic training regime, a moderate intensity (60% of maximum heart rate) aerobic training regime or a strengthening and stretching regime which served as an attention-placebo control. All three regimes were equated in frequency (one supervised and three unsupervised sessions per week) and duration (10 weeks). Dependent measures included a battery of psychological and physiological measures. The psychological measures were the POMS scale and a measure of perceived coping ability and well-being, while the physiological measures were a 12-min walk/run test and a sub-maximal cycle ergometer test during which oxygen consumption was measured. The main finding was that psychological benefits (reductions in tension/anxiety and an increase in coping ability) were evident for the moderate aerobic exercise condition, but not for the other two training regimes. The results for coping ability are depicted in Fig. 6.2.

The design employed by Moses et al. (1989) allows a more confident conclusion that the exercise caused the noted effects. In addition, the new dimension of exercise intensity has been added to the discussion of exercise and psychological effects. Moses et al. (1989) found the greatest improvements in the fitness measures in the high intensity group, while the greatest psychological gain was found in the moderate intensity group. This finding suggests that there is no straightforward relationship between fitness improvement and psychological benefit, which is contrary to what

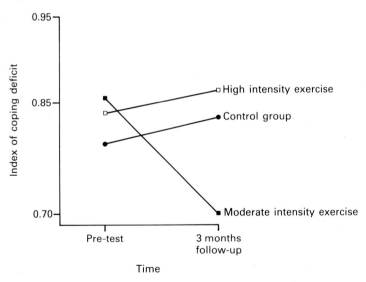

Figure 6.2. Index of coping deficit over a 3-month period for three different treatment groups. A reduction in coping deficit implies an increase in coping ability. (From Moses et al. (1989) reproduced with permission of Pergamon Press.)

previous researchers had suggested (Folkins et al. 1972; Brown et al. 1978; Martinsen et al. 1985). The question which remains is what kind of exercise (in terms of type of activity, frequency, duration and intensity) will produce the greatest psychological benefit? The attempt by Berger and Owen (1988) to answer this question for acute exercise failed to provide clear answers. Research on chronic exercise involvement and different exercise types is now needed.

The Effect of Exercise Deprivation

Another way of experimentally investigating the psychological effects of exercise is to take it away from regular participants. Baekeland (1970) deprived 14 regular exercisers of their usual exercise for 1 month and studied the effects of this on sleep patterns. The sex of the subjects was not stated. Changes in sleep patterns, such as increased wakefulness, were noted. The subjects also reported increased sexual tension and an increased need to be with others. It was concluded that this pattern of changes suggested an increase in anxiety during the time the subjects were deprived of their regular exercise. This study is limited by the fact that there is no control group and no account is taken of fitness levels, which Paxton et al. (1983) suggest are critical in sleep studies. Therefore, Baekeland's (1970) conclusions may not be valid.

Two other studies have looked at the effects of exercise deprivation. Tooman et al. (1985) measured mood profiles of both competitive and recreational runners after a normal training run, and then deprived them of running for 2 consecutive days. All runners experienced a positive mood swing after running, which was maintained into the first day without exercise. However, by the second day without exercise, mood scores had dropped to the level recorded before a regular run. This suggests that the positive effects of one exercise session may last up to 1 day. There was no difference between men and women in the pattern of these results. Morris et al. (1988) used a similar design on two groups of male runners (n = 40); one group was studied over a period of 6 weeks in which it completed regular training. The other group stopped running for weeks 3 and 4 of the study. The deprived runners showed more symptoms of anxiety and depression in comparison to the group having continuous training and this withdrawal effect lasted only during the period of deprivation. Both groups had similar scores by the end of the 6-week period.

The experimental paradigm of exercise deprivation is difficult to put into practice because not many exercisers who experience benefits from exercise are willing to give up their routines. Moreover, those exercisers who are willing to stop may be quite different from those who are not willing to comply with this experimental condition. Thus, a selection bias is likely to occur in exercise studies using this design. Similarly, the mechanisms of the withdrawal effect remain unclear. Negative mood shifts may be due to factors other than exercise withdrawal, such as a general change in normal daily routine.

The Effects of Exercise on Stress

Stress is a word in common every-day use which has a multitude of meanings. It is not usually considered to be a clinical problem. Most people use the word "stress" to describe the demands of commitments to work or family, dealing with travelling, resolving conflicts and other emotional issues. It is also true that pleasant situations such as holidays and weddings can be stressful. There is a growing volume of evidence to link stress with both physical and psychiatric ill health (Anisman 1984; Maier and Laudenslager 1985).

If we look at one possible model of stress, that of one of the most famous stress researchers, Selye (1956), we can see that it is not stress itself which may cause problems but lack of recovery from a stressful experience. According to Selye we all experience stress in our daily lives, and our bodies respond to the demands of these stresses in the same way. The natural process of the body is to create a recovery period in which our body systems return to normal. Most people find this recovery at home, taking a break, going away for the weekend, in leisure pursuits and in relaxation. In fact a recent survey of sources and effects of stress on executives (British Market Research Bureau 1989) revealed that over 60% of the respondents viewed taking holidays and taking regular exercise as the two principal means of coping with stress. Stress only becomes a problem when the recovery process is not allowed to occur. Without time to recover, the body arrives at a stage of exhaustion.

Certain types of social situation or personality disposition are perhaps more likely to lead to adverse health changes. It is also recognised that the amount of control a person has on his or her situation is a critical variable (see Chap. 4 on perceptions of control). Other researchers (Lazarus and Folkman 1984) suggest that the most important factor in the stress–health equation is the degree to which a person perceives threat in the stressful situation. Certain life events, such as divorce, becoming unemployed or moving house, are also recognised as being more stressful than routine daily living, and these life events can lead to an increased incidence of illness. Definitions of stress, and theoretical models used to explain its effects, are far from unified. Spielberger (1987) points out that there is a need to differentiate between the emotional responses, such as anxiety and anger, that people have in stressful situations. At best we have a developing area in medicine; it could be that exercise could play a role in combating stress. The link between exercise and stress theoretically proposes that the fitter the individual (usually aerobic fitness is referred to) the quicker the body systems return to normal after any stress-inducing experience (Hatfield and Landers 1987; Sinyor et al. 1983). Furthermore, aerobic fitness, it is proposed, may have a buffering effect on the extent to which the body responds to the stressful situations. This link between aerobic fitness and stress is based on the knowledge that both aerobic exercise and stress activate the sympathetic nervous system. Training for aerobic fitness causes adaptations which lead to greater efficiency of the systems involved; the more efficient the system the less a particular demand will affect it and the faster that system will recover to base-line levels.

The best evidence that aerobic fitness is associated with a buffering effect from stress is given by Crews and Landers (1987) who performed a meta-analysis on 34 studies. Meta-analysis is a statistical procedure which combines the size of effects found in different studies and is, therefore, a very useful way of gaining an overall picture of a research area. Crews and Landers' (1987) meta-analysis yielded 92 effects from 1500 subjects and showed that the overall effect size was 0.48, indicating that subjects who were aerobically fit had a reduced response to psychosocial stressors of about one-half of a standard deviation, compared to either control groups or base-line values. The evidence that fitter subjects have a faster return to normal after a stress-inducing experience is less clear. Unfortunately, the majority (26) of the studies reviewed by Crews and Landers (1987) were correlational, with fewer (8) employing a training design.

Brooke and Long (1987) tested the hypothesis that higher levels of aerobic fitness would lead to greater coping efficiency by asking 18 subjects to absail with a rope. The subjects were divided into high and low fitness groups by the median split method. Dependent measures, which included anxiety (via a self-report scale), heart rate and catecholamines, were taken at base-line levels, prior to the descent and after the descent. The results showed only weak support for the hypothesis because although the higher fitness group maintained lower heart rates throughout and recovered (in terms of anxiety levels and adrenaline levels) more quickly than the lower fitness group, the recovery pattern was not the same for heart rate, cortisol and noradrenaline. Often the results of cross-sectional studies, such as this, are difficult to interpret; the median split on fitness levels may indicate many things other than fitness, including genetic predisposition. What is required is a study in which subjects are trained while controls remain unchanged.

Steptoe et al. (1988) used a prospective methodology to ascertain if 10 weeks of moderate aerobic training could positively influence perceived coping ability and physiologically measured coping ability. Subjects (n = 53) were randomly assigned to either an aerobic training condition or a control condition (strength and mobility exercise). These researchers found that the group taking moderate aerobic exercise showed greater improvements in perceived coping abilities than the control group. This finding was confirmed by Moses et al. (1989). However, this pattern was not evident for the physiological measures which were made in a laboratory setting. Again this provides only weak support for the hypothesis that becoming fitter will lead to a greater ability to cope with stress.

Using a longitudinal methodology, Brown and Siegel (1988) ascertained if the amount of exercise undertaken by a group of American female adolescents (n = 364) was related to the amount of stress-induced ill health over a period of 8 months. The researchers found that the negative effect of stressful life events on health decreased as exercise levels increased. The authors were careful not to make any causal connections but said (Brown and Siegel 1988, p. 349) that their results ". . . provide the most compelling evidence to date for the ability of exercise to buffer the adverse effects of life stress". Roth and Holmes (1985) and Tucker et al. (1986) also report studies which support the notion that fitness provides a moderating effect on stress.

However, other researchers are critical both of the theoretical links between stress reactivity and fitness and the methodology which has been employed to date in this area. van Doornen et al. (1988) examined critically the assumption that fitness should have an effect on reaction to stress because the exercise and stress responses are similar. After discussing in detail the differences between a response induced by exercise and a response induced by stress for the heart, the vessels and the adrenomedullar system, they conclude that the theoretical analogy between the response to exercise and stress was not valid. However, they do suggest that there may be other reasons, such as a person's perception of the situation and coping abilities, which could predict an advantage for the aerobically fit person.

The methodological criticisms are largely concerned with subject classification based on arbitrary distinctions between high-fit and low-fit subjects; knowing that a percentage of any aerobic power score can be explained by heredity weakens the argument that being "fitter" combats stress. Results of studies which divide subjects by a fitness score could also mean that stress reactivity has a degree of heredity involved or that those who react most to stressful stimuli are also those who are least attracted to activity which would promote fitness. In addition, heart rate is often used as an independent variable to predict the aerobic power scores on which classification to high-fit and low-fit groups is made; heart rate is then often used as a dependent variable measuring reactions to stress. This confounding of dependent and independent variables is problematic. It has also not been determined whether physical fitness or activity history is the most important variable.

These methodological problems can be over-ruled in studies which train subjects aerobically. It could well be that training programmes need to be considerably longer than that normally required to induce aerobic improvement if reaction to stress is to be altered. Similarly, more studies are required on the possible effects of exercise and/or fitness on an individual's ability to cope with prolonged stress (Crews and Landers 1987).

Harmful Effects of Exercise

It does seem from the literature reviewed so far that only psychological benefit, and not harm, can be associated with exercise. The early literature which looked at possible harmful effects of exercise focussed on the term exercise "addiction" (Hailey and Bailey 1982; Morgan 1979b; Sachs 1981). The issue under discussion was whether or not what appears to be compulsive exercise behaviour is harmful. Previously, Glasser (1976) had suggested that regular non-competitive running could be a *positive* addiction which gave a degree of psychological strength to the runner, but these other articles suggest that compulsive exercising is not a healthy state at all.

Glasser pointed out that any activity, physical or mental, can be addictive, providing the activity fulfils the six basic criteria listed in Table 6.2.

The term "addiction" has proved to be confusing. Are people who exercise 5 or 6 times each week, or who experience withdrawal symptoms when they do not exercise, psychologically unhealthy or addicted? New terms which seemed derogatory have appeared in the literature, such as "obligatory running" (Blumenthal et al. 1984), and "compulsive running" (Nash 1987). However, there was not much evidence to suggest that a high level of activity in itself was a problem. Morgan (1979b) suggested that there was a problem if the person continued to exercise against medical advice, or in preference to family, social or job responsibilities.

The most useful contribution to this area has come from de Coverley Veale (1987a) who recommended a set of criteria which describe "exercise dependence" as a state, similar to alcohol, drug or gambling dependence, in which the person displays patterns of behaviour entirely controlled by their dependence. de Coverley Veale has created a set of diagnostic criteria which describe exercise dependence (see Table 6.3).

Table 6.2. Glasser's (1976) Criteria for Classifying an Activity as Addictive

1. The activity is non-competitive and of one's own choice. About an hour each day is devoted to this activity
2. The activity requires little skill or mental effort
3. The activity is not dependent on others, and is mostly undertaken alone
4. There is a belief that this activity is of value
5. There is a belief that persistence in the activity will lead to improvement
6. The activity can be done without self-criticism

de Coverley Veale also makes a useful distinction between those people who are *primarily* dependent on exercise, and those who are dependent secondarily to eating disorders. This distinction is important because there has been speculation that there may be a link between excessive exercise and eating disorders such as anorexia nervosa (Yates et al. 1983; Nash 1987). This link suggests that people who display anorexic behaviour (such as obsession with weight, distortion of body image) have the same personality traits as people who appear addicted to exercise. The possibility of this link came through clinical observations of anorexics and compulsive runners (people who could not derive pleasure from areas of life other than running), but the comparison has received criticism because the runners were male and the anorexics female (Knight et al. 1987) and because of the methods of assessment used in the Yates et al. study (Blumenthal et al. 1984). Nevertheless, some authors have suggested common features between anorexic and athletic females (see Table 6.4), and recent evidence suggests a high incidence of pathogenic weight-control behaviours among young people involved in sport.

Dummer et al. (1987) concluded, from their study of over 900 9–18-year-old boys and girls involved in competitive swimming, that 15.4% of girls (24.8% of postmenarcheal girls) used some form of pathogenic weight-control strategy, such as fasting, self-induced vomiting, use of diet pills,

Table 6.3. Proposed Diagnostic Criteria for "Exercise Dependence" (de Coverley Veale 1987a). (Reprinted with permission.)

A.	Narrowing of repertoire leading to a stereotyped pattern of exercise with a regular schedule once or more daily
B.	Salience with the individual giving increasing priority over other activities to maintaining the pattern of exercise
C.	Increased tolerance to the amount of exercise performed over the years
D.	Withdrawal symptoms related to a disorder of mood following the cessation of the exercise schedule
E.	Relief or avoidance of withdrawal symptoms by further exercise
F.	Subjective awareness of a compulsion to exercise
G.	Rapid reinstatement of the previous pattern of exercise and withdrawal symptoms after a period of abstinence

Associated features

H.	*Either* the individual continues to exercise despite a serious physical disorder known to be caused, aggravated or prolonged by exercise and is advised as such by a health professional, *or* the individual has arguments or difficulties with his/her partner, family, friends, or occupation
I.	Self-inflicted loss of weight by dieting as a means towards improving performance

Table 6.4. Distinguishing and Shared Features of the Anorexic Female and Athletic Female. (Adapted from Dishman (1986a) and McSherry (1984))

Anorexic	Athlete
Distinguishing Features	
Aimless physical activity	Purposeful training
Poor exercise performance	Increased exercise tolerance
Poor muscle development	Good muscle development
"Flawed" body image	Accurate body image
Body fat below normal range	Body fat within normal range
Shared Features	
Dietary faddism	
Controlled calorie consumption	
Low body weight	
High physical activity	
High levels of body awareness	

laxatives and diuretics. Such behaviours were much less prevalent in the boys, with only 3.6% reporting that they used at least one of these strategies. Similar results were found in a survey of 42 female American college gymnasts (Rosen and Hough 1988). They found that 62% were using some form of pathogenic weight-control strategy, mainly fasting, self-induced vomiting and diet pills. Of those who were told that they were too heavy by their coaches, 75% resorted to such behaviours. Similarly, Rosen et al. (1986) found pathogenic weight-control behaviours practised by athletes in a survey of ten sports. The highest incidence was found in gymnastics (74%) and distance running (47%).

Such data require careful scrutiny by those involved in sports where body weight may affect performance and/or appearance, and also where there are a high number of adolescent participants. This is one area of physical activity where the mental health outcomes may not be positive.

Despite the limited amount of evidence to suggest that some extreme levels of exercise are harmful, the popular press continues to warn of the risks of addiction to exercise (Rees 1988). It would seem that the clinical literature on the occurrence of exercise dependence can now use de Coverley Veale's (1987a) diagnostic criteria to build knowledge of the incidence and treatment of the problem; to date the prevalence and significance of exercise dependence in terms of public health are unknown.

7

Psychological Effects of Exercise for Clinical Populations

The effects of exercise on the normal population have been discussed in the previous chapter. Here, the potential role of exercise in clinical settings will be reviewed. The review will include depression, anxiety and psychiatric illnesses.

The Use of Exercise as a Treatment for Depression

Kostrubala (1976) provided anecdotal evidence for the use of running as a therapy for depression. Kostrubala is a psychoanalytic psychotherapist who is also an enthusiastic runner. He described his use of running as a way of enhancing the communication between therapist and patient. The idea that running (or something associated with the running) could alleviate depression led to experimental research in this area.

Group Designs

Greist et al. (1979a) were among the first therapists to use an experimental design to quantify the effects of exercise (in this case running) on depression. They randomly assigned 28 subjects to one of three treatment groups: (a) 10 sessions of time-limited psychotherapy which was based on behavioural techniques; (b) time-unlimited psychotherapy which was based on cognitive techniques; or (c) running, with a group leader, for 30–65 min three times each week. All treatments lasted for 10 weeks. The subjects were 13 men and 15 women, from a private clinic, who were diagnosed as depressed.

The results indicated that the eight subjects assigned to the running treatment had at least as much improvement as those in the other two conditions.

While Greist et al. (1979a) had made an important step in beginning the experimental research in this area, they acknowledged that the design had several flaws which limited both the internal and the external validity of the findings.The internal validity was limited by the presence of only one running leader, but several psychotherapists, and by the fact that the running group had more contact than the other two groups with the therapist and other patients. In addition, it is not clear which aspects of running treatment were related to improvement; social interaction, mastery of a task, or fitness improvements are all possible agents in the observed changes. Thus, it is difficult to separate the effects of the running itself from the effects of an enthusiastic running leader or the effects of time in treatment. The external validity of this study was limited by the use of patients in private practice. The initial finding, that running may be as beneficial as more traditional (North American) treatments for depression, led Greist and his associates (Klein et al. 1985) to conduct a second study which equated time in contact with the therapist and provided a comparison condition (meditation-relaxation) which controlled for some of the possible extraneous variables of the previous design.

In this second study 74 subjects were randomly assigned to group psychotherapy, meditation therapy or running therapy. Comparisons between the three groups, after 12 weeks of treatment and at a 9-month follow-up, led to the conclusion that the three treatments were equally effective in reducing depression; this is consistent with the finding of Greist et al. (1979a). However,the design of Klein et al.'s (1985) study does not rule out the possibility that depression improves over time even without treatment; for ethical and practical reasons it is very difficult for researchers to control for recovery over time. Ethically, people who are seeking help for depression should not be deprived of potentially beneficial treatment for long periods of time, and in the practical world if people are left without prescribed treatment they are likely to use their own resources (e.g., friends or family) to help themselves.

The findings of Greist et al. (1979a) and Klein et al. (1985) have been supported by other research. Reuter (1979) randomly assigned 18 students, who had sought help for depression at a North American university mental-health clinic, to one of two treatment groups. One group received counselling therapy for 10 weeks; the other group received the same counselling therapy, but in addition ran three times per week with a running leader. The results indicated that the group receiving both running and counselling improved significantly more on scores on the Beck Depression Inventory (BDI; Beck et al. 1961) than the group receiving only counselling. This conclusion must be interpreted with caution as the running and counselling group had more time in treatment each week than the counselling-only group. de Coverley Veale and Le Fevre (1988) report a similar finding for British day-patients in a psychiatric hospital. These authors conclude that there is benefit for depressed patients in adding exercise to normal treatment, but acknowledge that the positive effects may be due to the social interaction in the group exercise and/or the extra attention received via the exercise leader. However, Fremont and Craighead (1987) expanded on the design used by Reuter (1979) and ensured that the hypothesis of improvements being caused by extra attention could be tested.

In a study conducted with 49 volunteers, Fremont and Craighead (1987) randomly assigned subjects to one of three treatments: (a) cognitive therapy only for 1 hour per week, (b) running with a group leader for 20 min three times each week, or (c) both cognitive therapy (1 hour per week) and running therapy (20 min three times per week). The volunteers, who had responded to media advertisements for depression therapy, all met standardised screening criteria for depression. The results indicated that all three treatments were associated with equal improvements in depression, as measured by the BDI. This result, that running is as effective as other psychotherapeutic treatments for depression, is consistent with the findings of Greist et al (1979a) and Klein et al. (1985), but not with those of McCann and Holmes (1984) who used relaxation as a placebo control.

McCann and Holmes (1984) produced a well-designed study with 43 women, who were mildly depressed (i.e., scoring above 11 on the BDI), randomly assigned to either aerobic exercise, relaxation exercises or a no-treatment condition for 10 weeks. Subjects in the relaxation and aerobic exercise conditions had similar expectations about how much the treatment would help their depressed moods. The results indicated that the aerobic exercise condition had more effect on lowering depression scores than either the relaxation exercises or the no-treatment control condition. In comparing these results to other studies which show similar effects on depression from both exercise and psychotherapy two points should be considered. Firstly, although relaxation appears similar to meditation (which was successfully used in Klein et al.'s (1985) study) it may have less effect on depressed mood and more effect on tension/anxiety, since it focusses mostly on muscle tension. Secondly, in the McCann and Holmes (1984) study, the aerobic exercise class met as a group twice each week, whereas the relaxation condition was carried out by each subject following written and verbal instructions. The apparent advantage of the aerobic exercise could be explained by the effect of meeting as a group.

The main hypothesis which has been tested in the studies reviewed to date is that *aerobic* exercise has a therapeutic effect on depression. However, it may be that activity of any kind can have the same positive effects which have been reported for aerobic activity.

Mutrie (1986) compared the effects on depression, mood, and fitness of three different 8-week exercise programmes. The subjects (n = 24) were diagnosed as depressed by general practitioners (GPs), and then referred to a fitness consultant. The GPs were working within the National Health Service of the United Kingdom. Subjects were randomly assigned to three groups. Group A (n = 9) received 8 weeks of aerobic exercise, with strengthening and stretching exercise introduced after 4 weeks. Group B (n = 8) received 8 weeks of strengthening and stretching exercise, with aerobic exercise introduced after 4 weeks. Group C (n = 7) had no treatment for 4 weeks, and then received 8 weeks of exercise which included aerobic, strengthening, and stretching exercise. Each subject met individually with a fitness consultant every 2 weeks and undertook the exercise prescription from home. This ensured that results could not be explained by the group interaction effect. The fitness consultant taught the fitness programmes, set appropriate exercise goals, and conducted fitness tests. The dependent measures were the BDI, the POMS, an aerobic step test, and a sit-up test.

After 4 weeks of aerobic exercise group A had lower scores on the BDI (mean = 9.46) than at intake (mean = 22.44, $p < 0.01$). Reductions on the BDI were not evident after 4 weeks of non-aerobic exercise (group B) nor after 4 weeks of no-treatment (group C) (see Fig. 7.1). It is, therefore, more likely that the reduction in depression was caused by aerobic exercise itself, rather than by spontaneous remission or by peripheral effects of the experimental situation. In particular, the result cannot be explained by any effects of group interaction and it is unlikely that the differences between the two exercise groups can be explained by the effect of the consultant, since four different consultants were used. No fitness improvements were noted for any group after 4 weeks. However, after 8 weeks of exercise *all* subjects reported lower levels of depression, and more positive moods, and were found to be physically fitter. These improvements were maintained 20 weeks after the 8-week programmes. There was no relationship between the physiological and psychological measures in this study.

From the results of this study it would seem that aerobic exercise may have greater benefits than non-aerobic exercise over a short period of time (i.e., 4 weeks). It could be possible that initially the aerobic prescription was easier and more pleasant to follow and made the subjects leave their homes to walk. This could have initial benefits over the non-aerobic prescription which encouraged the exercise to be completed in the home environment. By the end of the treatment period and in the follow-up period all subjects were doing the same mixture of aerobic, strengthening and stretching exercise. It is not surprising, therefore, that no further group differences were established. Doyne et al. (1987) also provide supportive evidence that it is not only aerobic exercise which can have a positive effect on depression.

Doyne and her colleagues recruited 40 women in an American town by inviting them, through the media, to participate in a study on the effects of exercise on depression. Subjects were diagnosed as depressed via the Research Diagnostic Criteria (Spitzer et al. 1978) and were randomly assigned to aerobic exercise (walking/running at 80% maximum heart rate),

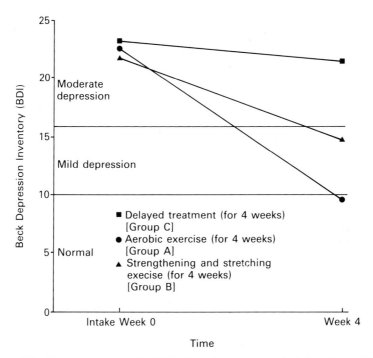

Figure 7.1. Mean scores on the BDI from intake to week 4 for three different treatment groups (Mutrie 1986).

or to weight-training exercise (standard exercises using "Universal" machines), or to a waiting-list control group. A standard exercise prescription of 3–4 sessions per week was used for an 8-week period. The results are shown in Fig. 7.2. Doyne et al. (1987) suggest that the results were consistent across all the measures used in the study (both psychometric and physiological) and showed (p. 752) "both statistically and clinically significant decreases in depression in the two exercise groups relative to the wait-list control. No significant overall differences in depression were found between the two exercise groups".

Interestingly, there were very small fitness improvements over the 8 weeks with no differential effect between the two treatment groups. The authors effectively argue that the fitness results are not caused by differential attrition between the groups or compensation by the weight-lifting group undertaking aerobic exercise at other times. It is acknowledged that errors may be present in estimating maximum oxygen uptake and in reporting intensity, frequency and duration of exercise, and that this may explain the lack of both reported change in fitness and difference between groups. However, it is also possible that a psychological effect occurs from exercise without necessarily being accompanied by a physiological effect. Further evidence for this possibility will be presented when the literature on

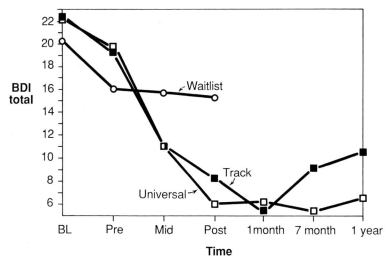

Figure 7.2. BDI scores from base line to 1 year follow-up for three different treatment groups in study by Doyne et al. (1987). (Copyright 1987 by The American Psychological Association. Reprinted by permission of the author.)

depressive patients who are hospitalised is reviewed. In conclusion, it can be seen that studies tend to show positive results in the use of exercise as a treatment for depression. The underlying mechanisms which could explain this conclusion are, as yet, unclear. For example, is it exercise itself or peripheral effects such as group interaction or charismatic leadership which cause the positive results?

Hospitalised Depressives

Conroy et al. (1982) used a quasi-experimental design, which compared hospitalised depressive patients (n = 9), who participated in a programme of aerobic exercise, with those who did not participate (n = 8). It was noted that the two groups did not differ on their scores on the BDI at the beginning of the programme. However, the group which had participated in exercise showed significant decreases on the BDI after 6 weeks, while the non-participants showed no change in depression. This finding could be related to differing expectations and motivations of the self-selected groups. A similar finding, however, is reported by Martinsen et al. (1985) who employed a stronger design. In this study 43 patients in hospital with depressive illnesses were randomly assigned to occupational therapy or aerobic exercise therapy. Depression scores (measured on the BDI) decreased more for the exercising group than the other group after a 9-week programme. Martinsen et al. (1985) also measured fitness improvements (via estimated maximum oxygen uptake scores) and noted that the biggest decreases in depression were associated with the biggest improvements in fitness.

More recent work from Martinsen et al. (1988), however, offers a different viewpoint. For the first time in a hospital setting the effects of aerobic and non-aerobic (weight-training) exercise were compared. The subjects in this study were 99 in-patients from a Norwegian hospital who were diagnosed has having a depressive illness. The exercise treatment lasted for 8 weeks and subjects were randomly assigned to treatment. The results of this study are illustrated in Fig. 7.3. It was found that both groups improved on psychometric measures of depression (Montgomery and Asberg's (1979) Rating Scale), but only the aerobic exercise group improved $\dot{V}O_{2max}$ scores over the experimental period. Thus it is clear that the exercise groups had different physiological outcomes, but the same psychological outcome. This finding provides evidence for a psychological rather than a physiological mechanism. This idea will be discussed later.

The findings from research designs employing contrasts between groups have been supported by case studies and small-n designs.

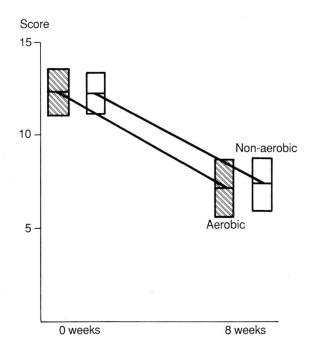

Figure 7.3. Mean scores, with 95% confidence intervals, on the Montgomery and Asberg Depression Rating Scale for psychiatric patients before and after 8 weeks of either aerobic or non-aerobic exercise. (From Martinsen et al. (1988), reproduced by permission of the author.)

Small-n Designs

Blue (1979) has reported alleviation of depression in two patients after 9 weeks of a jogging programme. Both of these patients had failed to respond to anti-depressant medication before starting the running programme. Doyne et al. (1983) employed a multiple base-line design on three women diagnosed as having a major depressive disorder. Expectancy effects were equal and exercise treatment was compared to a placebo condition. The exercise treatment induced improvements on depression scores which the placebo condition did not elicit. These gains were maintained to a 3-month follow-up test.

Another multiple base-line design, with five subjects, was reported by Buffone (1981). After 4-weeks recording of base-line data, subjects in this study were given a programme which combined cognitive therapy with running. While initial results indicated a decrease in depression scores (measured by the BDI), a 2-month follow-up evaluation revealed a recurrence of initial levels of depression and non-adherence to the running programme.

A strong design, which often allows rival explanations of effects to be ruled out, notes both treatment effects and the effects of taking treatment away. This is commonly known as a reversal design. This design was employed by Hartz et al. (1982) to examine the effects of aerobic exercise on seven clinically depressed hospital out-patients. There were two treatment phases and two non-treatment phases in the design. Improvements in depression scores were noted for three subjects after the aerobic exercise treatment. However, the scores did not return to base-line levels in the non-treatment phase as predicted. Hartz et al. (1982) concluded that a reversal design is not appropriate for studying the anti-depressant effects of exercise because these effects seemed to persist during the non-treatment phase. An alternative explanation could be that it was other factors, such as the attention of the therapist, which remained during the non-treatment phase, which caused the noted improvements to be maintained.

Measurement Concerns

Four major design problems appear in the literature which limit internal validity in the study of exercise and depression:

1. many designs lack a no-treatment control condition which would allow the hypothesis of spontaneous remission, without treatment, to be tested. Only McCann and Holmes (1984) and Mutrie (1986) included this control

2. most designs have not provided comparison placebo conditions which would allow alternative explanations of results, such as enthusiasm of

the exercise leader or the social interaction of the group, to be tested

3. the effect of exercise has often been confounded with time in contact with a professional (therapist or running leader), with runners often receiving more time than other groups

4. in many studies, subjects were aware of the exercise treatment, although they were not assigned to this group. This could lead to two problems: firstly, resentful demoralisation of the groups not receiving the running treatment may bias their scores; secondly, groups who are not receiving exercise treatment may begin exercise by themselves, thus confounding comparisons between the groups

There are fewer problems with external validity, since similar results have been obtained from volunteers, private patients and National Health Service patients, both in and out of hospitals. In addition, positive findings for the use of physical exercise as a treatment for depression have now been reported from North America, Scandinavia and the United Kingdom. The final criticism of the research to date is that it has been largely atheoretical. It has been difficult for readers to establish what underlying theory might predict the results obtained.

The Use of Exercise as a Treatment for Anxiety

In the literature which refers to the effects of exercise on anxiety, two kinds of exercise conditions can be differentiated. Firstly, the effects of *acute* exercise, that is a single bout of exercise, will be discussed, and secondly, the effects of *chronic* exercise, that is programmes of exercise lasting several weeks, will be discussed.

State anxiety has been a popular dependent measure in examining the acute effects of exercise. (Trait anxiety, by comparison, is relatively enduring and would, therefore, not be expected to change over short periods of time.) Several review articles (Folkins and Sime 1981; Mihevic 1982; Morgan 1985) have concluded that studies show that acute exercise has a tranquillising effect; this effect (according to Mihevic 1982) is evident a few minutes after the exercise ends and results in lower levels of state anxiety 20–30 minutes after exercise than before the start of exercise. However, many questions remain regarding these findings. Firstly, is the noted anxiety reduction anything more than a return to base line? Possible reductions in state anxiety after exercise can only be evaluated if several base-line measures are taken at various points prior to exercise. Anxiety may be increased immediately prior to treatment for experimental and control subjects alike due to anticipation; any reduction which is noted from this point may be a simple return to base line. This possibility is shown in Fig. 7.4. The effect may be particularly true for experiments involving exercise, since Morgan et al. (1980) have shown that state anxiety increases *during* laboratory exercise. Rather than exercise causing the reduction in anxiety, it could be argued that the *cessation* of exercise (or the experience of exercise on a treadmill) causes the higher than normal levels of anxiety to drop.

Secondly, is it clear that the subjects have abnormal levels of anxiety? Morgan (1979a) claimed that exercise has a tranquillising effect for clinically anxious persons, but offered no data to support this claim. The opposite effect has been suggested by Pitts and McClure (1967); they suggested that exercise will induce anxiety in those suffering from anxiety neurosis. Morgan (1979a) refuted this hypothesis, but only on the evidence of studies conducted on *normal* subjects.

Thirdly, what intensity of exercise is required to bring about a reduction in state anxiety? Morgan (1979a) has suggested that *vigorous* exercise is required to reduce anxiety levels for both male and female subjects; he cites studies which have shown that light exercise has no effect on anxiety, but the intensity (in terms of oxygen consumption or heart rate) is not specified. In direct contradiction to this finding, Steptoe and Cox (1988) have shown that a bout of high intensity exercise (cycling at 100 watts on

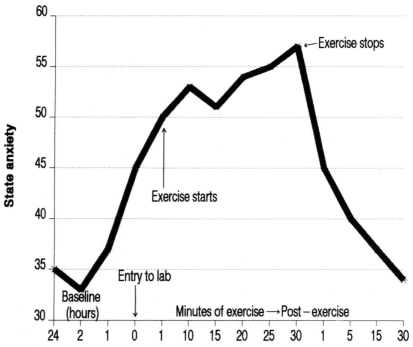

Figure 7.4. Hypothetical state anxiety scores from base line, through a 30-min exercise period, to 30 min post-exercise.

an ergometer) *increased* tension/anxiety scores both for subjects at an average and for those at a very high fitness level. Steptoe and Cox (1988) had more control in their experimental design than Morgan (1979a), including subjects who believed the experiment was about the effect of exercise on peripheral neurological symptoms. However, even this design could be improved upon since 100 watts will not provide exercise at the same intensity levels for all individuals. Indeed the perceived exertion rating recorded during the bout of high intensity exercise by Steptoe and Cox (1988) was only 13.1 for the group with the higher fitness levels and 14.5 for the group with the lower fitness levels. Both of these ratings are located between "hard" and "somewhat hard" on the Borg scale of perceived exertion (Borg and Noble 1974). It might be expected that high intensity exercise would elicit ratings of 16 or above which would be equivalent of "very hard". While intensity is clearly important in terms of understanding the effect of exercise on anxiety levels, what is required is a measure of intensity (e.g., oxygen consumption) which is comparable across studies.

Finally, are the effects of exercise on state anxiety the same for men and women? Most of the studies have used male subjects, but Wood (1977) did compare the effects of a 12-min run on both male (n = 62) and female (n = 44) students. He found that male and female students, who were classified as high-anxious, reduced their levels of state anxiety after the run, while male and female low-anxious students reported increased levels of state anxiety after the run. Since the pre-run anxiety scores were within the normal range, and the classification into high and low categories was made on an arbitrary basis, it is likely that these results could be explained by statistical regression to the mean rather than by the effects of exercise. Thus, it seems that the evidence for exercise having an acute effect on anxiety levels is far from convincing.

The effects of chronic exercise on anxiety levels are more difficult to find in the literature. Indeed, only one experimental study could be found. Steptoe et al. (1988) recruited 53 subjects who had higher than normal levels of anxiety. The subjects were matched for age, sex, habitual activity and anxiety levels and allocated to either moderate aerobic exercise or strengthening (using body weight for resistance) and stretching exercise. The second condition was seen as an attention-placebo control and subjects believed they were taking part in a health and fitness programme and were unaware that they had been selected on the basis of their anxiety scores. The exercise consisted of a 10-week programme in which subjects undertook one supervised and three unsupervised sessions each week.

Two physiological measures (a 12-min walk/run test and an estimated $\dot{V}O_{2\,max}$ from a cycle ergometer test) showed aerobic power improvements over the 10 weeks for the aerobic exercise group but not for the strengthening and stretching group. Thus the difference between the two modes of exercise was demonstrated. The aerobic exercise group also showed greater improvements, in comparison to the strengthening and stretching group, in tension/anxiety scores and confusion scores (measured by POMS), and coping assets (a measure derived by the researchers). This was a well-controlled study in which the results cannot be ascribed to peripheral experimental effects such as group interaction, expectations, or attention from the exercise leader. It is tempting to suggest that aerobic fitness improvements are the cause of the decreases in anxiety which were found, but in fact there was no correlation between the two measures. The dilemma of tracing a possible mechanism continues. While Doyne et al. (1987) and Martinsen (1988) found that training with weights had a similar positive effect on depression, this study found no such effect for strengthening and stretching on anxiety. Three possibilities exist to explain this apparent conflict.

Firstly, responses to different exercise modes may be quite different for those suffering from depressed moods and those suffering from higher-than-normal levels of anxiety. Secondly, the kind of weight training employed by Doyne et al. (1987) and Martinsen (1988), who both used machines with progressive resistance, may allow for progress and mastery to be perceived more easily than the strengthening and stretching programme employed by Steptoe et al. (1988), which did not use weights or machines. Thirdly, the positive results from other studies using non-aerobic exercise may be explained by social interaction or leadership effects; in the Steptoe et al. study there were more *unsupervised* than supervised exercise sessions for all groups.

In conclusion, there is relatively little experimental evidence that exercise has a positive effect on anxiety reduction; the area remains open for much future research. It should be noted that this conclusion is in direct contradiction to Morgan and Goldston's (1987, p. 156) statement that "exercise is associated with the reduction of stress emotions such as state anxiety". It is suggested that Morgan and Goldston's conclusion is based on poorly designed studies.

The Effect of Exercise on Psychiatric Patients

Several studies have indicated that hospitalised psychiatric patients are less physically fit than non-institutionalised normal people (Hodgdon and Reimer 1960; Martinsen et al. 1989; Morgan 1969; Zankel and Field 1959). It has been shown that such patients can make physiological gain from engaging in an exercise programme (Dodson and Mullens 1969; Levin and Giminio 1982). Four studies (Chamove 1988; Dodson and Mullens 1969; Hamilton 1984; Lion 1978) report positive psychological gains for psychiatric patients engaged in exercise and sport programmes, but, as these studies do not provide control groups, it is not possible to conclude that it was the activity (and not other effects such as extra attention) which caused the changes. However, Levin and Giminio (1982) also reported psychological benefits for schizophrenic patients in a 10-week aerobic exercise programme, and noted that control groups engaged in meditation and art did not improve.

As with other literature in this area, there is a need for more experimental research to support the claim that exercise can be beneficial for psychiatric patients (see Chamove 1988). Hesso and Sorenson (1982), in fact, noted the need for clearer evidence to support the use of exercise as part of the treatment of psychiatric patients. They suggested that when exercise or physical activity are voluntary options for patients it is very difficult to conduct systematic study of the effects of the activity. An alternative to this model is the situation in which the activity programme is seen as a natural part of treatment by all personnel involved. It is suggested by Hesso and Sorensen (1982) that this second model should be adopted by more institutions and that this would allow more systematic research to be carried out.

There are particular problems in suggesting an exercise programme for psychiatric patients. The first is that many such patients are taking some form of medication to control their illness. It is not yet clear whether or not exercise is a safe combination with all such medication. Martinsen (1987) has reported on his experience of using exercise as a regular part of treatment in a Norwegian psychiatric hospital. He says (p. 94), of patients who were taking psychotropic drugs while undertaking an exercise programme: "There have been no dangerous complications observed, such as cardiac diseases, and there have been no episodes of sudden death during exercise" and "some of the patients complained of common side effects of the medication, such as orthostatism, tachycardia, dry mouth, drowsiness and vertigo, but these side effects did not force them to reduce the intensity of the exercise, or drop out of the exercise programme".

Martinsen concludes that exercise is safe for psychiatric patients who are taking medication, if close medical supervision is provided.

Another problem for the researcher or clinician dealing with the psychiatric population is the wide range of possible illnesses which may be included in this category. The research is not yet at a stage where it can be said that exercise will have a positive effect on some of these categories and not on others. It may be, for example, that some illnesses, such as mania, do not respond well to exercise as a treatment.

Certain phobias have also responded to exercise as a treatment. Running has been used successfully to treat eight patients suffering from agoraphobia (Orwin 1981). The treatment involved asking the patients to run to the situation which they found fearful (e.g., public places such as supermarkets). Normally, in these situations, feelings of anxiety, such as increased respiration and heart rate, would be experienced by those suffering from agoraphobia. However, when they arrived at the feared situation breathless from running, the patients did not appear to feel anxious; they attributed increased respiration and breathing to the running and not to fear. Repeated treatments of this nature allowed all eight patients to recover from agoraphobia. Orwin (1981) reported similar success in using running for situational phobias.

There are other potential areas of psychological medicine in which benefits from exercise might be seen (see Dishman 1985, 1986a). These include schizophrenia (Chamove 1988), alcohol rehabilitation (Sinyor et al. 1983), drug rehabilitation (de Coverley Veale 1987b), tranquilliser withdrawal (Murdoch and Mutrie 1988) and psychological rehabilitation following cardiac arrest (Newton and Mutrie 1991).

8

Psychological Effects of Exercise: Possible Mechanisms

In this chapter of the section concerned with exercise and mental health, the possible mechanisms, which may operate when people perceive psychological benefit from exercise, will be reviewed. Human beings are complex organisms, and it is unlikely that any one of the mechanisms will provide a complete explanation of a particular behaviour. It is more probable that several mechanisms operate in a synergistic fashion to provide a psychological effect from exercise.

Effects of Exercise on the Central Nervous System

Reductions in electromyographic (EMG) recordings of muscle tension after exercise have been noted and replicated by de Vries (1968, 1981). The modality, intensity, frequency, and duration of exercise required to produce this tranquillising effect have been described by de Vries (1981, p. 53) as "rhythmic exercise such as walking, jogging, cycling, and bench stepping from 5 to 30 minutes at 30% to 60% of maximum intensities". Tooman (1982) failed to show decreases in muscle tension after habitual exercisers had completed a regular run. However, in Tooman's (1982) study, most runners exceeded the 30 min suggested by de Vries (1981). The duration of exercise may, therefore, be a crucial variable in determining reductions in muscle tension. Other objective measures of decreased arousal levels in the central nervous system (CNS) after exercise are decreased activity in the left hemisphere of the brain (Wales 1985) and decreased reflex responses (de Vries 1981).

Ellis (1973) suggested that exercise is a means by which we arrive at pleasurable levels of CNS arousal. Each person, according to Ellis (1973), has an optimal level of arousal, which he/she will find pleasurable. There are many different ways in which we can achieve optimal arousal states, but one benefit of exercise is that the reticular activating system is aroused without side effects such as those associated with chemical stimulants. It could be that this arousal is what makes people say that exercise makes them feel better.

Changes in biochemical activity during and after exercise may also affect the central nervous system. Acute bouts of exercise appear to cause increases in plasma levels of endorphins (endogenous, morphine-like chemicals; see Akil et al. 1984; Allen 1983; Grossman 1984; Steinberg and Sykes 1985). It has been speculated that these increases are associated with elevation of mood (Gambert et al. 1981), "runner's high" (Pargman and Baker 1980; Sachs 1984), decreased perception of pain in injured athletes (Moore 1982), addiction to exercise (Steinberg et al. 1988; Trotter 1984), and the anti-depressant effect of exercise (Greist et al. 1979b).

These speculations provide an endorphin hypothesis for the affective benefits associated with exercise (Morgan and O'Connor 1988). This hypothesis is appealing because endorphins have chemical properties which are similar to those of morphine (indeed the name "endorphin" is derived from endogenous morphine) and morphine has well-known analgesic and euphoric properties. Two strands of research literature support this hypothesis. First, post-exercise increases in plasma levels of the most powerful endorphin, beta-endorphin, have been noted by several researchers (Appenzeller et al. 1980; Carr et al. 1981; Colt et al. 1981; Farrell et al. 1982; Gambert et al. 1981; Howlett et al. 1984). Harber and Sutton (1984) summarised this effect as producing up to a five-fold increase in normal levels of beta-endorphin after exercise; they also noted that the post-exercise increase in beta-endorphin is present in both trained and untrained subjects. Second, attempts have been made to correlate changes in affect with beta-endorphin levels. These experiments involve either concomitant measures of mood elevation (Farrell et al. 1983; Markoff et al. 1982), or negation of responses, normally attributed to beta-endorphin, by the opiate antagonist naloxone (Haier et al. 1981).

To date, none of these experiments provide convincing evidence to support the hypothesis that exercise improves mood because it increases the production of beta-endorphin. Haier et al. (1981) did show that pain perception decreased after a run, and that this effect could be negated by injecting naloxone. Thus, there is some evidence that exercise-induced endorphin production is analgesic, but little evidence to suggest that it produces mood elevation.

The research related to the proposed endorphin hypothesis is in its infancy. Many questions can be posed at this stage. For example, exercise has been shown to increase plasma levels of endorphins in humans, but mood elevation, or anti-depressant effects, which are claimed to be associated with endorphins, are mediated within the CNS. Hawley and Butterfield (1981, p. 1591) summarised this criticism as follows: "only if central nervous system beta-endorphins are shown to be elevated in response to exercise can endogenous opioids be implicated in such subjective phenomena as the euphoria or anti-nociception frequently reported during exercise". It has not been shown that beta-endorphin crosses the blood–brain barrier, although Harber and Sutton (1984) note that plasma levels may be markers of CNS levels (see Sforzo 1988).

A second problem is that the increased levels of beta-endorphin which have been measured may not be enough to cause changes in affect (Harber and Sutton 1984). Indeed, Foley et al. (1979) showed that injecting 50 000 times normal levels of beta-endorphin into the bloodstream failed to cause changes in mood (affect). However, it has been shown that injections of beta-endorphin can improve the mood of hospitalised depressed patients (Gerner et al. 1980) and it is also known that electroconvulsive therapy (ECT), which can be used as a treatment for depression, increases plasma levels of beta-endorphin in depressives. The implication of these findings is that endorphins may play a role in producing an anti-depressive effect from exercise for depressives, but that endorphins are less likely to be involved in a mood-enhancing effect from exercise for non-depressed exercisers.

A third problem is that the literature has concentrated on the potential effects of beta-endorphin, but there are other endogenous substances, such as encephalins and dynorphins (Grossman and Sutton 1985; Hatfield and Landers 1987; Sforzo 1988) which also have morphine or opiate-like effects. It is possible that mood alterations may be caused by exercise-induced alterations in the levels of these less well-known opioids.

Despite the problems with the endorphin hypothesis for the anti-depressant and mood-enhancing effects of exercise, Morgan (1985) considered that it remains a tenable hypothesis.

This area of research, therefore, has many hypotheses which must be tested by future research. One major problem in the advancement of the endorphin hypothesis is the expense involved in researching these chemicals. Radioimmunoassays are very expensive and demand that samples are frozen immediately they are obtained.

Morgan (1985) also suggested that other neurotransmitters, and mono-amines in particular, might mediate the affective benefits which have been associated with exercise.

It has been noted (Riggs 1981) that circulating levels of noradrenaline and serotonin (two monoamines) increase with fairly intensive exercise, but that this response is reduced as the exercisers become fitter. This suggests that monoamines are involved in the stress response, making the CNS more able to cope with the demands of exercise. As fitness improves the exercise imposes less stress to the system, and thus the response is diminished. This parallels the stress response observed in the sympathetic nervous system (Schafer 1978).

An interesting addition to the monoamine hypothesis is that noradrenaline and serotonin levels tend to be low in depressed people (Morgan 1985). There have been no studies to date which directly link the two parts of this hypothesis in measuring the effect of exercise on noradrenaline levels of depressives. Morgan (1985) noted that many drugs which are used as anti-depressants increase noradrenaline levels.

These various effects may not be due to exercise itself, but to concomitant changes from homeostasis which exercise causes. For example, exercise of a sufficient intensity and duration will increase body temperature. Morgan and O'Connor (1988) suggest that increases in body temperature have been shown to affect central and peripheral neuron activity and the action of brain monoamines; in addition, both exercise-induced and passively-induced increases in rectal temperature have been associated with increased slow wave sleep (Horne and Staff 1983). It may be that exercise has an indirect effect on the central nervous system as a result of temperature increases.

Another example of indirect effects of exercise on the CNS is the possibility that cognitive function improves as a result of regular exercise. This effect may be caused by increasing oxygen and glucose transport to the brain (Young 1979).

In summary, research to date suggests that exercise may have a psychological effect by acting on the CNS. This action may involve decreasing levels of muscle tension, altering arousal levels, changing neurotransmission, or may be a result of increased temperature following exercise.

Effects of Exercise on the Sympathetic Nervous System

Both Schafer (1978) and Warshaw (1979) have suggested that running can be effective in helping people cope with the stresses of daily life. This coping mechanism can be broken down into two parts: (a) fitness being associated with attenuation of sympathetic responses from any given stressor, and (b) fitness being associated with a quicker return to normal levels for systems which are affected by stress. Research does support part (a) (Crews and Landers 1987), but support for part (b) is less convincing (see earlier discussion of the effects of exercise on stress, Chap. 6). The physiological adaptations which may associate increasing fitness with adaptations of the sympathetic nervous system (SNS) remain unclear (van Doornen et al. 1988), and it may well be that exercise has a positive effect on stress via other mechanisms. For example, in an excellent review of the effect of physical fitness training on mental health, Folkins and Sime (1981) have suggested that the theory of self-regulation as a means of coping with stress (Lazarus 1975) provided the best framework in which to place the concept of therapeutic exercise. Within this model exercise would be viewed, in a similar way to biofeedback, as a means of teaching self-regulation and coping. As yet, this theoretical framework has not produced much supportive research literature.

The Effects of Exercise on Self-esteem

Harris (1973) suggested that physical activity has great potential to affect self-esteem positively. Sonstroem (1982a, 1984) noted that body image and perceptions of physical ability were both highly correlated with measures of global self-esteem. Research has shown that fitness training improves self-concept, providing the participants perceive the fitness changes (Folkins and Sime 1981). Hughes (1984) reviewed a number of different psychological effects which had been cited as possible outcomes from regular exercise and concluded that self-concept was the only variable which has shown consistent improvement across studies.

Since depressed people have typically low estimates of self-worth, it seems reasonable to suggest that one mechanism explaining decreases in depression levels after a programme of exercise is related to improving how participants perceive themselves. Ossip-Klein et al. (1989) have shown that both aerobic exercise and weight training improved the self-concept of clinically depressed women. These authors suggest that the experience of mastery and perceptions of fitness improvements during the programme are the principal reasons for the improvements in self-concept.

Gruber (1986) conducted a meta-analytic review of the literature on self-esteem and exercise in children and concluded that in studies where children experienced physical activity interventions, self-esteem scores were nearly one-half of a standard deviation above those for children in the control groups, who did not exercise. The greatest effects were found for children with disabilities. As far as the type of physical activity was concerned, all of those studied showed positive effects, although aerobic fitness activities showed the most positive effect. It is likely that the type of activity is a subsidiary factor to the quality of the experience itself which, with children, may be heavily reliant on the teachers, coaches or leaders in structured activity and sport programmes.

In a review of exercise and self-esteem research, Sonstroem (1984) concluded that the methodological problems of the majority of studies prevented clear conclusions although the results do point towards the positive effects of exercise programmes on self-esteem scores. However, a number of factors related to the exercise programme and the measurement of self-esteem scores could account for this, such as increases in physical fitness, feelings of well-being, a sense of mastery or competence, or even experimental attention.

Recent developments in the multidimensional measurement of the physical aspects of self-perception (Fox 1988, 1990; Fox and Corbin 1989) should assist in the identification of the nature and extent of the effect of exercise on self-esteem. Fox (1990) has demonstrated that with college-age adults at least four types of physical self-perceptions can be identified. These are perceptions of sports competence, physical condition, physical appearance, and perceived strength. Depending on whether such perceptions are deemed to be important by individuals, these self-perceptions will affect feelings of physical self-worth and, ultimately, global self-esteem. This hierarchical model of physical self-perceptions is shown in Fig. 8.1.

A hierarchical and multidimensional approach to self-esteem may shed some light on the mechanisms of exercise and mental health.

The Effects of Exercise as a Mastery Experience

Sonstroem (1982a) suggested that one way in which exercise might improve self-esteem was by providing situations in which participants can master a task. Greist et al. (1981) made specific reference to mastering the skills of running as an important aspect of anti-depressant running. It seems particularly relevant to review this possible mechanism in the light of Seligman's (1975) "learned helplessness" theory of depression. This theory, as expanded by Abramson et al. (1978), suggested that depression resulted from the repeated experience of having no control over what happens in one's life, in conjunction with internal, stable and global attributions for failure (see also Alloy et al. 1988). Abramson et al. (1978) concluded that if people expect to be able to control both the good and bad things that

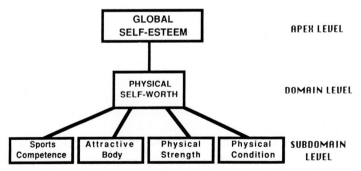

Figure 8.1. A hierarchical model of physical self-perceptions. (From "The physical self-perception profile: development and preliminary validation" by K.R. Fox and C.B. Corbin (1989) *Journal of Sport and Exercise Psychology*, 11: 414. Reprinted with permission of Human Kinetics Publishers.)

happen to them, then this expectation should immunise them against depression. While acknowledging that this theory does not provide a framework for all depressive states, it is useful to consider it in terms of the anti-depressant effect of exercise. If an exercise programme sets individualised goals for each participant, and if these goals are both realistic and challenging, then participants should gain a sense of achievement, and, eventually, of mastery. Furthermore, if fitness improvements are measured and offered as feedback, objective support is provided for the sense of improvement and mastery. Finally, if these changes are noted by the participant, it will be difficult to attribute them to external causes; it is hard for someone else, or something else, to be responsible for one's fitness improvements and physical skill development.

Support for the idea that exercise is beneficial because it provides a mastery experience has come from Robbins and Joseph (1985). These researchers hypothesised that one cause of negative affect which accompanies exercise deprivation is the loss of predictable feelings of success and self-fulfilment associated with running. Further discussion of this concept can be found in Chap. 4, which is concerned with perceptions of control.

The Effects of Exercise as a Distraction

Bahrke and Morgan's study (1978), which compared the effects of walking on a treadmill, meditating, and resting in a comfortable chair, on measures of state anxiety, has already been discussed under the heading of the effects of acute exercise involvement in Chap. 6, but discussion of this study is appropriate here also because Bahrke and Morgan (1978) suggested that one mechanism of the psychological benefits of exercise may be that it provides a distraction for the participant. It has already been suggested that the results of the study in question show a clear test–retest effect (since experimental and control groups all changed in the same way) rather than a distraction effect. However, although distraction from daily routine or problems does remain a tenable hypothesis which could explain why different kinds of exercise (Berger and Owen 1983; Doyne et al. 1987; Martinsen 1988; Mutrie 1986) can produce positive psychological effects, it has not been systematically tested as an independent variable in any of these studies. The work of Moses et al. (1989), which shows a psychological advantage for moderate aerobic exercise in comparison with high intensity aerobic exercise or strengthening and stretching exercise, would suggest that mechanisms other than distraction must be operating. Clearly, further research is required to test this hypothesis specifically: treatment groups which are exposed to something with the potential to distract in a similar way to exercise must be included in future designs.

The Effects of Exercise on Work Capacity

If chronic involvement in exercise leads to improvements in fitness, then participants should experience an increased capacity for physical work. The effects of this increased capacity might be felt by having more energy available for daily tasks, thus diminishing feelings of fatigue or lethargy. This increased sense of vigour could explain some psychological effects which have been reported. Early studies in this area suggested that there was a link between physiological and psychological improvements (Brown et al. 1978; Martinsen et al. 1985), but more recent research has established that physiological improvement (as measured by standard tests) is *not* a requirement of psychological improvement and that physiological and psychological changes are not necessarily correlated (Doyne et al. 1987; Mutrie 1986; Martinsen 1988; Steptoe et al. 1988). Two points should be noted for future research from this section.

Firstly, it may be that the standard exercise prescription for fitness, as described by the American College of Sports Medicine (ACSM 1978, 1986, 1990), is not necessarily the prescription required to achieve psychological benefit. The ACSM guidelines recommend aerobic exercise for a duration of 15–60 min, at an intensity of 60%–90% of maximum heart rate, and a frequency of 3–5 times per week. It may be that psychological gain can be achieved by daily exercise sessions of very low intensity (e.g., 50% maximum heart rate) and of very short duration (e.g., 10 min). Secondly, it could be that researchers have focussed on standard physiological tests (such as maximal oxygen uptake) which are not the most relevant or most changeable aspect of the person's physiological response to exercise. Some thought has to be given to tests which reveal submaximal improvements and not only in the cardiorespiratory system. It may be that other physiological changes, such as local muscle endurance, *will* correlate with psychological changes.

The Effects of Addiction to Regular Exercise

It is possible that people can experience long-term benefits from regular exercise because they become addicted to it. Central to the concept of positive addiction, as already discussed, is that regular involvement in an activity which provides pleasure and satisfaction allows the participant to gain an increased sense of self-confidence or "strength", as Glasser (1976) suggested. Furthermore, the activity affords the individual an opportunity to experience a euphoric mental state or, to put it in Glasser's (1976) terms, the brain has a chance to "spin free".

Meditation and running were the most popular activities reported by respondents to Glasser's survey (1976) about positive addiction. He suggested that meditation is less likely than running to achieve positive addiction, but that it is easier to do than running. Glasser (1976) also surveyed readers of a running magazine and found many of them to be positively addicted to running. Carmack and Martens (1979) also found that many runners (both competitive and recreational) were positively addicted to running. It seems that addiction to running can take place over a few weeks or months, or that it may require many years to develop (Sachs 1981). Further discussion on the topic of exercise addiction, with cautionary comments on the possibility of exercise dependence, can be found in an earlier section of Chap. 6 entitled "harmful effects of exercise".

In summary, seven possible mechanisms for the psychological effects of exercise have been reviewed. Exercise has been associated with changes in both the CNS and the SNS, with improved self-esteem and feelings of mastery, and with increased work capacity. In addition, it has been suggested that exercise may be beneficial because it distracts people from other aspects of life, or that becoming addicted to exercise may provide psychological strength. It was noted that not all the psychological effects of exercise are positive. These mechanisms provide tenable hypotheses which should be tested in future research in this area. It is suggested that the mechanisms are likely to operate in a synergistic way; it is also possible that different mechanisms will explain different aspects of the psychological effects noted. For example, there may be mainly a biochemical explanation for exercise alleviating depression, but a physiological reason why exercise is associated with feeling less tense. Future research must address these possibilities in a systematic way, such as that described by Platt (1964).

INTERVENTIONS, APPLICATIONS AND FUTURE DIRECTIONS

9

Intervention Strategies: The Individual

This chapter outlines a number of ways in which health professionals can help people adopt and maintain exercise. The theoretical background to the topic of exercise adherence has been dealt with in previous chapters, and the aim here is to provide practical ideas. People who might need this kind of help include those who would like to take more exercise but never get round to it, those who have been advised for medical reasons to improve their fitness, those who used to be active and would like to regain the habit, and those whose motivation to exercise typically lasts for only a few weeks. The bigger question of how to reach the population who have never considered increasing activity levels will be addressed in the next chapter which deals with intervention strategies for the school, workplace, community and medical settings.

Whenever possible, research findings which support the use of a particular technique will be cited; however, some of the techniques have been developed in a trial-and-error fashion by professionals who are trying to encourage regular activity rather than by researchers who are establishing the efficacy of different techniques. The result is that we do not yet know which is the best technique for any particular person and professionals will have to use their own judgement in selecting from the various techniques which will be described.

The study of patient compliance to medical treatment provides a framework for categorising the various techniques which are available, although the comparison is imperfect since most people come to exercise from a "wellness" perspective rather than an "illness" perspective. Haynes (1976) provided a review of strategies for increasing compliance to medical treatments and suggested that the options could be classified as behavioural, educational or combined (i.e., strategies which had both behavioural and educational components). Most psychology literature now refers to cognitive and behavioural strategies together and so this chapter will review cognitive-behavioural and educational techniques which are available to help people become active and stay active.

Cognitive-Behavioural Strategies

The use of cognitive-behavioural interventions in promoting participation in exercise is a logical extension of the use of such techniques in other areas of behaviour change. Reviews of traditional studies of behaviour modification in physical activity are now available (Buffone et al. 1984; Donahue et al. 1980; Kirschenbaum 1987; Knapp 1988; Lee and Owen 1985b, 1986; Martin 1981; Serfass and Gerberich 1984).

A good starting point for anyone seeking ways to improve exercise adherence is a sound knowledge of the various techniques of behaviour modification, although as Dishman (1990, p. 87) points out, we do not yet know how effective such techniques are in all areas of exercise behaviour: "Behavior modification techniques are collectively associated with an increase of 10%–25% in frequency of physical activity, but their impact on changes in intensity and duration of activity is less clear". What is clear is that the vast majority of cognitive-behavioural techniques which will be described focus on helping people find reinforcement from one exercise experience which encourages another exercise experience to take place. (See also Chap. 5 on self-confidence, as well as Kaplan et al. 1984.) The various techniques will now be described.

Positive Reinforcement

A consistent message from the discipline of behavioural psychology is that behaviours are repeated under the influence of positive reinforcement (e.g., praise, a reward, perceiving success). Negative reinforcement (e.g., terminating something unpleasant) can also be successful in encouraging a particular behaviour to be repeated, but punishment (e.g., presenting something unpleasant or taking away privileges) is a less effective strategy in trying to promote a particular behaviour. Ultimately, with the goal of helping people to become independent exercisers, the exercise itself must be intrinsically rewarding (see Chap. 2: reinforcement through positive affect) since there is some evidence to suggest that reliance on external motivators may act as a disincentive in the long run (see Chap. 4 and Weinberg 1984). With that caveat in mind, the general principle is that exercise professionals must find ways of positively reinforcing exercise behaviour. This means that the emphasis on this technique is in helping people to praise themselves, to provide their own rewards and to recognise their successes. In addition, if people are involved in exercise programmes they should look for teachers who use these techniques. Here are some suggestions for a positive approach to reinforcement.

Praise

Teachers should praise individuals as much as possible. Martin and Dubbert (1982) found that individual praise and feedback was more important than group praise and feedback in enhancing long-term adherence; 3 months after an exercise programme 54% of those receiving individual praise had continued exercising compared with 17% of those receiving group praise. It is very common, however, for teachers and exercise leaders to make their comments of a critical nature, for example "that's not bad, now try to run faster". Much of the educational training of these individuals involves analysing and correcting mistakes, so it is perhaps not surprising that this style is common. However, in terms of health-related fitness there is no sound reason, other than injury prevention, for improving technique. We would, therefore, suggest that critical comments are confined to aspects of technique that could lead to injury. The majority of comments should be in praise of something done well. Helping people to praise themselves really comes under positive self-statements and will be dealt with later in this chapter.

Rewards

Providing tangible rewards may help people get started into an exercise lifestyle, but it is not recommended for long-term adherence, since the ultimate goal is to help people to find the exercise experience rewarding in itself. However, any reward which enhances a person's sense of competence, while allowing that person to feel that the reward is not the only reason he or she is participating, is likely to enhance motivation (Deci and Ryan 1985). These techniques include: awarding T-shirts after the completion of a certain amount of exercise, listing names in a "club" list after a certain amount has been achieved (see Fig. 9.1), or making access to classes cheaper the more frequently people have attended in the past. Martin et al. (1984) used a lottery system of prizes in an effort to enhance adherence, but the strategy did not work; this serves to remind us that unless prizes (or rewards) reflect an element of increased competence they are unlikely to work as motivators (Deci and Ryan 1985). This is discussed more fully in Chap. 4.

Success

Feeling success from the completion of a task is an important motivator. At the start of an exercise plan it is very important to specify exactly what is manageable, otherwise it is easy for the novice exerciser to feel a sense of failure. If the expectation is to complete a whole class on the first attempt or to run as far as a companion who has been active for some time, then failure may ensue. Achieving feelings of success is clearly related to setting goals correctly and this will be discussed in more detail in the next section.

Another element of success is feeling a sense of progression or improvement. Helping people to feel that they are capable of more than they managed last month or that their heart rates are lower for the same amount of work can help participants feel success. Good examples of progressions are running or swimming programmes that have 4 different levels (and objectives) depending on fitness level (see Fig. 9.2).

A fitness assessment service is another method of providing feelings of success. Having a base-line score which can be improved upon may be motivating for some individuals (Nutbeam 1984; Mutrie and Grant 1985). However, scores obtained must be treated with caution. Comparing scores with norms (i.e., above average, average, below average) may be a very negative experience since for genetic or mechanical reasons some people may never get beyond the initial category (e.g., "below average"). Even if these norms are built from a population similar to those who are being assessed, the logic of the normal distribution implies that 50% of those being assessed will be below average; obviously this may not operate to motivate these people. Norms based on fitness scores may be inappropriate anyway if the objective is to convey a message about health. This is considered in more detail in Fox and Biddle (1988) and Whitehead et al. (1990). It would, therefore, seem more appropriate, in terms of motivation, to compare individuals with their own scores at base line; the major

---

****

CONGRATULATIONS!!

in the past month
the following people have all accumulated 300 minutes of swimming

Jane Fish

Peter Smith

Barry Jones

Edith McAnn

****

Figure 9.1. An example of positive reinforcement via a club list.

****
Pick up details of one of the following programmes; select the colour code that best describes your current fitness level.

Green programme

A walk/jog or swim programme to prepare the unfit for regular exercise.

Pink programme

A jogging or swimming programme intended for those with a low level of fitness.

Yellow programme

Intended for those with a reasonable level of fitness or who can comfortably complete the Pink programme suggestions.

Gold programme

An advanced programme for those who are fit; check that the Yellow programme suggestions are easy for you to manage before proceeding to the Gold suggestions.

****

Figure 9.2. An example of progressions in programmes.

problem in this situation is to establish that any changes noted are beyond those which can be expected by chance, or by the reliability of the equipment and the person conducting the assessments. Thus it is critical for an organisation offering fitness assessment to maintain a high standard of equipment calibration and to have well-trained personnel.

Terminating Unpleasantness

The experience of having something unpleasant stop is also reinforcing (technically it is referred to as negative reinforcement and is often confused with punishment). If this experience occurs after exercise it should increase the likelihood of the exercise behaviour being repeated. Thus if a person feels low in spirits or lethargic and finds that an activity session improves mood or energy levels then that person is likely to keep exercising.

Punishment

Punishment involves presenting something unpleasant or taking away something regarded as a pleasure. In educational contexts punishment follows behaviour that is undesirable (e.g., more homework or being kept in detention). Unfortunately, exercise itself has often been used as a punishment. Can you remember anyone from your own school experience being made to do some extra laps around the track as punishment for some misdemeanour? This has created an idea that exercise is no fun for some people ("you won't catch me getting all hot and sweaty!") and that may have to be overcome in order to keep people active; thus helping individuals to find enjoyable activities is an essential start in trying to achieve long-term adherence.

There are potentially punishing aspects to exercise that must be taken into consideration; too much activity for an untrained body will result in muscle soreness and feelings of fatigue. This is just the kind of punishment that results in early drop-out from over-vigorous programmes. In addition, it is often true that people have to give up something pleasurable to find the time to be active; being denied the chance to watch television, or go for a drink after work, or have extra sleep at the weekend, because of a new exercise plan, are potentially punishing experiences. Plans must, therefore, take these conflicting pleasures into account and exercise must be scheduled at times when minimal conflict with alternative activities exists.

Finally, teachers must be aware that critical comments, sarcasm and making people feel embarrassed will also act as punishment; there is perhaps no more important factor than a skilful and sympathetic teacher in creating an environment which is likely to keep people coming back. A surprising number of exercise promoters and leaders have made punishment a preferred style . . . "going for the burn" and "no pain no gain" are not uncommon phrases in exercise studios, but, we suspect, the punishment philosophy is essentially detrimental; most people will not maintain exercise under such conditions.

Self-reinforcement

The ultimate goal is to help people find exercise reinforcing. A step towards that is to find ways of self-reinforcement for exercise. One successful method of introducing self-reinforcement is to ask participants to list items that they would find rewarding (e.g., a new jogging suit) and to state the criteria needed before this reward could be received (Keefe and Blumenthal 1980; Blumenthal et al. 1982). Atkins et al. (1984) used a similar technique; they asked participants to note highly probable daily behaviours (e.g., taking morning coffee, watching a favourite television programme) and to make these events contingent upon completing the prescribed exercise.

Stimulus Control

This technique involves provision of a variety of cues which increase the likelihood of exercise. Reminders stuck into the diary, slogans posted on the wall, timetables with activity time written in are all examples of how cues to exercise can be placed. The kind of people who respond well to the time management strategies of listing priorities and noting them into a diary will probably respond well to stimulus control to help them keep exercise as part of their lifestyle. Brownell et al. (1980) showed that this technique can be successful in increasing activity in the workplace. They placed an eye-catching poster (see Fig. 9.3) at a lift, which suggested people could use the stairs instead. This stimulus resulted in almost 10% increase in stair-climbing over 2 weeks. A very powerful stimulus is having a friend who will call to check if you are going for that jog, or swim, or exercise work-out. Having a dog which needs exercise is also an important stimulus; it just might help some people to recognise that they should exercise as much as their dog. Professor Astrand, one of the world's most influential exercise physiologists, has suggested that you should take your dog for a walk every day, even if you don't have one!

Individualised Exercise Prescriptions

Whenever possible, plans for activity should be tailored to individual needs. The prescription which is often used is based on the American College of Sports Medicine guidelines (1990) and tends to be very general (e.g., three sessions of 30 minutes each week). The first thing that can be individualised is exercise intensity and taking time to explain individual targets for heart rate can be worthwhile, although inaccuracies will occur (Dishman 1988b). Secondly, the exact amount of time available should be established and the kind of activities which the person is likely to find enjoyable listed. Then the programme can be planned to that person's needs.

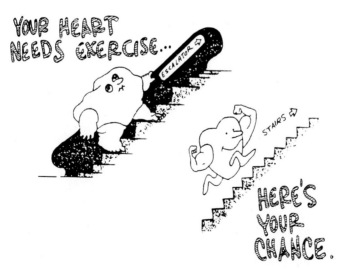

Figure 9.3. An example of stimulus control to increase stair-climbing. (From Brownell et al. (1980). Reproduced with the permission of the *American Journal of Psychiatry*.)

Goal-setting

Goal-setting has been used in industrial settings to increase and maintain
motivation (Naylor and Ilgen 1984). The use of this technique in sport
and exercise settings has also been described (Harris and Harris 1984;
Mutrie 1985; Locke and Latham 1985). The essence of this technique is
to set clear, realistic tasks for participants, which bring about a sense of
achievement on completion; this feeling of success is the motivator to
continue with the next set of goals. The difficulty is to set goals which are
specific rather than general (e.g., "I want to be able to complete a 10 km
fun run" rather than "I want to be fitter"). Goals also have to be realistic
and yet challenging.

The goal-setting process starts with the identification of long-term
objectives which are often very general (e.g., "by next summer I would like
to feel fitter and to have lost some weight"). These long-term goals then
have to be translated into intermediate and short-term goals. The
intermediate goals are set for 1–2 months ahead and are much more
specific (e.g., "I would like to be able to swim continuously for 20 minutes
in two months time"); the short-term goals are the small steps which will
help participants reach the intermediate and long-term objectives. Short-
term goals suggest what can be achieved each week until the intermediate
goal is reached (e.g., Mondays: go to swimming class to improve technique;
Wednesdays: swim for 15 minutes taking a rest every 2 lengths). Fig. 9.4
shows how the goal-setting plan can be laid out.

Martin et al. (1984) have studied two different goal-setting techniques
for use in exercise adherence. In their first study, they exposed a small
group of sedentary adults to shaping and maintenance strategies by
allocating them to one of two feedback conditions and one of two goal-
setting conditions. The feedback was given either individually or in a group,
whereas the goals were set for either the distance or the time of the
walk/run. Analyses revealed a significant interaction between goal-setting
and feedback such that the lowest attendance at the run/walk sessions
occurred for the subjects who were set the distance goals and received
group feedback. These results could be explained by the time goals allowing
for better time management and thus a better chance of reducing one of
the common barriers to exercise.

In an extension to this study, Martin et al. (1984) allowed the subjects
greater participation in the goal-setting process, and also incorporated a
"lottery" system of prizes according to their adherence. This strategy,
however, failed to affect adherence, where the goal-setting procedures were
shown to be effective. Subjects who were encouraged to modify their own
goals (flexible goal-setting) had a greater adherence rate than those with
fixed goals. This was supported in a follow-up study by Martin et al.
(1984).

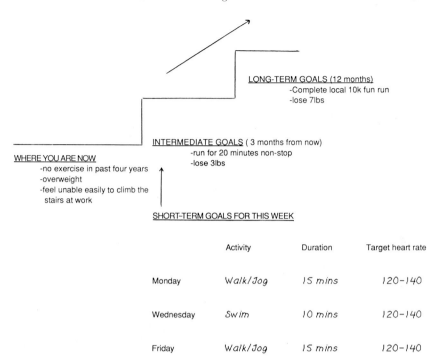

Figure 9.4. A goal-setting plan.

Attaching initial goal-setting to a contract has proved to be an effective
way of establishing exercise (Atkins et al. 1984; Epstein et al. 1980; Kau
and Fischer 1974; Wysocki et al. 1979). With this system the beginning
participant writes a "contract" which he or she signs with the exercise
leader (or another person with whom the contract seems important). By
declaring goals in this public way it is believed that people take them more
seriously, increase their commitment, and therefore increase the likelihood
of adherence to their plans. For example, Oldridge and Jones (1983) found
significantly better adherence from 'a group who agreed to sign a 6-month
contract for regular activity compared with a group who would not sign
such an agreement. This result may reflect initial differences in self-
motivation as well as the potential value of declaring targets. The contracts
can involve contingency clauses; for example, personal items or money
deposited at the start are returned on completion of weekly or intermediate
goals (Epstein et al. 1980). Eventually, the reinforcements need to be
thinned out to the point at which the exercise behaviour is being maintained
with reinforcement coming from the exercise experience itself (Kau and
Fischer 1974).

Along with establishing the potential gains from increasing activity (the
long-term goals) it is useful to prompt a recognition of the barriers that

may prevent goals being achieved (Knapp 1988). Offering individuals the chance to complete a decision balance sheet (Wankel 1984) or a decision matrix (Marlatt and Gordon 1985) will help people weigh up the advantages and disadvantages of increasing their levels of activity. The decision balance sheet asks people to consider, and write down, the potential gains and losses to self and to other important people as a result of increasing participation in exercise. It is then possible to discuss what strategies might help tip the balance to make the advantages outweigh the disadvantages. An example of the headings for a decision balance sheet is shown in Fig. 9.5. A decision matrix, on the other hand, asks participants to list short- and long-term consequences of both adhering to the plan for activity and failing to adhere to the plan. It would seem that such a matrix can be easily incorporated into the goal-setting procedure and an example of a format for completing a matrix is outlined in Fig. 9.6. Knapp (1988) points out that there have been no studies on the use of the decision matrix in exercise settings, but she sees it as potentially useful in helping people to recognise barriers (such as failing to return to regular activity after a holiday) and plan ways to overcome them.

A very successful example of goal-setting is Cooper's (1982) aerobic points system. The basis of the system is that points are allocated for different activities according to duration and intensity. The weekly goal is to achieve a total of 30 points. A varied programme can then be worked out for each individual. An example of the Cooper system is shown in Fig. 9.7.

One problem with goal-setting is that it can become inflexible. Good goal-setting technique should provide success on all short-term goals. If this is not happening then goals should be reset to an achievable level. At the other extreme it is possible that some people may become obsessive about achieving their targets and get themselves into a spiral of needing to achieve constant improvements. This situation will ultimately lead to feelings of failure. To help prevent this obsessive spiral the long-term goals should be clear and then goals which can *maintain* the desired effect can be set. Managing goal-setting is something which can be taught to

GAINS	LOSSES
To self	To self
To important others	To important others
Approval from others	Disapproval from others
Self-approval	Self-disapproval

Figure 9.5. The headings for a decision balance sheet.

	Adhering		Dropping-out	
	Plus	Minus	Plus	Minus
Short-term consequences				
Long-term consequences				

Figure 9.6. The format for a decision matrix.

ACTIVITY	POINTS
Monday	
Cycling 10 miles in 55 minutes	8.5
Tuesday	
Walk to work (1 mile) in 18 minutes	1
Wednesday	
Squash 50 minutes	7.5
Thursday	
Walk to work (1 mile) in 18 minutes	1
Friday	
Squash 50 minutes	7.5
Saturday	
Rest	1
Sunday	
Soccer 40 minutes	6
	31.5

Figure 9.7. The Cooper (1982) aerobic points system. The weekly goal is to achieve 30 points. Cooper (1982) has allocated points for different activities and so the points total can be achieved in a variety of ways. Here is one example.

participants; they may find it spilling over into other areas of life since it is likely to be a very transferable skill.

Self-monitoring

Self-monitoring is usually described as a cognitive-behavioural technique and has been used successfully used in enhancing exercise adherence (Martin et al. 1984; Oldridge and Jones 1983; Perkins et al. 1986). The basic principle of this technique is to raise awareness of the occurrences of the desired behaviour. When a person observes that he or she is completing exercise at a desired level this will be reinforcing; on the other hand, observing a failure to exercise in a particular way is punishing and may act to help the individual to change. In this sense self-monitoring goes along with goal-setting; monitoring occurs to check if the goals have been reached.

Sport has often been the setting for self-monitoring in the form of training diaries in which athletes record training/performance times, distances, efforts, and subjective appraisals. Sports psychologists have also used this technique to help athletes become more aware of particular aspects of their performance (e.g., Kirschenbaum and Wittrock 1984).

Typically, self-monitoring occurs via a written activity diary in which details of exercise completed are noted. An example of a page from such an activity diary is shown in Fig. 9.8.

This task may prove too onerous for some people. Unfortunately, as with many of the techniques discussed in this chapter, research cannot yet tell us which technique will work and which will not for any given person. Completing an activity diary may just not be feasible and require yet more motivation from a person who is struggling to maintain exercise motivation. An alternative is to get people to monitor aspects of exercise behaviour without having to write them down. Taking pulse counts or effort ratings or noting improvements (e.g., number of sit-ups completed) from the last exercise session may also operate as reinforcement without the burden of completing a diary. Rejeski and Kenney (1988) suggest that self-monitoring a single session of exercise, in terms of thoughts and feelings, is a very useful way to analyse negative thought patterns which may eventually cause drop-out.

Other people will respond very positively to an activity diary and will gain a great deal of reinforcement from reviewing their achievements over a period of months or even years. Juneau et al. (1987) report high levels of adherence (>90% for men and >75% for women) to a 24-week home-based exercise programme which included self-monitoring of heart rate and an activity diary. Results sheets from successive fitness assessments can operate in this way and an example is shown in Fig. 9.9. If staff time is available then activity can be centrally monitored in an easily accessible

WEEK NUMBER			DATE ....
DAY	ACTIVITY	DURATION	COMMENTS
MONDAY	Walked the dog	20 mins	quite brisk H.R. = 120
TUESDAY			
WEDNESDAY	Swam	15 minutes continous	felt good. 1st time I have managed 15m H.R. = 135
THURSDAY			
FRIDAY	Went to aerobics	30 minutes	A bit hard. Had to stop for breath H.R. = 150
SATURDAY			
SUNDAY			

Figure 9.8. An example of an activity diary for self-monitoring.

system for reference by exercisers and staff alike. Scherf and Franklin (1987) have described a sophisticated data documentation system which they have used effectively as a motivational tool in adherence to a cardiac rehabilitation programme.

Time Management

It has been noted (Chap. 2) that many people claim that they have no time to exercise. Shephard (1985) suggested that the problem was not so much lack of time, but making better use of available time. Godin et al. (1986b) have studied the problems of those who intend to exercise but do not and concluded that a perceived lack of time is a main concern. They suggest that these people have difficulty because their weekly schedules are poorly organised. Time management techniques might help people find a way to make exercise part of their lifestyle.

FITNESS ASSESSMENT RECORD

Name: A. Robic

Test number	1	2	3	4
Weight (kg)	69	67	65	
Max VO₂ (ml/kg per min)	35	40	42	
% body fat	29	28	27	
Sit-ups in 60 seconds	28	34	38	
Flexibility (cm)	31	32	32	

Figure 9.9. Using fitness assessment results as self-monitoring.

The first of these techniques would be to establish a person's priorities for the time they have free for leisure activities. For example, a mother of two children at nursery school may only consider that she has 5 free hours in the week in which she wants some relaxation time, time to visit friends and time to exercise. It would be important for her to establish if exercise had more, less or equal priorities to her other concerns. A second time-management technique would be to establish if activity can be increased without large commitments of time. Exploring the possibilities of cycling or walking to work, of exercising before work or during lunch-breaks, or of increasing walking rather than taking public or private transport, may prove fruitful for those who feel they have no free time. A third technique, which has been noted already in the section on goal-setting, would be to note down the exact time and day for exercise in a personal diary (e.g., Wednesday 5.15 squash with Jane) and to agree with oneself that these appointments are just as important as work engagements or other social engagements. Keefe and Blumenthal (1980) advised subjects that they should keep their exercise appointment with themselves or others at the same time each week in order to create a fixed pattern to the management of exercise time.

Social Support

As noted (Chap. 2), drop-out from exercise is often related to lack of support from spouse, family or friends, although the importance of this support may differ for men and women (Godin and Shephard 1985). If a person has a partner who feels that exercise is time away from shared time, that exercise is dangerous (Taylor et al. 1985), or that exercisers are slightly crazy, then the comments which may ensue will act as negative reinforcements, stopping exercise. In such a situation it may be easier to give up and stay at home rather than endure the anti-exercise environment. For someone in this situation there are a few positive ideas to pursue. First of all the person could encourage the partner or another member of the family to spend some time exercising with him or her. For example, going to the swimming pool or taking a walk at the weekend together. Secondly, this kind of person could enlist the help of several friends who have positive attitudes to exercise so that social support may come from work colleagues or other friends even if it is lacking at home. Creating this kind of network of support will help keep motivation going after holidays, injuries or illnesses, after which it is often easier to return to a less active lifestyle (Robertson and Mutrie 1989). One advantage of attending a class meeting as part of an exercise plan is that a network of support is easily created (Thow and Newton 1990). Further discussion of social influence factors can be found in Chaps 2 and 3.

Positive Self-statements

It has been recognised that maladaptive self-statements can limit gain and cause drop-out from therapeutic programmes (Buffone et al. 1984). In the exercise scenario such statements take the form of "I'm just not the active type" or "I've got no will power for exercise" or "I feel so stupid doing these kinds of things". Faced with this type of person the help should come in the form of changing negative statements to positive ones. For example "I get better at this each week" or "I can walk to work at least once each week" or "I feel good after I've been exercising". This particular technique has been used successfully by Atkins et al. (1984) to increase compliance to a walking programme. The task of changing negative to positive is, however, easier said than done as it is common for people lacking in self-confidence to have a trait of negative statements which is difficult to alter. Reinforcers for the use of positive statements will help change the natural thinking style. Encouraging people to provide their own praise for successful completion of some part of an exercise plan will start them on the process of making positive self-statements. For example, it is usually not too difficult to get people to agree that they can feel pleased with themselves on completing a jog, arranging a game of tennis, or managing a month of regular activity.

Association or Distraction

The idea that participation might be encouraged by teaching people to associate with thoughts and feelings during exercise has led to some contradictory findings. Associating to one's perceived level of exertion ("rating of perceived exertion" or RPE) is the basis of teaching people to maintain appropriate intensity levels and self-pacing, thus avoiding the negative consequences of fatigue or injury. However, Martin and Dubbert (1982) reported greater adherence from a group trained to focus on distracting thoughts (e.g., the smell of the flowers on a jogging route), than a group trained to focus on bodily sensations. Music in exercise classes provides an enjoyable distractor (see Boutcher and Trenske 1990) and can result in high levels of work rate for relatively low levels of perceived exertion (Sutherland et al. 1990). This kind of distraction could either increase adherence because the negative aspects of feeling fatigue are minimised, or it could decrease adherence because people work harder than necessary and the negative aspects of muscle soreness or even injury are increased. Boutcher and Trenske (1990) report that effort ratings were attenuated with music but only under light exercising conditions, suggesting that in more intense bouts the physiological cues dominate. Conversely, positive affect was reported to be higher in the moderate and high exercise conditions when music was playing. They concluded that since the influence of music on RPE and affect was dependent on the workload, the mechanisms underlying these changes remain unclear. Further research is required to help clarify this confusing picture.

Cognitive Rehearsal and Imagery

Cognitive rehearsal and imagery are standard techniques which sports psychologists have used to enhance performance (Bunker and Williams 1986; Vealey 1986b). Buffone et al. (1984) suggested that these techniques could also be used to increase exercise adherence. This technique would involve participants in rehearsing mentally aspects of exercise behaviour which need improvement. For example, if an office worker avoids going for a jog after work because she finds it difficult to say "no" to a relaxing cup of coffee with her co-workers, she could rehearse the scenario in which she says that today she would like to go for a jog instead. Or there may be certain images which a person can use to help him or her stay with the exercise plan. For example, the images of completing a 30-minute run with ease, or gaining more muscle tone, or having more energy to play with the kids, might just keep some people going when they feel like giving up. There appears to be no research evidence to support the use of these cognitive techniques in exercise adherence, but judging by the success of mental rehearsal and imagery in sport psychology (Feltz and Landers 1983) it seems worthwhile exploring these techniques with exercise behaviour.

Relapse Prevention

The use of the word relapse to describe a failure to maintain regular activity has become commonplace in the literature (Knapp 1988; Dishman 1990) and has been discussed already in Chap. 2. A more applied approach will be taken here. The concept of relapse is located in the literature which is concerned with overcoming addictive behaviours such as alcohol and drug abuse (Brownell et al. 1986; Marlatt and Gordon 1985). The concept can easily be applied to the scenario of relapse back into a sedentary lifestyle from an active one, but the analogy is somewhat strained since a sedentary lifestyle is not as immediately serious as a return to a life-threatening addiction. As Knapp (1988, p. 221) points out the goal with addictive behaviours is "to reduce a high-frequency, undesired behavior whereas in the promotion of physical activity the goal is to increase a low-frequency, desired behavior". *Lapses* from regular activity may describe more accurately the experience of many people, with *relapse* applying only if a long period of inactivity ensues. Rather than relying on the terminology from another field, for those working in health-related exercise the phrase "start/stop syndrome" may be more applicable. Nevertheless there are important points to learn from the relapse concept which can be applied to the area of exercise adherence.

The first point is that strategies are available to help people overcome the inevitable barriers (or high-risk situations – see Chap. 2) which life presents in the quest for continued activity (e.g., moving house, recovering from an illness, changing job, taking a holiday, emotional issues). If a decision balance sheet is used (see section on goal-setting) then people can often identify these barriers in advance and plan how to cope with them. The coping strategies should be selected from the techniques already listed according to what appears to suit an individual's style. For example, if social support seems to be important for a participant who has a start/stop exercise history, then planning how to maximise social support for a barrier, such as recovering from an illness, would seem appropriate. As Marlatt (1985) points out, it is possible to identify and predict situations which present high risk for relapse.

The second point which can be learned from the relapse model is that missing planned activity can lead to feelings of failure, loss of self-esteem and other damaging thoughts. In Marlatt's (1985) model this has been labelled the Abstinence Violation Effect, but that phrase does not seem to describe adequately the parallel exercise scenario. Perhaps a better phrase is the start/stop effect; guilt is probably the central emotion experienced when people fail to carry out their exercise plans. Guilt may motivate a person to return to activity. However, if the guilt leads to the person seeing himself or herself as a drop-out or someone lacking in willpower then strategies such as cognitive restructuring or more flexible goal-setting could be used.

Cognitive Restructuring

Cognitive restructuring would involve the person in analysing the reason for the lapse. Attributing the cause to something that can be changed allows the person to plan how to cope better in the future with that situation. It is important that the person maintains a feeling of control over the situation and recognises that although that particular situation (e.g., a family commitment) caused a lapse from activity this time, the same situation can be dealt with differently the next time. King and Frederiksen (1984) report the successful use of cognitive restructuring, coupled with immediate rescheduling of the missed session, in adherence to a jogging programme. (See Chap. 4 for a more detailed discussion of attributions and perceptions of control.)

Flexible Goal-setting

Creating more flexible goals might be particularly important for those who do not respond well to tightly structured plans. Thus each exercise session which appears to have a high lapse possibility should have a contingency plan. For example, if rain presents a high risk of lapse to a jogger then alternatives, such as a swim or a home-based routine can be planned. Alternatively, using flexible, intermediate goals (e.g., 5 weeks hence) may be more successful than fixed short-term goals, because there is less chance of failure than in weekly goal-setting (Martin et al. 1984).

Support for the relapse prevention approach has also come from Belisle et al. (1987). In their first study, 178 subjects who participated in a university sports centre programme in Canada acted as the experimental group and 172 as the control group. The experimental group received 10–15 minutes of information in each of their twice-weekly exercise sessions, as did the control group. However, the control group received "standard" health education material on jogging techniques, injury, food choices, stress management, smoking etc. The experimental group received material more related to relapse prevention and included self-management, high-risk situations, and the management of temporary lapses. Results showed that for both short-term (frequency) and long-term (3-month follow-up) adherence to the exercise classes was greater for the experimental group. These results were supported by a follow-up study 1 year later.

The research of Belisle et al. (1987) suggests that adherence can be improved by the use of relapse prevention strategies. Such intervention techniques were found to be cost-effective with a good return on adherence for a small amount of professional input.

Educational Strategies

The issues of how to define, provide and evaluate health education and promotion are a current concern in public health. Downie et al. (1990) suggest that the standard approach to health education has been to inform people of how to prevent ill-health, but that a more modern approach is required in which *positive* health is promoted. These authors define positive health as having two clear components, namely true well-being and fitness. If this definition becomes commonly accepted, health education campaigns will have more focus on the positive aspects of enhancing fitness. As we have pointed out in Section C, the process of enhancing fitness may also contribute to an increased sense of well-being. Thus educational strategies which aim to increase and sustain regular activity must be seen in the context of positive health promotion. In this context, exercise programmes which seek to involve participants in understanding the contribution of regular activity to health, while taking the individual's needs and perspectives into account, can have a major role to play in positive health promotion. This may be a particularly fruitful line for health promotors to follow because, as Shephard (1989b) points out, activity programmes have the potential to influence positively other health habits such as smoking and diet.

The topics which will be addressed in this section should be used in conjunction with many of the strategies already described. It is envisaged that this approach could form part of a mass media campaign or be part of group teaching or one-to-one counselling. What follows is a selection of topics which participants could learn about in order to increase the likelihood of having a lifestyle which involves regular activity.

What Is Fitness?

It has been suggested that improving patient understanding and recall of information can enhance compliance to medical treatment (Krantz et al. 1985). The same may be true for compliance to health promoting activity. There are many misconceptions about fitness and what people need to do in order to improve fitness. It is important to enhance participants' understanding of the components of health-related fitness, and the quantity and frequency of activity required to achieve and maintain fitness for health. Godin et al. (1986b) have established that many people who intend to exercise, but do not, are put off because they perceive that exercise would be tiring. To assist exercise promotion Godin et al. (1986b, p. 525) suggest: "the promotion of physical activity should at least stress the fact that one does not necessarily need to suffer and become exhausted from health-oriented exercise behaviour, thus counteracting the belief that exercising is too physically demanding".

Corbin et al. (1987a) suggested that the important elements of fitness for health are cardiovascular fitness, strength and muscle endurance, flexibility, and desirable body composition. In attempting to educate participants about these components several approaches may be used. For example, each week an educational theme can be high-lighted in an exercise class, leaflets which explain each component can be made available, or booklets with a comprehensive guide can be supplied. In addition, if a fitness assessment service is available locally this can provide an ideal focus for understanding the components of health-related fitness, since it is normal to have one test for each of the components mentioned above (Smith 1989). Dean (1987) completed a survey of perceptions about fitness tests and concluded that increased knowledge about fitness was the main motivator for increasing activity levels after undertaking fitness tests. However, other workers have claimed that increased knowledge will have limited impact on exercise intentions and behaviours (Dishman et al. 1985). More needs to be known about this. It is possible that a minimal threshold of knowledge is required, after which gains in knowledge will have little impact. Finally, a system of allowing participants to check their understanding should be built into the educational programme. This could take the form of consultation times, or self-administered quizzes on specific topics.

What Are the Health Benefits of Regular Activity?

Research tells us that if we are to attract people into activity then the immediate rather than long-term benefits of exercise should be emphasised (Eadie and Leathar 1988; Dean 1987). This implies that traditional campaigns which focus on benefits which may be achieved at some point in the future (such as reduced risk of cardiovascular disease) may not increase activity. Instead, when promoting the benefits of regular activity immediate gains such as "the feel better effect", increased energy levels, being able to do a little more each week, increased social contact, and enjoyment should be stressed. The longer-term benefits of reducing percentage body fat or improving scores on fitness assessments, or reducing coronary heart disease risk need to be put into the perspective of additional gain if activity is maintained. A good example of this approach is the poster shown in Fig. 9.10. It is intended to encourage students into regular exercise by promoting the stress-reducing effects of activity.

How to Avoid the Start/Stop Syndrome

We all must realise that the majority of people will face the situation in which regular exercise becomes a lower priority and a more sedentary

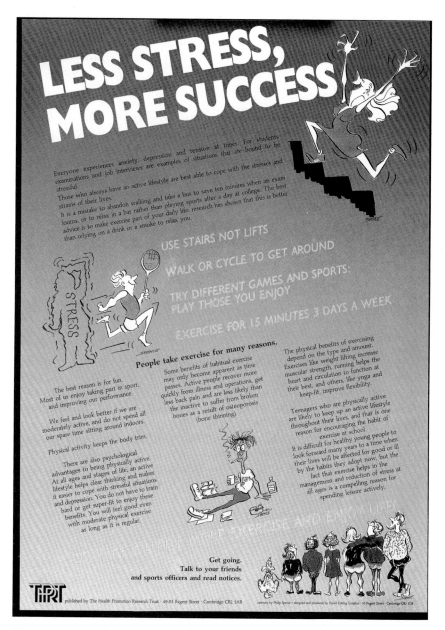

Figure 9.10. "Less stress, more succcess" poster encouraging participation through the promotion of well-being. (Reproduced with permission of the Health Promotion Research Trust. Cartoons by Philip Spence.)

existence will follow. Participants can be taught how to cope with this problem and, more importantly, how to get back to a regular exercise routine. Many of the techniques discussed under relapse prevention are important here. The main educational strategy is to help people understand this process and provide them with re-start opportunities.

Adult and Continuing Education Classes

Classes which intend to educate people about fitness for health often fail because the classes are focussed on activity rather than on making people independent exercisers. A class which runs for 10 weeks of a college or university term and leaves the participants without the knowledge of how to create their own exercise plan over the vacation is not achieving educational objectives. The same is true of school physical education programmes in which the topic of how to maintain activity after leaving school is rarely addressed. While the physical education profession is now attempting to address this problem (see Chap. 10 and Biddle (1987b)), the world of adult education is often faced with conflicts of educational versus commercial gain. For example, it may be commercially advantageous for a college to run exercise classes for adults, encouraging the same people to return each term; in the long run, the message of how to increase activity independently of the class environment is lost. Thus the educational impact on a local community is rather small compared with a campaign which focusses on how to be more active outside the classes. This conflict may not be easily resolved; it is lucrative to offer exercise classes, as many commercial and educational establishments have found out. At a minimum these classes must be on offer every week of the year, and not only in term-time, if regular participation is to be encouraged. In addition, information and guidance on alternative forms of activity should be made available to class participants even if this seems not to be in the commercial interest; not everyone in the local population will want to exercise in a class environment, so supervised exercise must be seen as a step in the direction of creating independent exercisers.

Self-help Tools for Starting and Continuing Activity

Clearly, many of the strategies which have been outlined in this chapter can be most easily applied in a one-to-one setting in which the exerciser can speak to someone with skills in exercise and counselling. In most unsupervised or "free living" situations such help is not readily available. In the long run, local health authorities may consider it cost-effective to employ community specialists in exercise to provide advice, fitness assessments or personal exercise programmes. In the short term, self-help packages could be made available through health promotion literature, wellness clinics, general practices, sports injuries clinics and sports shops. Based on the contents of this chapter, here are ideas for the contents of four self-help packages which those responsible for promoting activity can adapt to local situations:

Package 1 *Getting started with exercise*

Contents
1. Matching reasons for exercising with appropriate activities
2. A decision balance sheet
3. Enlisting support

Package 2 *Keeping going with regular activity*

Contents
1. Goal-setting
2. Self-monitoring
3. Self-reinforcement
4. Arranging cues for exercise

Package 3 *Avoiding the start/stop syndrome*

Contents
1. Contingency planning
2. Finding a way around the problems
3. Everyone has a little time to exercise

Package 4 *Improving your fitness knowledge*

Contents
1. The components of fitness
2. Simple home tests for each component
3. How much exercise is enough?
4. The physiological and psychological effects of regular exercise
5. Self-tests on the contents of package 4

Combined Strategies

It may seem obvious to state that it is likely that simultaneous use of more than one of the strategies outlined above will maximise the chance of creating an active lifestyle for those in need of such help. However, selecting the exact combinations to use in any particular situation is not easy to do, since, from the research completed to date, we do not yet know what strategies are most effective for any given person. An eclectic viewpoint is required to try and match the various techniques available with the person seeking help. For example, someone who feels that lack of time is his or her worst enemy, perhaps needs some time-management strategies and some educational input about how much time is required for health-related exercise. For someone who finds that his or her friends all feel that exercise is not important, finding alternative social support, while reinforcing exercise behaviour, might be the best starting point.

Research based on group designs has helped our understanding of the combinations of strategies which seem most effective. For example, Atkins et al. (1984) compared five different methods of increasing adherence to a therapeutic walking programme. The methods were behaviour modification, cognitive modification, attention control, no-treatment control, and a combination of cognitive and behaviour modification. It was found that the most effective method was the combined cognitive and behaviour modification. The results of this study are shown in Fig. 9.11.

It is interesting to reflect that the majority of opportunities to influence exercise behaviour on a one-to-one basis in the UK probably occur through brief instructions about exercise prescription or through fitness assessment. These scenarios are typically those which researchers have used as "control" conditions (Atkins et al. 1984; Noland 1989). These control conditions have been shown to have little effect on adherence. There is an obvious need for physical educators, exercise leaders, and physiologists to understand

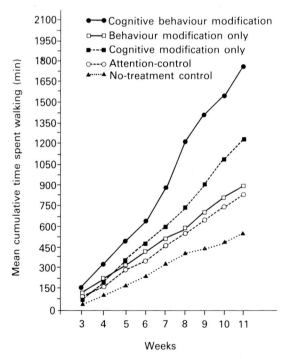

Figure 9.11. Cumulative weekly walking resulting from different adherence techniques (Atkins et al. 1984). (Copyright 1984 by The American Psychological Association. Reprinted by permission of the author.)

how they can influence positively long-term involvement in regular activity. As Noland (1989, p. 223) concludes: "Minimal contact such as a brief instruction period and pre- and post-physiological assessment appears to be inadequate when used as behavioral assistance to sedentary individuals".

Evaluating Programme Effectiveness

Any programme which seeks to change behaviour should include evaluation of how effective the selected strategies have been (Kazdin 1975). If the programme is part of a research project, then group designs which involve random assignment of subjects to various conditions can be employed. Such designs provide the strongest evidence for comparative effectiveness of the strategies involved. However, much of the work in exercise adherence occurs outside research projects. In these situations it is still important to log how effective a strategy has been in changing exercise behaviour. Individual progress can be monitored on a standard chart. Whenever possible it is desirable to establish base-line behaviour before implementing

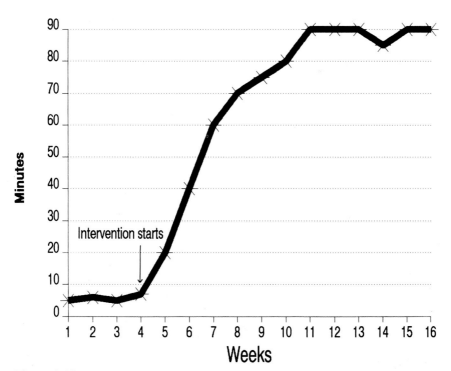

Figure 9.12. An example of a standard chart for monitoring changes in exercise behaviour.

a particular strategy. An example of such a recording chart is shown in Fig. 9.12.

A more sophisticated approach is to employ an experimental design, even if small numbers are involved. Two such designs will now be described.

Reversal Design

The reversal design is frequently used to evaluate psychotherapy interventions. In this situation the base-line rate of the targeted behaviour is noted (in our case exercise) and described as phase A. A reinforcement is then presented and the effect on the target behaviour noted (phase B). The reinforcement is then taken away, and target behaviour is again noted (phase A). Finally, the reinforcement is repeated, giving a typical ABAB design. If more exercise occurs during the B phases than during the A phases, it is concluded that the reinforcement has been effective. An example of a hypothetical ABAB design is shown in Fig. 9.13.

Multiple Base-line Designs

In this design the strategy to affect behaviour is introduced at different points in time for different people after a stable base line has been

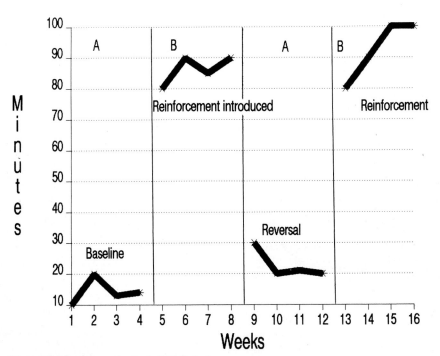

Figure 9.13. A hypothetical ABAB design.

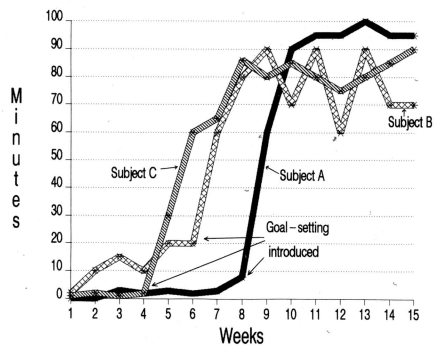

Figure 9.14. Hypothetical results from a multiple base-line study.

established. If the exercise behaviour increases on the introduction of the strategy for each of the individuals then the experimenter can have more confidence in the strategy under investigation. An example of hypothetical results from a multiple base-line study is shown in Fig. 9.14.

Conclusion

It is clear that people who want to increase their own or other people's exercise behaviour have many strategies available to help with this task. To date, research on these techniques is limited, but it does seem clear that attempting to put any strategy into operation is better than leaving people to find their own motivation for regular activity. The next stage for researchers is to establish the efficacy of the various techniques and to find out the characteristics of those who are likely to respond positively to any given technique.

10

Intervention Strategies: Organisations and Institutions

The previous chapter discussed interventions based on psychological principles which enable the individual to modify levels of physical activity. However, in addition to individual changes, there is a need to intervene at a macro level. Indeed, some would argue that the pervasive approach of individualism in health promotion is too simplistic and that more progress will be made with the adoption of a macro, societal approach (Sparkes 1989). It is our belief that the two approaches are complementary. In this chapter, four major organisations and settings will be discussed from the viewpoint of psychology and exercise promotion: school, workplace, community, and medical settings. The main emphasis will be on the school, given the clear potential for early interventions that is possible here. Less will be said about medical settings as the literature concerning this area, from a psychological point of view, has already been covered (Chaps 2 and 5).

The School

In commenting on the promotion of physical activity in the American population, Iverson et al. (1985, p. 219) said ". . . one community organisation – the schools – underpins the whole effort to achieve the goal of national fitness". Similarly, interest in the potential of schools to promote physical activity has been stated in policy documents in the USA and in Great Britain. For example, the American College of Sports Medicine (ACSM 1988, p. 422) opinion statement on "Physical Fitness in Children and Youth" stated the following recommendation: "School physical education programmes are an important part of the overall education process and should give increased emphasis to the development and maintenance of lifelong exercise habits and provide instruction about how to attain and maintain appropriate physical fitness".

This statement mirrors the current concern in Great Britain about the apparent lack of regular physical activity in children (see Chap. 1 and Armstrong 1987, 1990). In fact, the Sports Council (1988) factsheet on children's exercise, health and fitness recommends that "schools . . . should seek to ensure that children understand the importance of frequent, appropriate exercise, good eating habits, and the maintenance of the right bodyweight".

Judging by these statements, there would appear to be a need to look closely at the promotion of physical activity and exercise in schools. This has important implications from the point of view of socialising children into healthy lifestyles. The central part of a school that is identified with the promotion of exercise is that of physical education (PE), although the more generic health promotion activities can, and should, combine across curriculum areas.

The Role of Physical Education in Exercise Promotion

The discussion paper produced by Her Majesty's Inspectorate, "Physical Education from 5 to 16" (HMI 1989), lists 11 aims of physical education and these are shown in Table 10.1.

Interestingly, from a psychological viewpoint, four of these aims contain "psycho-motor" (physical) aims, four contain cognitive (knowledge) aims and five contain affective (attitudinal) aims. (Some contain more than one of these.) From the standpoint of promoting health-related physical activity and exercise, aims 2 and 3 are directly related to physiological changes, while aim 11 perhaps makes the assumption that changes in knowledge or value will change behaviour. These aims should include a statement about the behavioural skills required to adopt and maintain an exercise programme. Aims 9 and 10 clearly focus on psychological outcomes and are dealt with in more detail in Sections B and C of this book.

From a British perspective, there has been a tremendous growth in interest in the teaching of "health-related fitness" in physical education courses in schools since the early 1980s. The USA has a longer history of attempting such work, but the changes in British PE have been well documented (Biddle 1987b). Much of this work has concentrated on providing a rationale for teaching health-related work, of which prevention of disease has often been the most prominent. Relatively little has been documented on "model" programmes, and even less on programme evaluation.

Table 10.1. Aims of Physical Education for Ages 5 to 16 years (HMI 1989)

1.	To develop a range of psycho-motor skills
2.	To maintain and increase physical mobility and flexibility
3.	To develop stamina and strength
4.	To develop understanding and appreciation of the purposes, forms and conventions of a selection of physical activities
5.	To develop the capacity to express ideas in dance forms
6.	To develop the appreciation of the concepts of fair play, honest competition and good sportsmanship
7.	To develop the ability to appreciate the aesthetic qualities of movement
8.	To develop the capacity to maintain interest and to persevere to achieve success
9.	To foster self-esteem through the acquisition of physical competence and poise
10.	To develop self-confidence through understanding the capabilities and limitations of oneself and others
11.	To develop an understanding of the importance of exercise in maintaining a healthy life

Note. These aims are numbered for ease of identification in the text and are not in order of priority or importance.

Health-Related Fitness and a Health "Focus"

Since the rapid expansion of health-related fitness programmes in British schools in the 1980s there has developed a debate about the best way of implementing work on health and exercise in PE. The original approach, stemming largely from the USA (e.g., Corbin and Lindsey 1988), is what could be called a "direct approach" to educating children about the benefits and implementation of an exercise ("fitness for life") programme. This approach (see Biddle 1989b) advocates teaching units of work which are based around each of the major components of health-related fitness and exercise – i.e. cardiopulmonary exercise, muscular strength and endurance, and flexibility, with additional possibilities including body composition and stress management (see Corbin et al. 1987a; Fox and Whitehead 1987; Fox et al. 1987). Little systematic evaluation of the success of these types of programmes has been reported. However, since this approach requires teachers to change the content of their curriculum, others have advocated the "health focus" approach whereby the teaching of "health" knowledge and skills is performed through existing PE activities, such as track and field athletics, games, gymnastics and swimming. However, the focus has changed from the predominant skill-oriented approach to one in which "health" and fitness are emphasised. However, the variety of approaches that this focus offers may well be a weakness since one could question the likely impact of such approaches if the health message is lost within activities where it is more usual to use a skill-oriented approach. Equally, one could argue that when teaching, say, swimming, time would be better spent on skill acquisition, especially for younger children. In fact, the all-encompassing definitions sometimes given to health may prove useless from a curriculum planning point of view. For example, the British Association of Advisers and Lecturers in Physical Education (BAALPE 1988, p. 3) has stated that "by sharpening the focus on health, primary school pupils *will gain these benefits*: a positive feeling of self-esteem . . . a better understanding of how to look after oneself . . . wider communication skills . . . greater ability to handle personal responsibilities . . . better social skills . . . better physical skills" (*our emphases*). Two key points emerge here. First, the phrase "will gain these benefits" is clearly a naive overstatement. Second, the benefits they are suggesting are so broad that they refer to sound educational aims rather than to "health" objectives *per se*.

Some writers have argued that a change in teaching styles or emphasis produces a "health focus" (Health and Physical Education Project Newsletter 1986, 1987; Smith 1988). This could be challenged where, in gymnastics for example (see Smith 1988), a rather forced and potentially incorrect relationship between "health", "fitness" and "skill" could be established. Some gymnastic movements are potentially problematic from a health perspective anyway (Biddle 1989b), as are some other sports. Both these approaches to teaching health and fitness within PE require rigorous evaluation. Similarly, longitudinal studies are required to test the outcomes of different programmes. These outcomes could include health and fitness measures, participation rates, and attitudinal factors.

Health and Fitness Research with Children: Behavioural Issues

The Effects of Physical Education Programmes

There is an expanding literature supporting the role of physical activity and exercise in the promotion of health and well-being. In a review of the effects of physical education programmes, Vogel (1986) suggests that a large number of reported outcomes from PE have yet to be confirmed through appropriately designed research studies. In his summary, Vogel (1986) concludes the following from a review of physiological and motor performance outcomes:

1. There is convincing evidence that participation in physical education programmes can improve aerobic fitness, student physical activity levels, motor performance, muscular endurance, muscular power, and muscular strength, even though some of these parameters can decline during the teenage years (Bailey 1973). However, such predictable outcomes reported by Vogel (1986) are likely to be partly a function of the time committed to such activities. Longitudinal data are not available and it is the longevity

of physical change that is important from the point of view of health.

2. There is evidence that participation can improve balance, flexibility, selected measures of perceptual-motor performance, and movement speed.

3. There is little or no evidence that participation in physical education programmes improves agility, coordination, anaerobic fitness, alters height, weight or girth, alters nutritional practices, or retards the maturation process (see also Malina 1989).

In terms of psychological outcomes, Vogel (1986) reports the following:

1. There is evidence that participation in physical education programmes can contribute to academic performance. However, Vogel suggests that this link may be an indirect one. In fact, the more detailed evidence presented in his chapter does not provide convincing evidence at all. Of the five studies reported, only two showed significant effects, one of which was for reading "readiness" rather than actual achievement. The other study which found positive results was based on grading by teachers – a process open to considerable bias. Similarly, additional studies on daily physical education programmes, reported later in this chapter but omitted by Vogel, show that, *at best*, academic performance does not decline with extra PE and a reduction in classroom contact time.

2. There is evidence that participation in PE programmes can positively influence how children feel about physical activity and health/fitness. However, as discussed in Chap. 3, attitude-behaviour links are complex. Simple changes in global attitudes may not predict behaviour very well at all. The behavioural significance of Vogel's conclusion, therefore, may be limited.

3. There is convincing evidence that participation in PE programmes can improve knowledge related to healthy lifestyles. Although this is a positive finding, the research using the Health Belief Model and other models of attitudes, suggests that knowledge will contribute only small amounts of behavioural variance (see Godin and Shephard 1986b). Dishman et al. (1985) report that evidence is not available that shows that *changes* in knowledge affect activity levels.

4. There is no evidence that participation in PE programmes can improve self-concept or personality. This is in direct opposition to the conclusion reached by Gruber (1986) in his meta-analysis of self-esteem and exercise involvement in children. One of the problems with this area of research is the measurement of self-esteem. This has been discussed in Chap. 8 (see also Fox 1988, 1990; Fox and Corbin 1989). The consensus in the exercise science literature is that, despite research problems, self-esteem can be positively influenced by appropriate physical activity (see Sonstroem 1984; Sonstroem and Morgan 1989). The influence of physical activity on personality is more problematic due to measurement variability, the stability of some personality traits, and poor research designs (see Morgan 1980a).

In short, the measurement of outcomes from physical education programmes is difficult, and the review by Vogel (1986) high-lights the fact that while studies may show effects, the quality of research data in many of these studies is very limited. However, there remains a need for well-controlled, multi-variate, longitudinal research studies of physical education programmes and their outcomes (Malina 1989).

Childhood–Adulthood Links

One of the key aims in the teaching of health and fitness programmes in schools is that children should be taught how to become active adults. Very few studies, however, have adequately tested whether participation in childhood actually affects adult patterns of physical activity. The research problems associated with such a question are, of course, very large, but Powell and Dysinger (1987) have reviewed a small number of studies that have a bearing on this issue.

Powell and Dysinger (1987) reported only six studies related to the issue of childhood participation and adult activity levels. One of these was a cross-sectional survey, two were cohort studies, and three were case control studies. The 1972 National (USA) Adult Fitness Survey reported by Powell and Dysinger did provide some evidence that those who had participated in school sports teams were more likely to become active adults than those not participating at school. Similarly, those who took PE classes at school were more likely to be active in adulthood than PE non-participants. (The American education system does not guarantee that PE is taken by all pupils in some States, hence the participant/non-participant dichotomy that would generally not be found in British schools.) These results, however, are quite likely to be confounded by age, gender and availability of physical education programmes.

Paffenbarger's well-known epidemiological study of Harvard University alumni (see Paffenbarger and Hyde 1988), while being primarily an investigation of health outcomes from habitual physical activity, did, according to Powell and Dysinger (1987), provide some support for active college students also being active in their later adult years. However, this is not support for the childhood–adulthood link that many people seek. The habits adopted by the time young adulthood is reached may be quite different from those of the child.

Of the four other studies reviewed by Powell and Dysinger, two showed no relationship between child and adult physical activity patterns. The two that did suggest a link had methodological problems that severely weakened the conclusions.

Powell and Dysinger (1987) tentatively concluded that, at best, there was a suggestion of a relationship between childhood and adulthood activity levels. They suggest five points to be considered in future studies in this area. First, clearer and more consistent definitions are required of the key terms physical activity, exercise and sports (see Bouchard et al. 1990; Caspersen et al. 1985, and Chap. 1). Second, greater emphasis on the analysis of possible confounding variables is required. Third, bias in the recall of physical activity needs careful scrutiny. Fourth, more care is needed with selection bias in sample construction. Fifth, there is a need to investigate the quality and content of school PE programmes in relation to adult patterns of activity.

Dennison et al. (1988) looked at whether test scores of childhood fitness predicted participation in physical activity as an adult. They obtained the self-reported physical activity levels of 453 men aged 23–25 years and compared them with fitness test scores completed during their school years, either at 10–11 years or 15–18 years. Discriminant analysis revealed that performance on the 600-yard run/walk test was the best discriminator between active and inactive adults, with faster times predicting greater activity as an adult. Performance on a sit-up test, reported parental encouragement of exercise, participation in organised sports after leaving school, and reported spouse support all contributed, in the expected direction, to discrimination between the high- and low-activity groups. Early maturation may account for these results in so far as the early maturing children are likely to gain the most success and reinforcement from such tests. However, these results do suggest that childhood experiences may affect participation in adulthood.

Behaviour Change Programmes

Parcel et al. (1987) suggest that schools may need to implement changes based on the principles of social learning theory (see Chap. 3) and organisational change. Four schools in the USA were assessed on dietary habits and physical activity in PE and break times. The base-line data suggested that, in comparison with national recommendations, the school lunch was excessive in its provision of fat and salt, whereas in PE and break time, physical activity levels were low. The activity data mirror those of Armstrong and his co-workers from British children (Armstrong 1990). Parcel et al. (1987) were particularly concerned about the lack of continuous aerobic exercise undertaken in their base-line assessments. From such data, they suggest that a model for school intervention should involve principles of social learning theory, such as modelling, behaviour reinforcement and cognitive change, in addition to organisational changes in the school. In particular, they suggest that change must involve four stages: institutional commitment, structured alterations in school policies and practices, changes in the role and practices of staff, and the implementation of learning activities for students. The interventions suggested for aerobic physical activity by Parcel et al. (1987) based on these four stages are shown in Fig. 10.1.

Parcel et al. (1987) provide an interesting model that now requires testing. But one of the problems, at least as far as the physical activity intervention is concerned, is the extent to which PE lessons should become merely "physical training" sessions. The aims of PE, as identified in Table 10.1, point to many factors far beyond physiological development. This debate has recently been fuelled by three issues. First, the increased emphasis on health-related programmes in school PE has inevitably led to support for more fitness-type activities, but second, the data from recent research (e.g., Armstrong 1990; Parcel et al. 1987) show that children are inactive from the point of view of fitness development, and this can include PE lessons. Third, the call for more emphasis on physiological development of children in PE has been muted by the likely *reduction* in time for physical education as a result of the introduction of the National Curriculum in the

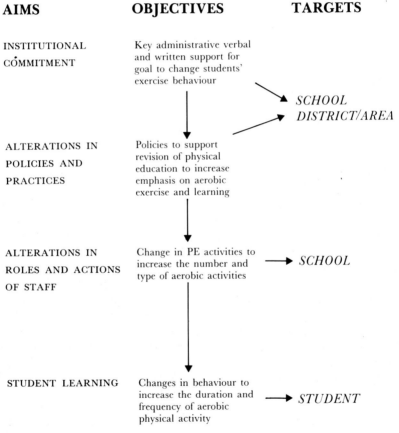

Figure 10.1. A school health promotion model applied to aerobic exercise. (Adapted from Parcel et al. 1987.)

UK, even though PE is a "foundation" (compulsory) subject. Similarly, in Scotland the introduction of an examinable course in PE (Standard Grade) has led to a situation in which some children can opt out of compulsory PE before the age of 16 years, and there is a similar erosion of time allocated to PE across the whole age range (Physical Education Association 1987). All of these issues centre on the role of PE in health education: is it PE's role to foster physiological change or is it more realistic, given the constraints, to give PE the role of creating desirable changes in behavioural skills such that children are more likely to be willing and able to adopt the appropriate activity patterns in their leisure time, both as youths and adults? In reality, the latter alternative is the only one available since the majority of schools have such limited time in which to attempt physiological change. Indeed, if changes of this nature were attempted with such limited class time, potentially negative exercise experiences could result. Perhaps a radical re-think is required of how physical education can fulfil both roles. Is it possible that motor and behavioural skills can be taught in small classes, while fitness activities could be taught in rather larger classes, thus reducing staff and curricular time? For example, intramural fitness-oriented games or other aerobic activity could be taught to large groups, perhaps twice per week, to enhance physiological development. Physical education must also consider initiating "homework" activity to make up for lack of curricular time.

Corbin et al. (1987a) suggest that PE objectives should be based on a "stairway" approach. First, students should be taught how to exercise which, in turn, may lead to changes in fitness. However, a more important step would be achieved if children could adopt their own exercise patterns, without the direct support of the teacher. This is referred to as "fitness independence". The modified stairway approach is illustrated in Fig. 10.2.

Another intervention programme, similar to that of Parcel et al. (1987), is described by Downey et al. (1987). Again, no intervention results are available, but the programme "Heart Smart" is a cardiovascular health promotion programme in schools as part of the larger Bogalusa (Louisiana, USA) epidemiological study. One of the goals of the "Heart Smart" programme is to develop an effective programme for cardiovascular risk reduction and health promotion; one that "positively influences predisposing factors (knowledge, attitudes, beliefs, values) and enabling factors (skills)" (Downey et al. 1987, p. 99). Part of the programme is to promote the adoption of regular exercise to increase cardiovascular fitness. The full model proposed by Downey et al. (1987) is shown in Fig. 10.3. Future studies will need to test the extent to which the "determinants" of behaviour actually do predict subsequent behaviour.

These authors suggest three forms of assessment of the intervention: process, impact and outcome evaluation. The process evaluation will involve a qualitative form of assessment of the overall intervention. The impact

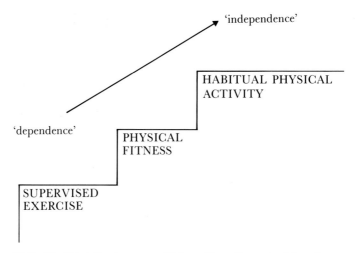

Figure 10.2. Modified "stairway to lifetime fitness" emphasising the move from dependence to independence. (Adapted from Corbin et al. 1987a.)

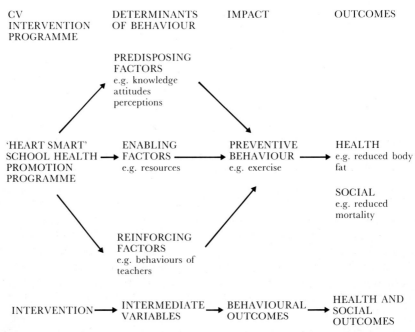

Figure 10.3. Cardiovascular health promotion for school age children. (A.M. Downey et al. (1987) "Implementation of 'Heart Smart': a cardiovascular school health promotion programme". *Journal of School Health*, 57 (3): © 1987 American School Health Association, PO Box 708, Kent, OH 44240. Reprinted with permission.)

evaluation documents short-term changes in factors such as attitudes and fitness. Outcome evaluation assesses long-term changes such as CHD risk reduction.

In relation to the point made earlier concerning the function of PE (physiological and behavioural change), a call has been made recently to implement daily PE, particularly in primary schools. The School Sport Forum (1988, p. 15) recommends: "As part of a school health policy, there should be a daily session of vigorous physical activity in each primary school as part of the physical education programme or as a supplement to it. A local education authority should be asked to set up a pilot scheme to determine the value of a similar policy in the secondary school".

Daily PE Studies

The evaluation of daily PE interventions is very difficult and fraught with potential methodological problems. However, some interventions have been evaluated (Dwyer et al. 1983; Pollatschek and O'Hagan 1989; Williams et al. 1982).

Dwyer et al. (1983) conducted a study of daily PE in Australian primary schools (pupils aged 10 years). In phase I they looked at seven schools, in each of which were randomly assigned a "fitness" class, a "skill" class and a control group. The fitness class participated in daily fitness activities, the skill class had daily skill-based physical education, while the control group participated in more "traditional PE" for three 30-min periods each week. Physiological and academic measures were taken before and after a 14-week intervention period. Results suggested positive fitness changes for the fitness group compared with the other two groups, as expected. Academic performance was unaffected. A measure of classroom behaviour showed positive changes for both the fitness and skill groups, but this is probably due to teacher expectancy effects rather than the intervention itself.

Phase II involved the investigation of 216 students who had experienced 2 years of the daily PE programme, although this time they had a combined fitness and skills emphasis. However, although positive physiological measures were observed in this group, no control group was used. Also, the observers from phase I were also used in phase II, thus leading to the conclusion that changes could be influenced by observer bias. The arithmetic test results showed no change from the figures elicited by the previous group in phase I.

Although this study points to beneficial physiological changes as a result of daily PE, this is highly predictable. The key issues here centre on long-term change in behaviour as a result of such intervention, and the methods adopted by Dwyer et al. (1983) were not able to demonstrate this. It was a pity that no psychological measures were taken. Similarly, daily PE could, unless the teacher is particularly innovative and imaginative, become repetitive and uninspiring to the pupils.

Pollatschek and O'Hagan (1989) reported results from an intervention in Scotland that involved a "quality daily physical education" programme in primary schools. Based on a Canadian programme, Pollatschek and O'Hagan (1989, p. 342) list the following aims of their intervention:

"(i). to develop and maintain the physical fitness of pupils;

(ii). to develop efficient and effective motor skills in pupils and enable the children to apply these skills to a variety of physical activities;

(iii). to develop knowledge and understanding of factors involved in attaining competence in, and appreciation of, physical activity;

(iv). to develop natural links, using physical activity as a learning medium, with other curricular areas in order to maximise coherent learning situations for children;

(v). to develop and maintain positive personal attributes, interpersonal relationships, and a positive attitude towards participation in physical activity".

Few of these aims were directly tested in the study reported here, but the Pollatschek and O'Hagan (1989) paper was a report of only part of a wider project. However, it was unclear whether the reported research was attempting to study the health and fitness or skill outcomes of a daily PE programme.

A daily PE group (n = 222) was compared with a group experiencing "normal PE" (i.e., one period/week) (n = 83) on physical, academic and attitudinal measures before and after the intervention. Physical tests included a shuttle run, standing long-jump, sit-ups, flexed arm hang from a beam, 50-metre sprint, and endurance run. Some of these tests showed superior effects for the daily PE group after the intervention, although these differences occurred in only 5 of 12 post-intervention analyses (there were 6 tests for boys and girls separately). Indeed, the test item most relevant to health outcomes (endurance run) showed no difference between the daily and "normal" PE groups for boys or girls, despite the stated aims of the programme. This is probably a reflection of the maturational and motivational variability of the children (Malina 1989; Fox and Biddle 1988), the association between cardiovascular fitness and heredity, and the inconsistent validity of endurance run tests in testing cardiovascular performance (Safrit et al. 1988).

Unfortunately, the conclusions drawn by Pollatschek and O'Hagan are rather more optimistic than the data suggest. First, they concluded that the daily PE group was superior in motor fitness to the normal PE group in "most items" when, in fact, it was only just over 40% of the items, and second, Pollatschek and O'Hagan (1989, p. 347) concluded that "at a time of concern about the inactive lifestyles and lack of fitness in young people, the results from this action research project reinforce the benefits of a specially designed programme". However, as already stated, one of the key fitness tests (the endurance run) showed no change.

Pollatschek and O'Hagan found no difference in academic test score between the two groups after the intervention. The daily PE group had more positive attitude scores (attitudes to school) both pre- and post-test. The only "evidence" cited by these authors for positive affective change was anecdotal teacher reports, but these are likely to be affected by a response bias, or halo effect, as the teachers were aware of the intervention.

Williams et al. (1982) studied the effect of daily physical education on primary school children in New Zealand on the attitudes children held towards physical activity. After a 10-week intervention no difference was noted between an experimental and control group similar in socio-economic background. However, a more positive attitude was found after the programme for an experimental group that was lower in socio-economic status and who had low pre-test attitude scores.

From the studies related to daily physical education, it can be concluded that while cardiorespiratory fitness may be improved through such regular involvement in exercise, there is little evidence supporting the view that physical activity levels are increased (see Bryant et al. 1984a, b; Coates et al. 1981; MacConnie et al. 1982; Perry et al. 1987; Shephard et al. 1980).

In summary, the daily PE studies reported have failed to provide the necessary evaluative rigour to conclude about the benefits of daily PE, other than the obvious (and probably transitory) physical changes. Daily PE requires greater scrutiny and evaluation, including longitudinal study, before judgements can be made about its effectiveness or desirability in promoting children's health.

Children, Exercise and Public Health

The "public health" approach is one that concentrates on the level of functioning and well-being in a community rather than in any one individual (Powell 1988; see Chap. 1). It is an approach that is relevant to the application of psychological principles to the promotion of exercise in the school, workplace and community, although many interventions will, of course, include more individually-based strategies. Schools clearly are an important vehicle for promoting public health, including exercise and habitual physical activity.

Simons-Morton et al. (1987) discussed the interface between public health, children and exercise. They concluded that while children are probably the fittest section of society, at least in terms of cardiorespiratory fitness, the limited data available suggest that children are very inactive in their leisure time (see Armstrong 1990). Similarly, Simons-Morton et al. (1987) report that observational studies of PE lessons often show very little sustained activity suitable for the enhancement of cardiorespiratory fitness, with over a third of lesson time being devoted to management and organisational issues. In addition, these authors addressed the important public health issue of whether children's activities had a "behavioural carry-over" into adulthood (see section on childhood–adulthood links, earlier in this chapter).

Simons-Morton et al. (1987) concluded:

1. children's cardiorespiratory fitness requires better assessment across the population
2. children's physical activity patterns require better assessment, including the use of more consistent definitions of levels of physical activity
3. assessment is required of the amount of time spent in moderate to vigorous physical activity (MVPA) in school PE time
4. studies are required which investigate the effects of PE programmes that are oriented towards the use of MVPA on the MVPA of youth in leisure time and the carry-over into adulthood

The paper by Simons-Morton et al. (1987) brought a series of rebuttals (Bar-Or 1987; Corbin 1987; Cureton 1987; Lee et al. 1987; Sallis 1987; Seefeldt and Vogel 1987) and a subsequent reply from Simons-Morton et al. (1988a) (see also the extended discussion by Simons-Morton et al. 1988b).

Bar-Or (1987) concluded that the school should be used as the primary target for promoting public health through exercise. However, he put the emphasis on the need for physical educators to change their programmes to cater for a greater emphasis on health. Drawing on successful intervention programmes for weight control in schools, Bar-Or (1987) suggested that a successful programme requires multidisciplinary input across exercise, nutrition and behaviour modification, regular structured physical activity opportunities, a team approach across the school staff, and parental involvement.

Cureton (1987), in his rebuttal to the Simons-Morton et al. (1987) paper, supported Bar-Or's call for a shift in emphasis in school physical education. Cureton (1987, p. 318) says "The fact that school physical educators have not responded more rapidly to alter traditional curricula in order to place more emphasis on teaching physical fitness and health concepts and exposing children to physical activity and skills that can be used throughout life to promote health and fitness is discouraging".

Lee et al. (1987), however, question whether it is feasible to redesign PE curricula to improve cardiovascular fitness and, at the same time, still achieve important objectives such as skill development; a point echoed by Corbin (1987) and Seefeldt and Vogel (1987). The latter researchers question whether sufficient time is available in the PE curriculum to achieve the fitness and health objectives stated by Simons-Morton et al. (1987).

Similarly, time expended on such a singular objective, according to Seefeldt and Vogel, is questionable. Lee et al. suggested that health/fitness attitude change was more important. Similarly, Sallis (1987) thought that transient fitness changes were not as important as longer-term changes in behaviours, and suggested (pp. 328–329): "school physical education programmes must affect physical activity outside class and over time if they are to be considered successful ... It is clear that the current generation of school physical education programmes are not serving the public health needs of children, but it is not apparent what the characteristics of the next generation of physical education programmes should be".

Simons-Morton et al. (1988a) concluded that they believed that a major goal for physical education was to increase the proportion of children receiving appropriate physical activity, which they defined as MVPA with carry-over value for adulthood. They recognised the time constraints, but suggested two strategies. First, class time should have a greater proportion of MVPA than is usually the case, and second, physical educators must encourage children to adopt physical activity in their leisure time by making it enjoyable and fostering appropriate knowledge and skills.

This public health perspective has been mirrored by developments in Britain, some of which were discussed at the beginning of this chapter. Much remains to be done, but recognition that the school has the potential to be a major catalyst for important public health initiatives needs to be stronger, and a greater use of well-controlled longitudinal studies of the outcomes of such health programmes is also required.

The school has been discussed in some depth as it is the institution that has such a clear role in promoting exercise and health through the curriculum, and in particular physical and health education. However, recent developments have also led to exercise and health being promoted in other settings, such as the workplace.

The Workplace

An area that has seen considerable expansion in the field of health/fitness promotion is that of worksite or "corporate" fitness programmes. They are often more extensive than just exercise and fitness programmes and are sometimes referred to as "wellness" programmes. This expansion is particularly evident in North America and Japan, although European initiatives also exist (Fielding 1984; Shephard 1986). This section of the chapter, therefore, will consider the rationale behind such programmes and the claims made about cost effectiveness. In addition, an example programme will be outlined and the associated psychological issues of corporate promotion of fitness, particularly adherence to such programmes, will be discussed.

Rationale for Corporate Wellness Programmes

The motivations and rationale behind the development of health and fitness programmes at the worksite can be quite varied and need not necessarily be economic. Some of the major benefits thought to accrue from such programmes include improved corporate image and recruitment, better productivity, lower absenteeism and worker turnover, and reduced medical costs and incidence of industrial injuries (Shephard 1986, 1989a).

Corporate Image and Recruitment

It has been argued that the type of person attracted to a company offering a comprehensive wellness programme will be a high achiever, have a low absenteeism record and good productivity. This is difficult to quantify although the improved company image that may stem from such an intervention should enhance recruitment prospects. In addition, an appropriate advertising theme may centre on health and fitness, such as the "strength", "fitness/leanness", or "power" of the company. All of these factors may, directly or indirectly, increase worker satisfaction.

Productivity

Subjective reports have indicated favourable changes in productivity with the introduction of a company fitness or wellness programme. However, many of the studies have examined the impact on white-collar workers where the measurement of productivity is difficult. In addition, it is problematic to measure productivity of blue-collar or shop-floor workers; they are unlikely to support a wellness programme with productivity improvements as a key outcome. However, in a review by Shephard (1989a), ten of eleven studies showed increases in productivity, measured in a variety of ways, after a fitness intervention. However, few studies are able to control for Hawthorn effects when conducting research in this environment.

Absenteeism

Similarly, studies on absenteeism and corporate fitness programmes are favourable, and Shephard (1989a) reports such a trend in 18 of 19 studies. It is possible, however, that a self-selection process is at work here with only the conscientious workers choosing the health and fitness programmes. However, anecdotal evidence also suggests that some workers will volunteer to participate in fitness programmes, if conducted in work time, in order to avoid their work commitments.

Turnover

There is little systematic evidence on the effects of fitness programmes on staff turnover. However, if the previous suggestions concerning recruitment, company image and worker satisfaction are true, one could expect a reduced turnover of staff with such a programme. This, of course, is not always positive as all corporations will want some turnover to maintain a freshness of approach and to generate new ideas.

Most of the apparent benefits so far mentioned have yet to be compared with other interventions, such as increased holiday entitlement, better pay and conditions, and other factors.

Medical Costs

The upsurge of health and fitness programmes in industrial companies in North America could, at least in part, be attributed to the huge costs incurred for health insurance. However, a similar trend towards private health insurance for British workers in some companies means that industrial concerns may increase their investment in fitness programmes. Recent research suggests that medical costs can be reduced substantially through appropriate interventions to encourage health and fitness (Shephard 1989a).

Industrial Injuries

British estimates suggest that over two million people consult their GP about back pain in any one year with the peak occurring in the 45–65-year-old group – often the most valuable people to industry. Back pain also accounts for nearly 10% of the days lost through certified incapacity for work (see Wells 1985).

Health and fitness interventions could reduce this burden on industry and on the individual. Exercise may be an appropriate strategy for some back-pain sufferers (see Nachemson 1990; Patton et al. 1986; Powell 1988, and Chap. 1), although other interventions are also possible, such as classes in posture and methods of lifting objects, stress management, and ergonomic considerations in the workplace.

Positive results have been reported from a small number of studies investigating fitness programmes and industrial injuries (Shephard 1989a).

Evaluating the Outcomes of Corporate Wellness Programmes

So far, a case has been made for the benefits of industrial wellness programmes that has been based primarily on economic indicators, either directly or indirectly. This reflects a cost benefit analysis (CBA) approach whereby an evaluation of the effectiveness of the programme is performed.

However, recent work suggests that other approaches could be used, such as a cost effectiveness analysis (CEA) or a cost utility analysis (CUA). These are summarised in Table 10.2. It is likely that companies interested in developing a wellness programme will go beyond a CBA and look towards CEA whereby competing resources are considered. However, ultimately, a CUA may be used whereby the quality of life of the employees may be the prime consideration (Everly et al. 1987; Smith 1985).

Johnson and Johnson "Live for Life" Programme

The Johnson and Johnson pharmaceuticals company established their "Live for Life" wellness programme in the late 1970s (see Wilbur and Garner 1984). A number of interventions took place, but two are of particular interest here: the "core action programmes" and environmental changes.

The core action programmes consisted of a number of courses on offer to the staff. These included: smoking cessation, weight control, exercise, stress management, yoga, nutrition, and "personal power" (a stress-control and assertiveness course). Such programmes are likely to suffer from poor adherence rates and thus the impact, when averaged across all employees, could be quite low. However, in addition to structured and supervised programmes, Johnson and Johnson also made a number of environmental changes in an effort to promote a healthier lifestyle. These included fitness and exercise changes (installation of locker and shower facilities on site, as well as exercise equipment), nutrition information in food areas, healthier foods in vending machines and cafeterias, weighing scales in toilet areas, and a referral service for stress management. Additional stress management interventions included the introduction of flexible working hours, the encouragement of car sharing for travelling to and from work, and blood-pressure checks. A smoking policy was formulated for the company and greater publicity to the wellness programme was available through increased use of notice boards, newsletters etc.

Evaluation of the "Live for Life" programme shows positive results across

Table 10.2. Economic Measures of Health and the Effectiveness of a Corporate Wellness Programme. (Adapted from Smith 1985)

Type of Evaluation	Question Attempted to be Answered
Cost Benefit Analysis (CBA)	Does the programme pay off?
Cost Effectiveness Analysis (CEA)	How effective is the programme compared with investment in other resources?
Cost Utility Analysis (CUA)	How does the programme affect the length and quality of life?

a number of health and lifestyle factors. In addition, evaluation is ongoing for other indices, such as attitudes, as well as economic markers such as turnover and productivity (see Wilbur et al. 1986; Wilbur and Garner 1984).

Psychological Issues in Corporate Wellness Programmes

One of the most important issues associated with corporate wellness programmes is that of adherence. The investment in staff, facilities and other aspects of the programme may affect only a small percentage of the workforce if there is a high drop-out rate. Factors affecting adherence to exercise have already been discussed at some length in this book (see Chap. 2). However, in this section the issue of adherence will be considered briefly as it relates to research conducted in industrial settings. More detailed discussion can be found in Baun and Bernacki (1988), Gettman (1988) and Shephard (1988).

Davis et al. (1984) studied the factors likely to influence the intention to participate in worksite health promotion activities. Investigating a variety of health behaviours, including exercise, with a sample of over 800 State employees in South Carolina, Davis et al. found that perceptions of being at risk from lack of exercise were related to the intention to participate in a worksite health promotion programme. This is an important issue as quite often researchers and health promoters will find that programmes are attended by those already partly adopting the behaviour in question (see Bailey and Biddle 1988) or who are at low risk. The people who need the intervention the most are often those least likely to get involved (Dishman et al. 1985). Davis et al. (1984) also found that perceptions of low self-efficacy in exercise were predictive of an intention to change their behaviours and to be dissatisfied with their current activity levels (see Chap. 5). This led Davis et al. to propose a psychosocial model of health promotion in the workplace.

Steinhardt and Carrier (1989) expanded on this approach by investigating the social-environmental, physical-behavioural, and psychological factors influencing both early and continued participation in a worksite fitness programme. They studied 403 employees of the Conoco World Headquarters in Houston, Texas. Measures were taken, or were available, on:

1. participation rates at one and six months
2. psychological data: specifically measures of estimation of physical ability and attraction to physical activity, self-motivation, and attitudinal commitment to exercise
3. physical data: cardiovascular fitness, body fat, and recent participation
4. social-environmental: youth participation, social support, and convenience of the facility

Results were analysed by dividing the subjects into two groups: "adherers" (more than six visits per month) and "non-adherers" (fewer than six visits per month). At 1 month the groups could be seen to be clearly different such that adherers reported greater convenience of the exercise facility, a higher attitudinal commitment, and greater recent participation. Additionally, adherers were more likely to be males. However, predictors of adherence at 6 months were slightly different. Convenience of the facility and attitudinal commitment were still significant predictors of adherence, but in addition so was estimation of physical ability. Higher body fat also predicted drop-out – a finding reported elsewhere (Dishman and Gettman 1980; Dishman et al. 1985). Overall, the Conoco health and fitness programme was successful in attracting over 60% of the employees to enrol at the fitness centre. However, the adherence rates were not better than 50%, although this is typical of supervised exercise programmes (Dishman 1990; Dishman et al. 1985), and is similar to the adherence rate reported by Farrally et al. (1988) with workers in a Scottish company.

Wier and Jackson (1989) reported that employees participating in the NASA Johnson Space Centre fitness programme were best predicted by prior activity patterns and higher aerobic fitness. This suggests that corporations need to implement strategies that are likely to appeal to the sedentary and "unfit" worker so that the benefits of the programme accrue across as wide a sample of the company's workforce as possible.

In a study of a small sample of police officers, Gettman et al. (1983) reported better adherence rates for those in an unsupervised exercise condition. The major reason for drop-out was perceived lack of time. These results suggest that fitness programmes in corporations need to be flexible and not always supervised, so that the problem of formally arranged times for exercise is reduced. Fitness programmes may need to be part of the normal working day to avoid these problems. Wanzel and Danielson (1977) also reported factors associated with inconvenience as major reasons for drop-out from a Canadian corporate fitness programme.

In a review of the effectiveness of fitness promotion programmes in modifying exercise behaviours, Godin and Shephard (1983) suggest that the workplace offers a convenient and cost-effective environment in which to promote physical fitness. However, they also recognise that changes must occur in society at large, such as an acceptance of exercise as a societal norm, before physical activity and fitness promotion, in the workplace or elsewhere, becomes more successful than the current adherence rates suggest.

In conclusion, Shephard's (1985) main comments on the establishment of a corporate fitness programme are high-lighted:

1. only 20% of employees will take up the offer of a regular exercise programme; half will have dropped out within a few months

2. physicians (GPs) should be contacted for support of the company programme
3. blue-collar workers and people at the "low end" of the white-collar organisations need to be targeted
4. the most frequently pursued activities (e.g., jogging, walking, swimming) require little organisation, equipment and no partner
5. the main perceived barrier is lack of time
6. a fairly slow rate of progression in exercise programmes should be adopted in order to avoid injury, discomfort etc
7. graded classes should be provided to accommodate varying ability/fitness levels
8. the reasons why employees will want to become active are: looking good, feeling good, making social contacts, and being in better health

The Community

The changes in patterns of physical activity in Western societies are now becoming more extensively documented at the community level (Canada Fitness Survey 1983a, b; Collins 1987; Fenner 1987; McIntosh and Charlton 1985; Stephens 1987). However, there remain many problems with the evaluation of appropriate "outcomes" in community campaigns in exercise promotion (Iverson et al. 1985; Wankel 1988). This section of the chapter will address the promotion of exercise in the community and make specific reference to psychological factors that have received some attention in research studies with community samples. Details of participation patterns will not be dealt with in detail here but can be found in Chap. 1 and some studies on community samples that have a bearing on specific psychological issues are also addressed in other chapters.

Factors Affecting Community Exercise Participation

The determinants of physical activity and exercise in the community are potentially vast in number and would require a truly multidisciplinary perspective to reveal anything like a "true" picture and would include social, demographic, environmental, economic and cultural factors. Given the theme of this book, therefore, a more restricted view will be outlined here and will concentrate on the motivations and attitudes of participants and drop-outs from community programmes (see Iso-Ahola 1980; Wankel 1988). Wider issues of public health campaigns and exercise will be considered where appropriate.

Why Do People Participate?

Although this issue has been dealt with in the chapter on exercise adherence, the reasons identified through community surveys will be high-lighted with a view to providing guidelines for community promotion of exercise.

One of the most extensive surveys of involvement in physical activity across the community was carried out by the Canadian government through the Canada Fitness Survey (1983a). Over 23 000 Canadians over the age of 10 years were investigated. When compared with other health-related behaviours, this sample placed physical activity as being less important to their health than adequate sleep, good diet, medical/dental care, not smoking, maintaining weight, and control of stress. Nevertheless, 46% of the sample rated physical activity as "very important to their well-being", although predictably this figure fell to 26% for those categorised as sedentary. When people were asked to rate ten different reasons for being active in their leisure time a trend towards health and well-being was quite evident. Fig. 2.2 in Chap. 2 shows the results for the five highest rated reasons across all subjects with the graph showing the percentage of cases rating the reason as "very important". Although one might expect age differences here, the results of the Canadian Youth and Physical Activity study of the Canada Fitness Survey (1983b) are similar for the 10–18-year-old group as across the full age range (see Fig. 10.4). However, unpublished data of our own suggest that participants in sports and exercise at a selected group of British leisure centres do differ by age in their motives for participation. The younger participants tended to be more motivated by challenge and skill-learning whereas the older participants reported stronger motivation for health, relaxation and social factors (Ashford and Biddle 1990).

Fig. 10.5 illustrates the main obstacles to exercise identified in the 20-years-and-over age group in the Canada Fitness Survey (1983a). This shows that the main obstacles are related to perceived lack of time and poor motivation. This is supported by studies of supervised exercise programme drop-outs (Dishman et al. 1985) and local community surveys (Butler 1987; Lawrence et al. 1988) and suggests that a lack of community facilities is not necessarily such a problem as is sometimes thought.

The results of the Canada Fitness Survey suggest that the time factor is greater for men whereas the effort and motivation factor is greater for women. This requires further investigation from the point of view of remedial strategies and community provision. Whether these gender differences are related to lifestyle *per se* remains to be seen. Also, a more detailed understanding of the meaning attached to these terms is required. "Effort" may reflect inconvenience and time factors in arranging exercise or could apply equally to the physical effort needed in more vigorous programmes. As reported in Chap. 2, sex-role perceptions and prior experience of exercise intensity may affect ratings of perceived effort during

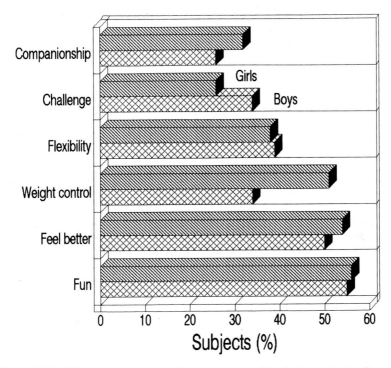

Figure 10.4. Main reasons rated as "very important" for being active by Canadian youths aged 10–19 years. (Adapted from Canada Fitness Survey 1983b.)

prolonged exercise, as may other non-physiological factors (see Dishman and Landy 1988; Williams and Eston 1989).

Given these results, it is predictable that when these subjects were asked about factors that might encourage them to become more active, the factor of time was dominant (see Fig. 10.6). Two particularly important results are evident here. First, 20% said that "nothing would increase activity" for them, suggesting that a hard core of non-exercisers poses a particular problem as far as change is concerned. Second, only 6% said that more information on the benefits of physical activity would encourage them to become more active. This supports the summary findings reported by Dishman et al. (1985) that information *per se* does not provide the necessary motivation for change in behaviour, although the source of the information can be an important factor (see Eadie and Leathar 1988). It is likely that many people already know the potential benefits of exercise but that changing behaviour requires the learning of new behavioural skills, reduction of perceived barriers, increased social support, and other factors.

It is widely believed that Western societies have experienced an "exercise boom" since the early 1980s. Unfortunately, the data do not provide for easy comparisons over time, although it is thought that a greater interest

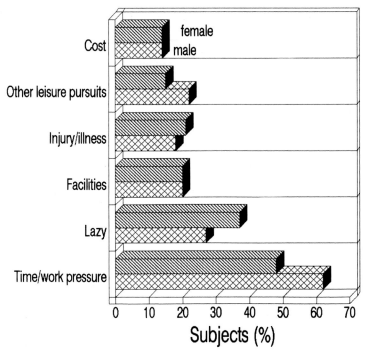

Figure 10.5. Main obstacles to increased physical activity for Canadian adults. (Adapted from Canada Fitness Survey 1983a.)

in exercise for health reasons currently exists than previously (Blair et al. 1987b; Collins 1987; Stephens 1987).

A study commissioned for the Sports Council (Schlackmans 1986) highlights the nature and extent of women's involvement in community health and fitness programmes. They studied just under 2000 active and inactive women in ten towns in England in both exercise and non-exercise settings. A variety of exercise classes were identified, ranging from "traditional" keep-fit classes, jazz dance groups, and "American stretch" classes, to aerobic exercise to music ("aerobics") classes. From a psychological perspective it is informative to note that six different clusters of participants were identified (see Table 10.3).

The "sporty socialisers" represented those who were interested in the social aspects of the exercise class, and yet, at the same time, seemed to be quite fit, good at other sports and interested in their own progress in exercise. The "weight conscious" group reported being interested in the exercise primarily for weight loss, and were more likely to perceive themselves as being overweight and were less likely to take part in other sports.

The "keen exercisers" showed opposite trends to the "weight conscious" group. The "keen exercisers" reported being particularly interested in the physical fitness benefits of the class but not the social aspects, and they were concerned about the quality of instruction. They tended to be good at other sports and perceived themselves to be fit. The majority were in full-time work and without children.

The other three groups were clearly associated with different stages in the life cycle. The "get out of the house" group was the youngest and represented those who had little interest in the social or physical benefits of the exercise class, but used the class as a means of merely getting away from the house. The group labelled "modern mothers" was slightly older, keen on sport and quite fit. The majority had given up work, they were interested in their exercise progress, and did not attend classes merely to get away from the house. Finally, the "social contact" group was older than the "modern mothers" and seemed to represent women who either lived alone or whose children had left home. They were interested in the exercise classes from a social contact perspective. The adherence to these classes tended to be very good.

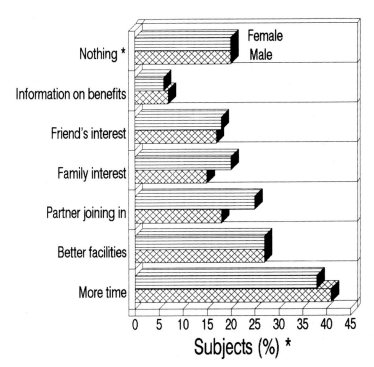

Figure 10.6. Main changes that would encourage more activity in Canadian adults. (Adapted from Canada Fitness Survey 1983a.) *Note: percentages for the changes include those who identified at least one change and exclude those who said "nothing".

Table 10.3. Clustering of Women's Exercise Classes. (Adapted from Schlackmans 1986)

Group	Estimated Percentage of Women's Exercise Market
Sporty Socialisers	25%
Weight Conscious	18%
Keen Exercisers	17%
Get Out of the House	8%
Modern Mothers	16%
Social Contact	15%

These data, in addition to previous studies that have investigated participation motivation in community samples (Canada Fitness Survey 1983a, b), demonstrate the importance of understanding the variety of motives people may have in adopting and maintaining involvement in community exercise settings. The Schlackmans (1986) report also showed that the women's exercise market is a volatile one and that women will drop out and re-enter this market fairly frequently. This needs consideration by exercise promoters.

Attitudes towards Exercise and Public Health Campaigns

The relationship between attitude and behaviour has been discussed in Chap. 3, along with research data on the nature of attitudes towards exercise. Although there are few data on the extent of attitude *change* in relation to exercise, the increased levels of participation in recent years suggests that a similar shift in attitude has also occurred. However, recent data from the Heartbeat Wales (1987) project reveal that changes in knowledge, attitude and beliefs are still needed for quite a large number of people.

One of the few studies to investigate attitudes about exercise and fitness, using qualitative techniques, was undertaken by Eadie and Leathar (1988). These researchers specifically set themselves two objectives: (1) to ascertain what people understand by the terms "health" and "fitness" and what factors are thought to influence health and fitness; (2) to understand how media campaigns might influence people's ideas about fitness and health.

Qualitative group discussions were used and approximately 140 subjects were involved, all from Glasgow and Edinburgh. In terms of the respondents' understanding of the terms fitness and health, at least six dimensions could be differentiated: perceptual emphasis (positive or negative), level of complexity (simple or complex), level of importance (high or low), measurability (easy or difficult), behavioural objectives (improvement or maintenance), and amount of control (high or low).

Regarding the perceptual emphasis, subjects viewed fitness as a physical ability helping them to carry out their daily routine. It was also associated with positive leisure activity, such as sport and exercise. Health, on the other hand, tended to be viewed negatively, for example in terms of illness and problems.

Fitness was also seen as a physical concept whereas health was viewed as physical and social. Health tended to be viewed in a more complex way and was seen to be more important than fitness, yet more difficult to measure.

Views were expressed about the difference between maintenance and improvement. Fitness was seen as a concept involving improvement whereas health was viewed more in terms of maintenance. Interestingly, although many respondents thought fitness could be controlled, few exercised this control. Physical activity perceived as requiring effort and commitment was labelled unenjoyable. Finally, health was largely seen to be uncontrollable, with some exceptions.

These data provide interesting insight into the different perceptions associated with fitness, exercise and health in a Scottish sample. Eadie and Leathar (1988) concluded that their respondents viewed fitness as an element of health and as a means to health, and also that health was a pre-condition to fitness. However, the majority viewed themselves as healthy but unfit. Only in exceptional circumstances was the view expressed that someone could be fit but unhealthy.

The terms "sport", "exercise" and "active recreation" were viewed differently. Sport was associated with aggressive, active, interpersonal competition whereas exercise was seen primarily in terms of developing physical abilities such as endurance and strength. Active recreation described the overlap between sport and exercise, such as walking. These distinctions are shown in Fig. 10.7.

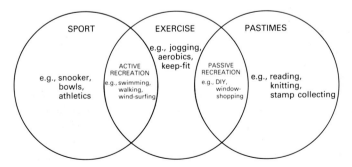

Figure 10.7. Perceptions of sport, exercise and leisure. (From Eadie and Leathar 1988. Reprinted with kind permission of The Scottish Sports Council.)

Not surprisingly, Eadie and Leathar (1988) found that television was perceived as the most powerful source of information about community health and fitness, and, for women, the use of magazines was also seen as appropriate for the dissemination of information. Social advertising (i.e. information/persuasion campaigns) was viewed as potentially effective as long as it was interesting and attractive, not negative or over-persuasive, was new or unique, and attempted to extend existing attitudes rather than change them outright. Some views were expressed that suggested that "authoritarian" messages were disliked, as were those originating from central government. Local messages and campaigns were viewed as creating greater identification with the campaign theme and were thought to be more likely to produce effective changes.

In summary, Eadie and Leathar's (1988) research suggested that fitness marketing in the community should observe four main guidelines. First, it should have a positive appeal. Fitness was seen as relatively unimportant to many of the subjects in this study. Therefore, appeals to exercise based on fear of negative events are likely to be rejected. Marketing should emphasise the more immediate social and mental benefits. Second, a greater emphasis on "universal representation" is required to make fitness and exercise a socially acceptable activity for all and not just for those fit and good at sport. However, and third, campaigns must recognise individuality by suggesting a wide range of opportunities for people to choose from. Finally, fitness marketing should high-light the informal nature of participation, since many people appear to be put off highly structured and professionalised activities. These recommendations resemble those of Olson and Zanna (1981).

Fitness Testing and Exercise Promotion

A technique that has been used extensively to promote health and fitness is physical fitness testing (Bailey and Biddle 1988; Crowe 1987; Godin and Shephard 1983). Two types of strategies have been used: a mobile unit travelling to particular locations, such as worksites, and a fitness-testing station at a community "health fair". Crowe (1987) reports positive, although largely anecdotal, evaluations of fitness tests at health fairs, and there is generally very little information available on the effectiveness of such promotional strategies, although the results of fitness tests in rehabilitation settings have shown some positive results from a motivational perspective (Bruce et al. 1980; Oldridge and Spencer 1985). Godin and Shephard (1983) were unable to draw definitive conclusions from their review of studies on the effectiveness of fitness promotion programmes in modifying exercise behaviours. Of the 15 studies reviewed only five evaluated long-term cost effectiveness and cost-benefit. The others were "impact" studies which evaluated only the immediate effects of the promotion.

Bailey and Biddle (1988) reported data from the health fair located at the 1986 British National Garden Festival at Stoke-on-Trent where over 13 000 people participated in health-related physical fitness tests. However, the data revealed that the less fit were most reluctant to take part although a small follow-up study did show that the fitness testing had a positive motivational effect on those who did undergo the initial test battery.

In concluding this section on community issues in health and fitness promotion, it is clear that public health campaigns and community promotional strategies must account for the wide variations in motivations and perceptions that are associated with the concepts of health, fitness, sport and exercise. Nevertheless, both the Canadian and the Welsh data do at least suggest that health-related motives are strong in the intent to be physically active (Canada Fitness Survey 1983a; Heartbeat Wales 1987).

Medical Settings

The psychological factors associated with the promotion of health-related activity in medical settings centres primarily on cardiac rehabilitation, particularly in respect of adherence (Oldridge 1988). In addition, Mutrie (1986) has reported success in developing improved mental health through exercise in a medical setting. This is supported by Prosser and his co-workers (Prosser et al. 1978, 1981, 1985; see also Biddle 1989c). The literature relevant to exercise-based cardiac rehabilitation adherence is reviewed in Chap. 2, and mental health studies are described in Chaps 6–8. Similarly, Taylor et al. (1985) have shown that self-efficacy can be enhanced in both men who have suffered a myocardial infarction and their wives, following appropriate exercise intervention in medical settings. This study was reviewed in Chap. 5.

The dominant resource allocation in British hospitals is towards curative rather than preventive measures, with the National Health Service (NHS) accounting for over 90% of annual British health expenditure (Chew 1986). Nevertheless, it is possible that a greater orientation towards preventive medicine may include the promotion of exercise through medical personnel. For example, Iverson et al. (1985) suggest that the family practitioner is well placed to provide advice about exercise although the education of medical doctors may not always include contemporary research from the exercise sciences. Indeed, the content of Sherin's (1983) paper on the health benefits of exercise and appropriate exercise prescription suggests that some medical practitioners are not well informed of the basics of these topics. Similarly, Calnan and Johnson (1983) suggest that general practitioners

(GPs) can be effective health educators, but that more research is required to consider the best ways.

Thow and Newton (1990) reported their experience of establishing an exercise intervention both within and outside the hospital setting. Their programme was aimed at cardiac rehabilitation in the first instance, but overall they had a five-stage approach ranging from cardiac rehabilitation in the hospital to community health education promotions. Even though the initial emphasis was on post-MI patients, others were encouraged to attend, such as spouses and other hospital workers.

The evaluation of the impact medical practitioners have on the exercise habits of the community is not well documented. Wallace and Haines (1984) surveyed the attitudes of over 3000 patients in two areas of London. The results showed that 72% thought that their doctor should be interested in physical fitness, yet only 38% thought that their doctor actually had been interested. This discrepancy between patients' expectations and perceptions of interest taken by the GP was also evident for smoking, drinking and body weight.

Despite this discrepancy, Campbell et al. (1985) have reported a successful intervention in exercise promotion in a village community in southern England which involved the local doctor (see also Browne 1986). This is consistent with the philosophy emanating from recent government legislation, since the 1990 National Health Service and Community Care Act puts a greater emphasis on preventive health practice, including physical activity. For example, the Department of Health's (1990) pamphlet on the NHS reforms, which was sent to all households in the UK, states on p. 4 that "good health care is not just about treating you when you are ill, but also giving help and advice so that you stay fit and well". The pamphlet states explicitly that "lifestyle" check-ups will be available, including professional advice on exercise, and that GPs will be encouraged to provide more health promotion clinics (see Thow and Newton 1990).

Iverson et al. (1985) give the following points concerning exercise promotion in medical settings:

1. the majority of exercise programmes in medical settings are associated with cardiac rehabilitation
2. health personnel in medical settings are in an excellent position to offer advice on exercise, and this is particularly true for family practitioners who are more likely to be in regular contact (see Calnan and Johnson 1983)
3. advice from a doctor is frequently cited as a possible motivating factor to exercise
4. evidence appears to show that relatively few family practitioners counsel their patients about exercise
5. it appears that doctors can be effective in changing patient behaviours, thus providing an important source for exercise promotion

It appears, however, that despite recent legislation in the UK (see Department of Health 1990), there is some way to go before promotion of physical activity becomes a widely practised feature of medical care settings other than as part of rehabilitation and curative programmes.

11

Conclusions and Future Directions

There is little doubt that the majority of health-related research in the exercise and sport sciences has been from a biological perspective. The state-of-the-science book produced from the 1988 International Conference on Exercise, Fitness and Health, held in Toronto, Canada (Bouchard et al. 1990) contains 62 chapters. Only 6 of these could be classified as "behavioural" in orientation and include substantial reference to psychological or social issues associated with exercise behaviours. In short, we are in a much better position to answer the question "what happens to our body when we exercise?" than we are to answer the questions "what determines whether someone adopts a physically active lifestyle?" or "what happens psychologically during or after participation in exercise?" However, as argued throughout this book, the latter questions require answers if we are to optimise the benefits to physical health of physical activity and exercise.

The purpose of this book, therefore, has been to present the current research knowledge on the psychology of physical activity and exercise.

Summary Issues in the Psychology of Physical Activity and Exercise

Psychological Antecedents

Given the evidence supporting the benefits of appropriate physical activity for health promotion and reduction of risk for chronic disease, it is important to understand the likely determinants, correlates or antecedents of exercise.

There is little doubt that progress in this area will be enhanced through a multidisciplinary approach, utilising perspectives outlined in Fig. 2.11. While the point has been made that the psychological issues of participation have not been studied as extensively as they might, this is not to say that psychology has all the answers. Psychological constructs may well prove to be the important "end points" immediately before decision-making about physical activity. However, such decisions are also likely to be influenced by prior factors of social history, social setting, economics, political factors and so on. It is possible that some of these potential influences are removed in time from immediate decision-making ("distal" antecedents), whereas the psychological issues dealt with in this book may be more "proximal" antecedents. This requires testing.

There is little doubt that research into exercise adherence has been restrictive in terms of studying primarily participating adults in supervised exercise programmes. Work on the psychological antecedents of exercise should involve a developmental approach whereby the factors influencing participation at different times in the life cycle are identified for both supervised and more spontaneous or "free-living" settings, thus allowing for a clearer picture of the psychological antecedents of both exercise *and* physical activity.

Similarly, Sallis and Hovell (1990) have suggested that the antecedents, or determinants, of exercise require investigation at several different points in the "natural history" of exercise. This is illustrated in Fig. 11.1.

The natural history model suggests four phases that require investigation in terms of three transition stages:

1. from sedentary behaviour to exercise adoption

2. from adoption to either maintenance or drop-out

3. from drop-out to resumption

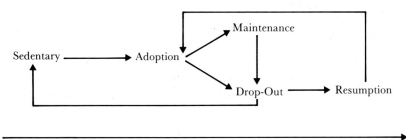

Figure 11.1. Four major phases of the natural history of exercise. (From "Determinants of exercise behaviour" by J. Sallis and M. Hovell (1990) *Exercise & Sport Sciences Reviews*, 18: 309. Reprinted with permission of the American College of Sports Medicine.)

We have more information on the maintenance of exercise than we do on either adoption or resumption.

Finally, it should be noted that this book has adopted psychological perspectives and models that have appeared most relevant to health and exercise behaviours, such as locus of control, self-efficacy etc. It remains to be seen in some cases whether these are the best models for studying exercise. An integration with biological factors, for example, may be required given the role of physical exertion in the behaviour under study.

Psychological Outcomes

The psychological or "mental health" outcomes of involvement in physical activity and exercise have proved elusive from a research perspective. This has been for two reasons. First, the measurement technology used for assessing outcomes has been varied and often inconsistent, and second, the experimental manipulations and control operated in research settings has not been optimal. However, one should not under-estimate the difficulty of research in this field, despite the frequently cited anecdotal reports of "feeling better" for exercise.

The effects of exercise may be different for different types of people, and for this reason we have separated "normal" from "clinical" populations. However, distinctions between other groups may also be required, such as age and gender. Indeed, Stephens (1988) found that the most pronounced benefits to mental health from physical activity in population surveys were reported by women and older subjects. Similarly, little is known of the effects of involvement in sport or exercise on children, despite the claims made about effects on self-esteem and "character" development. Although some evidence does support the potential for self-esteem enhancement in children through physical activity, it is likely that the *quality* of the experience, and in particular the leadership of teachers, parents etc, will be critical factors.

A consensus statement has been produced on exercise and mental health (Morgan and Goldston 1987). However, a number of issues remained unresolved. Although few workers would dispute the potential of exercise to increase feelings of well-being and mental health, more needs to be known about the mechanisms of such effects so that positive experiences can be maximised. This remains an important challenge for researchers since not only will it impact on mental health itself, but it is also likely to lead to greater adherence to exercise.

Interventions

Interventions can take place at the micro (individual) or macro (organisational) level. Both have been addressed here, although psychology has a longer history of looking at the individual's change in behaviour. Research suggests that behaviour modification strategies can have a significant impact on the adoption and maintenance of exercise, but this effect will weaken with time. The strategies, therefore, require to be learned from childhood rather than being seen as "special" interventions. For example, schools could teach children appropriate "lifestyle management" skills, such as goal-setting, self-reinforcement, time management, and other self-regulatory skills. These should be seen to be of equal importance to knowing about the effects of exercise on the body.

Interventions at the macro level have met with mixed success. The emphasis, at least in Britain, has tended to be in schools and in the community at large, with less emphasis being placed on exercise promotion in the workplace or in medical settings. However, this is now changing with governmental policy forcing a greater emphasis on health promotion in the National Health Service, and industry becoming more aware of the potential benefits of "corporate health" programmes. However, we need to know more about the mechanisms of behaviour change through such approaches.

Research Issues

Measurement

Two measurement issues require further work for the future. The first is measurement of the behaviour under investigation – physical activity and exercise. Adherence to supervised exercise programmes, while not easy to measure, does allow for the assessment of attendance, and possibly intensity and duration too. However, dropping out of a supervised programme may lead the researcher to classifying the individual as a non-adherer when the individual may choose to exercise elsewhere. Similarly, "adherence" to exercise should be seen as a process rather than a static or "all-or-none" behaviour.

The assessment of habitual physical activity is a more difficult problem because of its unstructured and sporadic nature. Methods such as heart rate telemetry and motion sensors have been used to quantify the level of activity throughout the day, but these methods do not inform us of the type of activity. Observational and self-report methods will be required to do this but some instruments have unknown properties of reliability and validity. In short, the assessment of physical activity is difficult, although expediency dictates that large-scale surveys of epidemiological significance will have to use self-report measures, although these should, of course, be validated against other measures.

The second measurement problem in this field concerns the assessment of the psychological antecedents and consequences of exercise. This problem is not unique to the behaviour under study in this book, of course, but has been an important issue in psychology from the earliest days of the discipline.

Antecedents. The following issues associated with the measurement of psychological antecedents of exercise require further attention.

1. The utility of general psychological trait measures in predicting exercise behaviour. Are more exercise-specific measures required? The discussion on locus of control (LOC) in Chap. 4 shows that the assessment of this construct has been made in terms of general LOC, health LOC and exercise/fitness LOC. However, the more specific measures for exercise have failed to predict exercise behaviours in a strong way. Similarly, the global trait of self-motivation, as measured with the SMI and reported in Chap. 2, may be a better predictor of exercise if questions in the inventory referred to exercise. At present the SMI assesses "general" self-motivation.

2. The utility of general psychological models. This has been alluded to earlier in this discussion. It remains to be seen how useful some models are in predicting exercise behaviours. It seems right, however, that one starting point should be a known and well-tested psychological theory. However, developments to include exercise-related factors may be required to improve the ability of models to predict exercise behaviour.

3. Research paradigms. To date, the psychological study of exercise and physical activity has adopted a positivistic approach, relying on experimental and quasi-experimental research designs. Other approaches are required to supplement this, such as case-study and single-subject designs, interview and qualitative methods.

Consequences. The following issues associated with the measurement of psychological consequences of exercise require further attention.

1. "Returning to base-line effect". It has yet to be demonstrated in some studies of the acute effects of exercise on mental health whether the reduction in, for example, anxiety after exercise is merely a return to a base-line level following the elevated levels of anxiety elicited by the testing situation.

2. Some standardisation in instruments is required, although the extensive use of just a few inventories, such as the State-Trait Anxiety Inventory, the Beck Depression Inventory, and the Profile of Mood States, has helped in this respect. Nevertheless, the large-scale survey data on exercise and mental health (e.g., Stephens 1988) report different instruments from those used in many laboratory studies.

3. The assessment of "mental health" is difficult and, to date, has been

restricted to anxiety, depression and self-esteem. Measures of quality of life and wider aspects of "well-being" are required to obtain a more complete picture.

Concluding Remarks

The major emphasis in research on exercise, physical activity and health has been in the physical and biological sciences, and this is also reflected in media coverage. Similarly, position statements, such as the New Case for Exercise (Fentem et al. 1988), give only passing mention to psychological aspects of exercise and health.

We hope, through this book, to have broadened this perspective by adopting a psychological perspective on health and physical activity, although we recognise that others must follow with their treatment of other potential influences. It is our belief that mental outcomes of exercise are equally as important as physical outcomes, and that without greater knowledge of the antecedents of exercise behaviours, they will not be achieved to the extent that we would wish from a public health perspective.

References

Abramson, L.Y., Seligman, M.E.P. & Teasdale, J.D. (1978). Learned helplessness in humans: Critique and reformulation. *Journal of Abnormal Psychology*, 87, 49–74.

Ajzen, I. (1988). *Attitudes, Personality and Behaviour*. Milton Keynes: Open University Press.

Ajzen, I. & Fishbein, M. (1980). *Understanding Attitudes and Predicting Social Behaviour*. Englewood Cliffs, NJ: Prentice-Hall.

Ajzen, I. & Madden, T.J. (1986). Prediction of goal-directed behaviour: Attitudes, intentions, and perceived behavioural control. *Journal of Experimental Social Psychology*, 22, 453–474.

Ajzen, I. & Timko, C. (1986). Correspondence between health attitudes and behaviour. *Basic and Applied Social Psychology*, 7, 259–276.

Akil, H., Watson, S.J., Young, E., Lewis, M.E., Khachaturian, H. & Walker, J.M. (1984). Endogenous opioids: Biology and function. *Annual Review of Neuroscience*, 7, 223–255.

Alexopoulos, G.S., Inturrisi, C.E., Lipman, R., France, R., Haycox, J., Dougherty, J.H. & Rossier, J. (1983). Plasma immunoreactive β-endorphin levels in depression. *Archives of General Psychiatry*, 40, 181–183.

Allen, M. (1983). Activity-generated endorphins: A review of their role in sports science. *Canadian Journal of Applied Sports Science*, 8, 115–133.

Alloy, L.B., Abramson, L.Y., Metalsky, G.I. & Hartlage, S. (1988). The hopelessness theory of depression: Attributional aspects. *British Journal of Clinical Psychology*, 27, 5–21.

American Alliance of Health, Physical Education, Recreation and Dance (AAHPERD) (1984). *Technical Manual: Health-related Physical Fitness*. Reston, Va: AAHPERD.

American Alliance of Health, Physical Education, Recreation and Dance (1988). *Physical Best: The American Alliance Physical Fitness Education and Assessment Program*. Reston, Va: AAHPERD.

American College of Sports Medicine (1978). Position statement on the recommended quantity and quality of exercise for developing and maintaining fitness in healthy adults. *Medicine and Science in Sports*, 10, vii–x.

American College of Sports Medicine (1986). *Guidelines for Graded Exercise Testing and Exercise Prescription*. Philadelphia: Lea & Febiger.

American College of Sports Medicine (1988). Opinion statement on physical fitness in children and youth. *Medicine and Science in Sports and Exercise*, 20, 422–423.

American College of Sports Medicine (1990). Position stand: The recommended quantity and quality of exercise for developing and maintaining cardiorespiratory and muscular fitness in healthy adults. *Medicine and Science in Sports and Exercise*, 22, 265–274.

American Psychiatric Association (1980). *Diagnostic and Statistical Manual of Mental Disorders* (3rd edn). Washington, DC: American Psychiatric Association.

Ames, C. & Ames, R. (1984). Goal structures and motivation. *The Elementary School Journal*, 85, 39–52.

Andrew, G.M. & Parker, J.O. (1979). Factors related to dropout of post myocardial infarction patients from exercise programmes. *Medicine and Science in Sports and Exercise*, 11, 376–378.

Andrew, G.M., Oldridge, N.B., Parker, J.O. et al. (1981). Reasons for dropout from exercise programmes in post-coronary patients. *Medicine and Science in Sports and Exercise*, 13, 164–168.

Anisman, H. (1984). Vulnerability to depression: Contribution of stress. In R.M. Post & J.C. Ballenger (Eds.). *Neurobiology of Mood Disorders*. Baltimore: Williams and Wilkins.

Appenzeller, D., Standefer, J., Appenzeller, J. & Atkinson, R. (1980). Neurology of endurance training. *Neurology*, 30, 418.

Armstrong, N. (1987). Health and fitness programmes in schools: A physiological rationale. In S.J.H. Biddle (Ed.). *Foundations of Health-related Fitness in Physical Education*. London: Ling (PEA).

Armstrong, N. (1990). Children's physical activity patterns: The implications for physical education. In N. Armstrong (Ed.). *New Directions in Physical Education - Volume 1*. Champaign: Human Kinetics.

Armstrong, N., Balding, J., Gentle, P. & Kirby, B. (1990a). Patterns of physical activity among 11 to 16 year old British children. *British Medical Journal*, 301, 203–205.

Armstrong, N., Balding, J., Gentle, P., Williams, J. & Kirby, B. (1990b). Peak oxygen uptake and physical activity in 11 to 16 year olds. *Pediatric Exercise Science*, 2, 349–358.

Ashford, B. & Biddle, S.J.H. (1990). Participation in community sports centres: Motives and predictors of enjoyment. Paper presented at British Association of Sports Sciences conference, Cardiff.

Atkins, C.J., Kaplan, R.M., Timms, R.M., Reinsch, S. & Lofback, K. (1984). Behavioural exercise programmes in the management of chronic obstructive pulmonary disease. *Journal of Consulting and Clinical Psychology*, 52, 591–603.

B.A.A.L.P.E. (1988). *Health-focused Physical Education*. Leeds: BAALPE.

Baekeland, F. (1970). Exercise deprivation: Sleep and psychological reactions. *Archives of General Psychiatry*, 22, 365–369.

Bahrke, M.S. & Morgan, W.P. (1978). Anxiety reduction following exercise and meditation. *Cognitive Therapy and Research*, 2, 323–333.

Bailey, D.A., (1973). Exercise, fitness and physical education for the growing child: A concern. *Canadian Journal of Public Health*, 64, 421–430.

Bailey, C. & Biddle, S. (1988). Community health-related physical fitness testing and the National Garden Festival Health Fair at Stoke-on-Trent. *Health Education Journal*, 47, 144–147.

Bandura, A. (1977a). *Social Learning Theory*. Englewood Cliffs, NJ: Prentice-Hall.

Bandura, A. (1977b). Self-efficacy: Toward a unifying theory of behavioural change. *Psychological Review*, 84, 191–215.

Bandura, A. (1986). *Social Foundations of Thought and Action: A Social Cognitive Theory*. Englewood Cliffs, NJ: Prentice-Hall.

Bandura, A. (1989). Perceived self-efficacy in the exercise of personal agency. *The Psychologist: Bulletin of the British Psychological Society*, 10, 411–424.

Bandura, A. (1990). Perceived self-efficacy in the exercise of personal agency. *Journal of Applied Sport Psychology*, 2, 128–163.

Bandura, A. & Adams, N.E. (1977).Analysis of self-efficacy theory of behavioural change. *Cognitive Therapy and Research*, 1, 287–310.

Bandura, A., Taylor, C.B., Williams, S.L., Mefford, I.N. & Barchas, J.D. (1985).

Catecholamine secretion as a function of perceived coping self-efficacy. *Journal of Consulting and Clinical Psychology*, 53, 406–414.

Bandura, A., Cioffi, D., Taylor, C.B. & Brouillard, M.E. (1988). Perceived self-efficacy in coping with cognitive stressors and opioid activation. *Journal of Personality and Social Psychology*, 55, 479–488.

Bannister, D. & Fransella, F. (1971). *Inquiring Man*. Baltimore: Penguin.

Barker, D.J.P. & Rose, G. (1990). *Epidemiology in Medical Practice*. Edinburgh: Churchill Livingstone.

Bar-On, D. & Cristal, N. (1987). Causal attributions of patients, their spouses and physicians, and the rehabilitation of the patients after their first myocardial infarction. *Journal of Cardiopulmonary Rehabilitation*, 7, 285–298.

Bar-Or, O. (1987). A commentary to children and fitness: A public health perspective. *Research Quarterly for Exercise and Sport*, 58, 304–307.

Bar-Or, O. & Ward, D.S. (1989). Rating of perceived exertion in children. In O. Bar-Or (Ed.). *Advances in Pediatric Sport Sciences: III. Biological Issues*. Champaign: Human Kinetics.

Barrell, G., High, S., Holt, D. & MacKean, J. (1988). Motives for starting running and for competing in full and half marathon events. In *Sport, Health, Psychology and Exercise Symposium proceedings*. London: The Sports Council/Health Education Authority.

Barrell, G., Chamberlain, A., Evans, J., Holt, J. & MacKean, J. (1989). Ideology and commitment in family life: A case study of runners. *Leisure Studies*, 8, 249–262.

Baun, W.B. & Bernacki, E.J. (1988). Who are corporate exercisers and what motivates them? In R.K. Dishman (Ed.). *Exercise Adherence: Its Impact on Public Health*. Champaign: Human Kinetics.

Beck, A.T., Ward, C.H., Mendelson, M., Mock, J. & Erbaugh, J. (1961). An inventory for measuring depression. *Archives of General Psychiatry*, 4, 561–571.

Becker, M.H., Haefner, D.P., Kasl, S.V., Kirscht, J.P., Maiman, L.A. & Rosenstock, I.M. (1977a). Selected psychosocial models and correlates of individual health-related behaviours. *Medical Care*, 15 (Supplement), 27–46.

Becker, M.H., Maiman, L.A., Kirscht, J.P., Haefner, D.P. & Drachman, R.H. (1977b). The Health Belief Model and prediction of dietary compliance: A field experiment. *Journal of Health and Social Behaviour*, 18, 348–366.

Becker, M.H., Radius, S.M., Rosenstock, I.M., Drachman, R.H., Schuberth, K.C. & Teets, K.C. (1978). Compliance with a medical regimen for asthma: A test of the Health Belief Model. *Public Health Reports*, 93, 268–277.

Belisle, M., Roskies, E. & Levesque, J-M. (1987). Improving adherence to physical activity. *Health Psychology*, 6, 159–172.

Bem, D.J. (1972). Self-perception theory. In L. Berkowitz (Ed.). *Advances in Experimental Social Psychology. Vol 6*. New York: Academic Press.

Bem, S.L. (1974). The measurement of psychological androgyny. *Journal of Consulting and Clinical Psychology*, 42, 155–162.

Benfari, R.C., Eaker, E. & Stoll, J.G. (1981). Behavioural intentions and compliance to treatment regimes. *Annual Review of Public Health*, 2, 431–471.

Bentler, P.M. & Speckart, G. (1981). Attitudes 'cause' behaviours: A structural equation analysis. *Journal of Personality and Social Psychology*, 40, 226–238.

Berg, K. (1986). Metabolic disease: Diabetes mellitus. In V. Seefeldt (Ed.). *Physical

Activity and Well-being. Reston, VA: American Alliance for Health, Physical Education, Recreation and Dance.

Berger, B.G. & Owen, D.R. (1983). Mood alterations with swimming: Swimmers really do 'feel better'. *Psychosomatic Medicine*, 45, 425–433.

Berger, B.G. & Owen, D.R. (1988). Stress reduction and mood enhancement in four exercise modes: Swimming, body conditioning, hatha yoga and fencing. *Research Quarterly for Exercise and Sport*, 59, 148–159.

Bialer, I. (1961). Conceptualisation of success and failure in mentally retarded and normal children. *Journal of Personality*, 29, 303–320.

Biddle, S.J.H. (1984). Motivational issues in health-related fitness: A note of caution. *British Journal of Physical Education*, 15(1), 21–22.

Biddle, S.J.H. (1986a). The contribution of attribution theory to exercise behaviour. In J. Watkins, T. Reilly & L. Burwitz (Eds.). *Sports Science*. London: Spon.

Biddle, S.J.H. (1986b). Incentive schemes in exercise: Saints or sinners? *Health and Physical Education Project Newsletter*, 3, 4–7.

Biddle, S.J.H. (1987a). Exercise and lifestyle. *Campbell's Institute for Health and Fitness Turnaround Lifestyle System*. Loughborough University of Technology.

Biddle, S.J.H. (1987b) (Ed.). *Foundations of Health-related Fitness in Physical Education*. London: Ling (PEA).

Biddle, S.J.H. (1988a). The other 'S' factor: Stress recognition and management. *Bulletin of Physical Education*, 24(1), 26–31.

Biddle, S.J.H. (1988b). Methodological issues in the researching of attribution–emotion links in sport. *International Journal of Sport Psychology*, 19, 264–280.

Biddle, S.J.H. (1989a). 'Innovation without change' and the ideology of individualism: A reply to Sparkes. *British Journal of Physical Education*, 20(2), 64–65.

Biddle, S.J.H. (1989b). Approaches to implementing health-related fitness in schools. *Perspectives*, 41, 26–36.

Biddle, S.J.H. (1989c). Exercise and the treatment of depression. *British Journal of Hospital Medicine*, 42, 267.

Biddle, S.J.H. & Armstrong, N. (1990a). *It Doesn't Have to Hurt!* London: BBC Continuing Education Publications.

Biddle, S.J.H. & Armstrong, N. (1990b). Children's physical activity patterns: An exploratory study of psychological predictors. Paper presented at British Association of Sports Sciences conference, Cardiff.

Biddle, S.J.H. & Ashford, B. (1988). Cognitions and perceptions of health and exercise. *British Journal of Sports Medicine*, 22, 135–140.

Biddle, S.J.H. & Bailey, C.I.A. (1985). Motives for participation and attitudes toward physical activity of adult participants in fitness programmes. *Perceptual and Motor Skills*, 61, 831–834.

Biddle, S.J.H. & Hill, A.B. (1988). Causal attributions and emotional reactions to outcome in a sporting contest. *Personality and Individual Differences*, 9, 213–223.

Bird, A.M. & Cripe, B.K. (1986). *Psychology and Sport Behaviour*. St. Louis: Times Mirror/Mosby.

Blair, S.N. (1984). How to assess exercise habits and physical fitness. In J.D. Matarazzo, S.M. Weiss, J.A. Herd, N.E. Miller & S.M. Weiss (Eds.). *Behavioural Health: A Handbook of Health Enhancement and Disease Prevention*. New York: Wiley.

Blair, S.N. (1988). Exercise within a healthy lifestyle. In R.K. Dishman (Ed.). *Exercise Adherence: Its Impact on Public Health*. Champaign: Human Kinetics.

Blair, S.N., Pate, R.R., Blair, A., Howe, H.G., Rosenberg, M. & Parker, G.M. (1980). Leisure time physical activity as an intervening variable in research. *Health Education*, 11(1), 8–11.

Blair, S.N., Kohl, H.W. & Goodyear, N.N. (1987a). Rates and risks for running and exercise injuries: Studies in three populations. *Research Quarterly for Exercise and Sport*, 58, 221–228.

Blair, S.N., Mulder, R.T. & Kohl, H.W. (1987b). Reaction to 'Secular trends in adult physical activity: Exercise boom or bust?'. *Research Quarterly for Exercise and Sport*, 58, 106–110.

Blair, S.N., Kohl, H.W., Paffenbarger, R.S., Clark, D.S., Cooper, K.H. & Gibbons, L.W. (1989a). Physical fitness and all-cause mortality: A prospective study of healthy men and women. *Journal of the American Medical Association*, 262, 2395–2401.

Blair, S.N., Clark, D.G., Cureton, K.J. & Powell, K.E. (1989b). Exercise and fitness in childhood: Implications for a lifetime of health. In C.V. Gisolfi & D.R. Lamb (Eds.). *Perspectives in Exercise Science and Sports Medicine, Vol 2. Youth, Exercise and Sport*. Indianapolis: Benchmark Press.

Blue, F.D. (1979). Aerobic running as a treatment for moderate depression. *Perceptual and Motor Skills*, 48, 228.

Blumenthal, J.A., Williams, R.S., Wallace, A.G., Williams, R.B. & Needles, T.L. (1982). Physiological and psychological variables predict compliance to prescribed exercise therapy in patients recovering from myocardial infarction. *Psychosomatic Medicine*, 44, 519–527.

Blumenthal, J.A., O'Toole, L.C. & Chang, J.L. (1984). Is running an analogue of anorexia nervosa? *Journal of the American Medical Association*, 252, 520–523.

Boothby, J., Tungatt, M.F. & Townsend, A.R. (1981). Ceasing participation in sports activity: Reported reasons and their implications. *Journal of Leisure Research*, 13, 1–14.

Borg, G. (1973). Perceived exertion: A note on 'history' and methods. *Medicine and Science in Sports*, 5, 90–93.

Borg, G. & Noble, G.J. (1974). Perceived exertion. *Exercise and Sport Sciences Reviews*, 2, 131–153.

Bouchard, C. (1988). Gene-environment interaction in human adaptability. In R.M. Malina & H.M. Eckert (Eds.). *Physical Activity in Early and Modern Populations*. Champaign: Human Kinetics and the American Academy of Physical Education.

Bouchard, C. (1990). Discussion: Heredity, fitness and health. In C. Bouchard, R.J. Shephard, T. Stephens, J.R. Sutton & B.D. McPherson (Eds.). *Exercise, Fitness and Health: A Consensus of Current Knowledge*. Champaign: Human Kinetics.

Bouchard, C., Shephard, R.J., Stephens, T., Sutton, J.R. & McPherson, B.D. (1990) (Eds.). *Exercise, Fitness and Health:A Consensus of Current Knowledge*. Champaign: Human Kinetics.

Boutcher, S.H. & Trenske, M. (1990). The effects of sensory deprivation and music on perceived exertion and affect during exercise. *Journal of Sport and Exercise Psychology*, 12, 167–176.

Brawley, L.R. & Roberts, G.C. (1984). Attributions in sport: Research foundations, characteristics and limitations. In J. Silva & R. Weinberg (Eds.). *Psychological Foundations of Sport*. Champaign: Human Kinetics.

Bray, G.A. (1990). Exercise and obesity. In C. Bouchard, R.J. Shephard, T.

Stephens, J.R. Sutton & B.D. McPherson (Eds.). *Exercise, Fitness and Health: A Consensus of Current Knowledge*. Champaign: Human Kinetics.

Brewin, C.R. (1988). Editorial: Developments in an attributional approach to clinical psychology. *British Journal of Clinical Psychology*, 27, 1–3.

Brewin, C.R. & Shapiro, D.A. (1984). Beyond locus of control: Attribution of responsibility for positive and negative outcomes. *British Journal of Psychology*, 75, 43–49.

British Market Research Bureau (1989). *Executive Stress*. London: British Market Research Bureau.

Brodie, D.A. (1988). Techniques of measurement of body composition: Parts I and II. *Sports Medicine*, 5, 11–40, 74–98.

Brody, E.B., Hatfield, B.D. & Spalding T.W. (1988). Generalisation of self-efficacy to a continuum of stressors upon mastery of a high-risk sport skill. *Journal of Sport and Exercise Psychology*, 10, 32–44.

Brooke, S. & Long, B.C. (1987). Efficiency of coping with a real life stressor: A multimodel comparison of aerobic fitness. *Psychophysiology*, 24, 173–180.

Brown, J.D. & Siegel, J.M. (1988). Exercise as a buffer of life stress: A prospective study of adolescent health. *Health Psychology*, 7, 341–353.

Brown, R.S. (1982). Exercise and mental health in the pediatric population. *Clinics in Sports Medicine*, 1, 515–527.

Brown, R.S., Ramirez, D.E. & Taub, J.M. (1978). The prescription of exercise for depression. *The Physician and Sportsmedicine*, December, pp. 35–45.

Browne, D. (1986). Prescribing exercise from general practice. In D.P. Gray (Ed.). *Medical Annual*. Bristol: Wright.

Brownell, K.D. & Stunkard, A.J. (1980). Physical activity in the development and control of obesity. In A.J. Stunkard (Ed.). *Obesity*. Philadelphia: W.B. Saunders.

Brownell, K.D., Stunkard, A.J. & Albaum, J.M. (1980). Evaluation of and modification of exercise patterns in the natural environment. *American Journal of Psychiatry*, 137, 1540–1545.

Brownell, K.D., Marlatt, G.A., Lichtenstein, E. & Wilson, G.T. (1986). Understanding and preventing relapse. *American Psychologist*, 41, 765–782.

Bruce, R.A., DeRouen, T. & Hossack, K. (1980). Pilot study examining the motivational effects of maximal exercise testing to modify risk factors and health habits. *Cardiology*, 66, 111–119.

Bryant, J.G., Garrett, H.L. & Dean, M.S. (1984a). Coronary heart disease: The beneficial effects of exercise to children. *Louisiana State Medical Journal*, 136, 15–17.

Bryant, J.G., Garrett, H.L. & Dean, M.S. (1984b). The effects of an exercise programme on selected risk factors to coronary heart disease in children. *Social Science and Medicine*, 19, 765–766.

Buffone, G.W. (1981). Psychological changes associated with cognitive behaviour therapy and an aerobic running programme in the treatment of depression. Paper presented at the Association for Advancement of Behaviour Therapy conference, Toronto, Canada.

Buffone, G.W., Sachs, M.L. & Dowd, E.T. (1984). Cognitive-behavioural strategies for promoting adherence to exercise. In M.L. Sachs & G.W. Buffone (Eds.). *Running Therapy: An Integrated Approach*. Lincoln: University of Nebraska Press.

Bunker, L. & Williams, J.M. (1986). Cognitive techniques for improving performance and building confidence. In J.M. Williams (Ed.). *Applied Sport Psychology*. Palo Alto, Ca: Mayfield.

Burton, D. (1989). Winning isn't everything: Examining the impact of performance goals on collegiate swimmers' cognitions and performance. *The Sport Psychologist*, 3, 105–132.

Butler, J.R. (1987). *An Apple a Day . . . ? A study of Lifestyles and Health in Canterbury and Thanet*. Canterbury: University of Kent.

Calabrese, L.H. (1990). Exercise, immunity, cancer, and infection. In C. Bouchard, R.J. Shephard, T. Stephens, J.R. Sutton & B.D. McPherson (Eds.). *Exercise, Fitness and Health: A Consensus of Current Knowledge*. Champaign: Human Kinetics.

Callen, K.E. (1983). Mental and emotional aspects of long-distance running. *Psychosomatics*, 24, 133–151.

Calnan, M.W. & Johnson, B.M. (1983). Influencing health behaviour: How significant is the general practitioner? *Health Education Journal*, 42, 39–45.

Campbell, M.J., Browne, D. & Waters, W.E. (1985). Can general practitioners influence exercise habits? Controlled trial. *British Medical Journal*, 290, 1044–1046.

Canada Fitness Survey (1983a). *Fitness and Lifestyle in Canada*. Ottawa: Canada Fitness Survey.

Canada Fitness Survey (1983b). *Canadian Youth and Physical Activity*. Ottawa: Canada Fitness Survey.

Canada Fitness Survey (1986). *Physical Activity among Activity-limited and Disabled Adults in Canada*. Ottawa: Canada Fitness Survey.

Cantu, R.C. (1982). *Diabetes and Exercise*. Ithaca: Mouvement.

Carmack, M.A. & Martens, R. (1979). Measuring commitment to running: A survey of runners' attitudes and mental states. *Journal of Sport Psychology*, 1, 25–42.

Carr, D.B., Bullen, B.A., Skrinar, G.S. et al. (1981). Physical conditioning facilitates the exercise-induced secretion of beta-endorphin and beta-lipoprotein in women. *New England Journal of Medicine*, 305 (10), 560–563.

Carron, A.V. (1980). *Social Psychology of Sport*. Ithaca: Mouvement.

Carron, A.V. (1988). *Group Dynamics in Sport*. London, Ontario: Sports Dynamics.

Carron, A.V., Widmeyer, W.N. & Brawley, L.R. (1988). Group cohesion and individual adherence to physical activity. *Journal of Sport and Exercise Psychology*, 10, 127–138.

Carter, J.A., Lee, A.M. & Greenockle, K.M. (1987). Locus of control, fitness values, success expectations and performance in a fitness class. *Perceptual and Motor Skills*, 65, 777–778.

Caspersen, C.J. (1989). Physical activity epidemiology: Concepts, methods, and applications to exercise science. *Exercise and Sport Sciences Reviews*, 17, 423–473.

Caspersen, C.J., Powell, K.E. & Christenson, G.M. (1985). Physical activity, exercise and physical fitness: Definitions and distinctions for health-related research. *Public Health Reports*, 100, 126–131.

Chamove, A.S. (1988). Exercise effects in psychiatric populations: A review. In *Sport, Health, Psychology and Exercise Symposium proceedings*. London: The Sports Council/Health Education Authority.

Champion, V.L. (1985). Use of the Health Belief Model in determining frequency of breast self-examination. *Research in Nursing and Health*, 8, 373–379.

Cherlin, A. & Bourque, L.B. (1974). Dimensionality and reliability of the Rotter I-E scale. *Sociometry*, 37, 565–582.

Chew, R. (1986). *Health Expenditure in the UK*. London: Office of Health Economics.

Chubb, M. (1990). Discussion: Determinants of participation in physical activity. In C. Bouchard, R.J. Shephard, T. Stephens, J.R. Sutton & B.D. McPherson

(Eds.). *Exercise, Fitness and Health: A Consensus of Current Knowledge*. Champaign: Human Kinetics.

Clough, P.J., Shepherd, J. & Maughan, R.J. (1988). Motivations for running. In *Sport, Health, Psychology and Exercise Symposium proceedings*. London: The Sports Council/Health Education Authority.

Coates, J.R., Jeffrey, R.W. & Slinkard, L. (1981). Heart healthy eating and exercise: Introducing and maintaining changes in health behaviours. *American Journal of Public Health*, 71, 15–23.

Collins, B.E. (1974). Four components of the Rotter internal-external scale: Belief in a difficult world, a just world, a predictable world, and politically responsive world. *Journal of Personality and Social Psychology*, 29, 381–391.

Collins, M. (1987). Sociology of sport and exercise in the United Kingdom. In *Exercise Heart Health*. Proceedings of Coronary Prevention Group conference, London.

Colt, E.W., Wardlaw, S.L. & Frantz, A.G. (1981). The effect of running on β-endorphin. *Life Science*, 28, 1637–1640.

Conroy, R.W., Smith, K. & Felthouse, A.R. (1982). The value of exercise in a psychiatric hospital unit. *Hospital and Community Psychiatry*, 33, 641–645.

Cook, T.D. & Campbell, D.T. (1979). *Quasi-experimentation: Design and analysis issues for field settings*. Chicago: Rand McNally.

Cooper, K.H. (1982). *The Aerobics Program for Total Well-being*. New York: Bantam.

Corbin, C.B. (1981). Sex of subject, sex of opponent, and opponent ability as factors affecting self-confidence in a competitive situation. *Journal of Sport Psychology*, 3, 265–270.

Corbin, C.B. (1984). Self-confidence of females in sports and physical activity. *Clinics in Sports Medicine*, 3, 895–908.

Corbin, C.B. (1987). Youth fitness, exercise and health: There is much to be done. *Research Quarterly for Exercise and Sport*, 58, 308–314.

Corbin, C.B. & Lindsey, R. (1988). *Concepts of physical fitness*. 5th Edn. Dubuque, Iowa: Wm C. Brown.

Corbin, C.B. & Nix, C. (1979). Sex-typing of physical activities and success predictions of children before and after cross-sex competition. *Journal of Sport Psychology*, 1, 43–52.

Corbin, C.B., Stewart, M.J. & Blair, W.O. (1981). Self-confidence and motor performance of preadolescent boys and girls studied in different feedback situations. *Journal of Sport Psychology*, 3, 30–34.

Corbin, C.B., Landers, D.M., Feltz, D.L. & Senior, K. (1983). Sex differences in performance estimates: Female lack of self-confidence versus male boastfulness. *Research Quarterly for Exercise and Sport*, 54, 407–410.

Corbin, C.B., Fox, K.R. & Whitehead, J.R. (1987a). Fitness for a lifetime. In S.J.H. Biddle (Ed.). *Foundations of Health-related Fitness in Physical Education*. London: Ling (PEA).

Corbin, C.B., Nielsen, A.B., Borsdorf, L.L. & Laurie, D.R. (1987b). Commitment to physical activity. *International Journal of Sport Psychology*, 18, 215–222.

Corbin, C.B., Whitehead, J.R. & Lovejoy, P.Y. (1988). Youth physical fitness awards. *Quest*, 40, 200–218.

Covington, M.V. & Omelich, C.L. (1979). Effort: The double-edged sword in school achievement. *Journal of Educational Psychology*, 71, 169–182.

Cox, B.D., Blaxter, M. et al. (1987). *The Health and Lifestyle Survey*. London: Health Promotion Research Trust.

Cox, R.H. (1985). *Sport Psychology: Concepts and Applications*. Dubuque, Iowa: Wm C. Brown.

Crews, D.J. & Landers, D.M. (1987). A meta-analytic review of aerobic fitness and reactivity to psychosocial stressors. *Medicine and Science in Sports and Exercise*, 19 (5, Supplement), S114–S120.

Crowe, P. (1987). *Health Fair Handbook*. London: Health Education Council.

Crowne, D.P. & Marlowe, D. (1960). A new scale of social desirability independent of psychopathology. *Journal of Consulting Psychology*, 24, 349–354.

Csikszentmihalyi, M. (1975). *Beyond Boredom and Anxiety*. San Francisco: Jossey-Bass.

Cureton, K.J. (1987). Commentary on 'Children and fitness: A public health perspective'. *Research Quarterly for Exercise and Sport*, 58, 315–320.

Davis, K.E., Jackson, K.L., Kronenfeld, J.J. & Blair, S.N. (1984). Intent to participate in worksite health promotion activities: A model of risk factors and psychosocial variables. *Health Education Quarterly*, 11, 361–377.

Dean, A. (1987). *Beliefs about Exercise and Patterns of Participation: Report of a Social Survey into Physical Activity and Fitness Testing*. Centre for Leisure Research, Dunfermline College of Physical Education.

Deci, E.L. & Ryan, R.M. (1985). *Intrinsic Motivation and Self-determination of Human Behaviour*. New York: Plenum.

de Coverley Veale, D.M.W. (1987a). Exercise dependence. *British Journal of Addiction*, 82, 735–740.

de Coverley Veale, D.M.W. (1987b). Exercise and mental health. *Acta Psychiatrica Scandanavica*, 76, 113–120.

de Coverley Veale, D.M.W. & Le Fevre, K. (1988). Aerobic exercise in the adjunctive treatment of depression: A randomised controlled trail. In *Sport, Health, Psychology and Exercise Symposium proceedings*. London: The Sports Council/Health Education Authority.

Dennison, B.A., Straus, J.H., Mellits, E.D. & Charney, E. (1988). Childhood physical fitness tests: Predictor of adult physical activity levels? *Pediatrics*, 82, 324–330.

Department of Health (1990). *The Health Service: The NHS Reforms and You*. London: HMSO.

Department of Health and Human Services (1980). *Promoting Health/Preventing Disease: Objectives for the Nation*. Washington, DC: US Government Printing Office.

Department of Health and Human Services (1986). *Midcourse Review: 1990 Physical Fitness and Exercise Objectives*. Washington, DC: US Government Printing Office.

Desharnais, R., Bouillon, J. & Godin, G. (1986). Self-efficacy and outcome expectations as determinants of exercise adherence. *Psychological Reports*, 59, 1155–1159.

de Vries, H.A. (1968). Immediate and long-term effects of exercise upon resting muscle potential level. *Journal of Sports Medicine and Physical Fitness*, 8, 1–11.

de Vries, H.A. (1981). Tranquilliser effect of exercise: A critical review. *The Physician and Sportsmedicine*, 9(11), 47–53.

Dishman, R.K. (1981). Biologic influences on exercise adherence. *Research Quarterly for Exercise and Sport*, 52, 143–159.

Dishman, R.K. (1982). Compliance/adherence in health-related exercise. *Health Psychology*, 1, 237–267.

Dishman, R.K. (1985). Medical psychology in exercise and sport. *Medical Clinics of North America*, 69, 123–143.

Dishman, R.K. (1986a). Mental health. In V. Seefeldt (Ed). *Physical Activity and Well-being*. Reston, VA: American Alliance for Health, Physical Education, Recreation and Dance.

Dishman, R.K. (1986b). Exercise compliance: A new view for public health. *The Physician and Sportsmedicine*, 14(5), 127–145.

Dishman, R.K. (1987). Exercise adherence and habitual physical activity. In W.P. Morgan & S.E. Goldston (Eds.). *Exercise and Mental Health*. Washington: Hemisphere.

Dishman, R.K. (1988a) (Ed.). *Exercise Adherence: Its Impact on Public Health*. Champaign: Human Kinetics.

Dishman, R.K. (1988b). Behavioural barriers to health-related physical fitness. In L.K. Hall & G.C. Meyer (Eds.). *Epidemiology, Behaviour Change, and Intervention in Chronic Disease*. Champaign: Life Enhancement Publications.

Dishman, R.K. (1989). Exercise and sport psychology in youth 6 to 18 years of age. In C.V. Gisolfi & D.R. Lamb (Eds.). *Perspectives in Exercise Science and Sports Medicine. Vol II. Youth, Exercise, and Sport*. Indianapolis: Benchmark Press.

Dishman, R.K. (1990). Determinants of participation in physical activity. In C. Bouchard, R.J. Shephard, T. Stephens, J.R. Sutton & B.D. McPherson (Eds.). *Exercise, Fitness and Health: A Consensus of Current Knowledge*. Champaign: Human Kinetics.

Dishman, R.K. & Dunn, A.L. (1988). Exercise adherence in children and youth: Implications for adulthood. In R.K. Dishman (Ed.). *Exercise Adherence: Its Impact on Public Health*. Champaign: Human Kinetics.

Dishman, R.K. & Gettman, L.R. (1980). Psychobiologic influences on exercise adherence. *Journal of Sport Psychology*, 2, 295–310.

Dishman, R.K. & Ickes, W. (1981). Self-motivation and adherence to therapeutic exercise. *Journal of Behavioural Medicine*, 4, 421–438.

Dishman, R.K. & Landy, F.J. (1988). Psychological factors and prolonged exercise. In D.R. Lamb & R. Murray (Eds.). *Perspectives in Exercise Science and Sports Medicine. I. Prolonged Exercise*. Indianapolis: Benchmark Press.

Dishman, R.K. & Steinhardt, M. (1988). Reliability and concurrent validity for a 7-d recall of physical activity in college students. *Medicine and Science in Sports and Exercise*, 20, 14–25.

Dishman, R.K., Ickes, W. & Morgan, W.P. (1980). Self-motivation and adherence to habitual physical activity. *Journal of Applied Social Psychology*, 10, 115–132.

Dishman, R.K., Sallis, J.F. & Orenstein, D. (1985). The determinants of physical activity and exercise. *Public Health Reports*, 100, 158–171.

Dishman, R.K., Patton, R., Smith, J., Weinberg, R.S. & Jackson, A. (1987). Using perceived exertion to prescribe and monitor exercise training heart rate. *International Journal of Sports Medicine*, 8, 208–213.

Dodson, L.C. & Mullens, W.R. (1969). Some effects of jogging on psychiatric hospital patients. *American Corrective Therapy Journal*, 23, 130–134.

Dohrenwend, B.S. & Dohrenwend, B.P. (1974). *Stressful Life Events: Their Nature and Effects*. New York: John Wiley.

Donahue, J.A., Gillis, J.H. & King, K. (1980). Behaviour modification in sport and physical education. *Journal of Sport Psychology*, 2, 311–328.

Downey, A.M., Frank, G.C., Webber, L.S. et al. (1987). Implementation of 'heart smart': A cardiovascular school health promotion programme. *Journal of School Health*, 57(3), 98–104.

Downie, R.S., Fyfe, C. & Tannahill, A. (1990). *Health Promotion Models and Values*. New York: Oxford University Press.

Doyne, E.J., Chambless, D.L. & Beutler, L.E. (1983). Aerobic exercise as a treatment for depression in women. *Behaviour Therapy*, 14, 434–440.

Doyne, E.J., Ossip-Klein, D.J., Bowman, E.D., Osborn, K.M., McDougall-Wilson, I.B. & Neimeyer, R.A. (1987). Running versus weight lifting in the treatment of depression. *Journal of Consulting and Clinical Psychology*, 55, 748–754.

Duda, J.L. (1987). Toward a developmental theory of children's motivation in sport. *Journal of Sport Psychology*, 9, 130–145.

Duda, J.L. (1988). The relationship between goal perspectives, persistence and behavioural intensity among male and female recreational sport participants. *Leisure Sciences*, 10, 95–106.

Duda, J.L. (1989). Goal perspectives and behaviour in sport and exercise settings. In C. Ames & M. Maehr (Eds.). *Advances in Motivation and Achievement. VI. Motivation Enhancing Environments*. Greenwich, CT: JAI Press.

Duda, J.L. & Tappe, M.K. (1988). Predictors of personal investment in physical activity among middle-aged and older adults. *Perceptual and Motor Skills*, 66, 543–549.

Duda, J.L. & Tappe, M.K. (1989a). Personal investment in exercise among middle-aged and older adults. In A. Ostrow (Ed.). *Aging and Motor Behaviour*. Indianapolis: Benchmark Press.

Duda, J.L. & Tappe, M.K. (1989b). Personal investment in exercise among adults: The examination of age and gender-related differences in motivational orientation. In A. Ostrow (Ed.). *Aging and Motor Behaviour*. Indianapolis: Benchmark Press.

Duffy, P.J., Shiflett, S. & Downey, R.G. (1977). Locus of control: Dimensionality and predictability using Likert scales. *Journal of Applied Psychology*, 62, 214–219.

Duke, M., Johnson, T.C. & Nowicki, S. (1977). Effects of sports fitness camp experience on locus of control orientation in children ages 6 to 14. *Research Quarterly*, 48, 280–283.

Dummer, G., Rosen, L., Heusner, W., Roberts, P. & Counsilman, J. (1987). Pathogenic weight control behaviours of young competitive swimmers. *The Physician and Sportsmedicine*, 15(5), 75–84.

Dweck, C.S. (1980). Learned helplessness in sport. In C. Nadeau, W. Halliwell, K. Newell & G. Roberts (Eds.). *Psychology of Motor Behaviour and Sport, 1979*. Champaign: Human Kinetics.

Dweck, C.S. & Leggett, E.L. (1988). A social-cognitive approach to motivation and personality. *Psychological Review*, 95, 256–273.

Dwyer, T., Coonan, W.E., Leitch, D.R., Hetzel, B.S. & Baghurst, R.A. (1983). An investigation of the effects of daily physical activity on the health of primary school students in South Australia. *International Journal of Epidemiology*, 12, 308–313.

Dzewaltowski, D.A. (1989). Toward a model of exercise motivation. *Journal of Sport and Exercise Psychology*, 11, 251–269.

Eadie, D.R. & Leathar, D.S. (1988). *Concepts of Fitness and Health: An Exploratory Study*. Edinburgh: Scottish Sports Council.

Edwards, W. (1954). The theory of decision making. *Psychological Bulletin*, 51, 380–417.

Eisen, M. & Zellman, G.L. (1986). The role of health belief attitudes, sex education, and demographics in predicting adolescents' sexuality knowledge. *Health Education Quarterly*, 13, 9–22.

Eisenman, P. (1986). Physical activity and body composition. In V. Seefeldt (Ed.). *Physical Activity and Well-being*. Reston, VA: American Alliance for Health, Physical Education, Recreation and Dance.

Eiser, J.R. (1982). Addiction as attribution: Cognitive processes in giving up smoking. In J.R. Eiser (Ed.). *Social Psychology and Behavioural Medicine*. Chichester: Wiley.

Eiser, J.R. (1986). *Social Psychology*. Cambridge: Cambridge University Press.

Eiser, J.R. (1987). *The Expression of Attitude*. New York: Springer-Verlag.

Eiser, J.R. & van der Pligt, J. (1988). *Attitudes and decisions*. London: Routledge.

Eiser, J.R., Sutton, S.R. & Wober, M. (1978). Smokers' and non-smokers' attributions about smoking: A case of actor-observer differences? *British Journal of Social and Clinical Psychology*, 17, 189–190.

Ellis, M.J. (1973). *Why People Play*. Englewood Cliffs, NJ: Prentice-Hall.

Epstein, L.H. & Wing, R.R. (1980). Aerobic exercise and weight. *Addictive Behaviours*, 5, 371–388.

Epstein, L.H., Wing, R.R., Thompson, J.K. & Griffin, W. (1980). Attendance and fitness in aerobic exercise. *Behaviour Modification*, 4, 465–470.

Everly, G.S., Smith, K.J. & Haight, G.T. (1987). Evaluating health promotions in the workplace: Behavioural models versus financial models. *Health Education Research: Theory and Practice*, 2, 61–67.

Ewart, C.E. (1989). Psychological effects of resistive weight training: Implications for cardiac patients. *Medicine and Science in Sports and Exercise*, 21, 683–688.

Ewart, C.E., Taylor, C.B., Reese, L.B. & DeBusk, R.F. (1983). Effects of early post myocardial infarction exercise testing on self-perception and subsequent physical activity. *American Journal of Cardiology*, 51, 1076–1080.

Ewart, C.E., Stewart, K.J. Gillilan, R.E. & Kelemen, M.H. (1986a). Self-efficacy mediates strength gains during circuit weight training in men with coronary artery disease. *Medicine and Science in Sports and Exercise*, 18, 531–540.

Ewart, C.E., Stewart, K.J., Kelemen, K.H. et al (1986b). Usefulness of self-efficacy in predicting overexertion during programmed exercise in coronary artery disease. *American Journal of Cardiology*, 57, 557–561.

Eysenck, H.J. (1967). *The Biological Basis of Personality*. Springfield, Il: C.C. Thomas.

Farrally, M., Docherty, G., Emery, M. et al. (1988). Promoting fitness in the workplace: Physical activity and exercise compliance. In *Sport, Health, Psychology and Exercise Symposium proceedings*. London: The Sports Council/Health Education Authority.

Farrell, P.A., Gates, W.K., Morgan, W.P. & Maksud, M.G. (1982). Increases in plasma β-endorphin and β-lipotropin immunoreactivity after treadmill running in humans. *Journal of Applied Physiology*, 52, 1245–1249.

Farrell, P.A., Gates, W.K., Morgan, W.P. & Pert, C.B. (1983). Plasma leucine enkaphalin-like radioreceptor activity and tension-anxiety before and after competitive running. In H.G. Knuttgen, J.A. Vogel & J. Poortmans (Eds.). *Biochemistry of Exercise*. Champaign: Human Kinetics.

Feltz, D.L. (1982). Path analysis of the causal elements in Bandura's theory of self-efficacy and an anxiety-based model of avoidance behaviour. *Journal of Personality and Social Psychology*, 42, 764–781.

Feltz, D.L. (1988a). Self-confidence and sports performance. *Exercise and Sport Sciences Reviews*, 16, 423–457.

Feltz, D.L. (1988b). Gender differences in the causal elements of self-efficacy on a high avoidance motor task. *Journal of Sport and Exercise Psychology*, 10, 151–166.

Feltz, D.L. & Landers, D.M. (1983). The effects of mental practice on motor skill learning and performance: A meta-analysis. *Journal of Sport Psychology*, 5, 25–57.

Feltz, D.L. & Mugno, D.A. (1983). A replication of the path analysis of the causal elements in Bandura's theory of self-efficacy and the influence of autonomic arousal. *Journal of Sport Psychology*, 5, 263–277.

Feltz, D.L., Landers, D.M. & Raeder, U. (1979). Enhancing self-efficacy in high-avoidance motor tasks: A comparison of modelling techniques. *Journal of Sport Psychology*, 1, 112–122.

Fenner, N. (1987). Leisure, exercise and work. In B.D. Cox, M. Blaxter et al. (Eds.). *The Health and Lifestyle Survey*. London: Health Promotion Research Trust.

Fentem, P.H., Bassey, E.J. & Turnbull, N.B. (1988). *The New Case for Exercise*. London: The Sports Council and Health Education Authority.

Fielding, J.E. (1984). Health promotion and disease prevention at the worksite. *Annual Review of Public Health*, 5, 237–265.

Fishbein, M. & Ajzen, I. (1975). *Belief, Attitude, Intention and Behaviour: An Introduction to Theory and Research*. Reading, Mass: Addison-Wesley.

Foley, K.M., Kourides, I.A., Inturrisi, C. et al (1979). β-endorphin: Analgesic and hormonal effects in humans. *Proceedings of the National Academy of Science of the USA*, 76, 5377–5381.

Folkins, C.H. & Sime, W. (1981). Physical fitness training and mental health. *American Psychologist*, 36, 373–389.

Folkins, C.H., Lynch, S. & Gardner, M.M. (1972). Psychological fitness as a function of physical fitness. *Archives of Physical Medicine and Rehabilitation*, 53, 503–508.

Forsterling, F. (1985). Attributional retraining: A review. *Psychological Bulletin*, 98, 495–512.

Forsterling, F. (1988). *Attribution Theory in Clinical Psychology*. Chichester: Wiley.

Fox, K.R. (1988). The self-esteem complex and youth fitness. *Quest*, 40, 230–246.

Fox, K. (1990). *The Physical Self-Perception Profile Manual*. DeKalb, Il: Office for Health Promotion, Northern Illinois University.

Fox, K.R. (1991). A clinical approach to exercise in the severely obese. In T.A. Wadden & T.B. Van Itallie (Eds.). *Treatment of Severe Obesity by Diet and Lifestyle Modication*. New York: Guilford Press.

Fox, K.R. & Biddle, S.J.H. (1988). The use of fitness tests: Educational and psychological considerations. *Journal of Physical Education, Recreation and Dance*, 59 (2), 47–53.

Fox, K.R. & Corbin, C.B. (1989). The physical self-perception profile: development and preliminary validation. *Journal of Sport and Exercise Psychology*, 11, 408–430.

Fox, K.R. & Whitehead, J.R. (1987). Student-centred physical education. In S.J.H.

Biddle (Ed.). *Foundations of Health-related Fitness in Physical Education*. London: Ling (PEA).

Fox, K.R., Whitehead, J.R. & Corbin, C.B. (1987). Getting started in health-related fitness. In S.J.H. Biddle (Ed.). *Foundations of Health-related Fitness in Physical Education*. London: Ling (PEA).

Franklin, B. (1988). Program factors that influence exercise adherence: Practical adherence skills for the clinical staff. In R.K. Dishman (Ed.). *Exercise Adherence: Its Impact on Public Health*. Champaign: Human Kinetics.

Fremont, J. & Craighead, L.W. (1987). Aerobic exercise and cognitive therapy in the treatment of dysphoric moods. *Cognitive Therapy and Research*, 11, 241–251.

Gale, J.B., Eckhoff, W.T., Mogel, S.F. & Rodnick, J.E. (1984). Factors related to adherence to an exercise programme for healthy adults. *Medicine and Science in Sports and Exercise*, 16, 544–549.

Gambert, S.R., Garthwaite, T.L., Hagen, T.L., Tristani, F.E. & McCartney, D.J. (1981). Exercise increases plasma beta-endorphins (EP) and ACTH in untrained human subjects. *Clinical Research*, 29, 429a.

Garfinkel, P.E. & Coscina, D.V. (1990). Discussion: Exercise and obesity. In C. Bouchard, R.J. Shephard, T. Stephens, J.R. Sutton & B.D. McPherson (Eds.). *Exercise, Fitness and Health: A Consensus of Current Knowledge*. Champaign: Human Kinetics.

Gatch, C.L. & Kendzierski, D. (1990). Predicting exercise intentions: The theory of planned behaviour. *Research Quarterly for Exercise and Sport*, 61, 100–102.

Gerner, R.H., Catlin, D.H., Gorelick, D.A., Hui, K.K. & Li, C.H. (1980). β-endorphin intravenous infusion causes behavioural change in psychiatric inpatients. *Archives of General Psychiatry*, 37, 642–647.

Gettman, L.R. (1988). Occupation-related fitness and exercise adherence. In R.K. Dishman (Ed.). *Exercise Adherence: Its Impact on Public Health*. Champaign: Human Kinetics.

Gettman, L.R., Pollock, M.L. & Ward, A. (1983). Adherence to unsupervised exercise. *The Physician and Sportsmedicine*, 11(10), 56–66.

Gill, D.L. (1986). *Psychological Dynamics of Sport*. Champaign: Human Kinetics.

Glasser, W. (1976). *Positive Addiction*. New York: Harper & Row.

Godin, G. & Shephard, R.J. (1983). Physical fitness promotion programmes: Effectiveness in modifying exercise behaviour. *Canadian Journal of Applied Sports Science*, 8, 104–113.

Godin, G. & Shephard, R.J. (1984). Normative beliefs of school children concerning regular exercise. *Journal of School Health*, 54, 443–445.

Godin, G. & Shephard, R.J. (1985). Psychosocial predictors of exercise intentions among spouses. *Canadian Journal of Applied Sports Science*, 10, 36–43.

Godin, G. & Shephard, R.J. (1986a). Importance of type of attitude to the study of exercise behaviour. *Psychological Reports*, 58, 991–1000.

Godin, G. & Shephard, R.J. (1986b). Psychosocial factors influencing intentions to exercise of young students from grades 7 to 9. *Research Quarterly for Exercise and Sport*, 57, 41–52.

Godin, G. & Shephard, R.J. (1990). Use of attitude-behaviour models in exercise promotion. *Sports Medicine*, 10, 103–121.

Godin, G., Shephard, R.J. & Colantonio, A. (1986a). Children's perception of parental exercise: Influence of sex and age. *Perceptual and Motor Skills*, 62, 511–516.

Godin, G., Shephard, R.J. & Colantonio, A. (1986b). The cognitive profile of those who intend to exercise but do not. *Public Health Reports*, 101, 521–526.

Godin, G., Colantonio, A., Davis, G.M., Shephard, R.J. & Simard, C. (1986c). Prediction of leisure time exercise behaviour among a group of lower-limb disabled adults. *Journal of Clinical Psychology*, 42, 272–279.

Godin, G., Desharnais, R., Jobin, J. & Cook, J. (1987a). The impact of physical fitness and health-age appraisal upon exercise intentions and behaviour. *Journal of Behavioural Medicine*, 10, 241–250.

Godin, G., Valois, P., Shephard, R.J. & Desharnais, R. (1987b). Prediction of leisure time exercise behaviour: A path analysis (LISREL V) model. *Journal of Behavioural Medicine*, 10, 145–158.

Godin, G., Vezina, L. & Leclerc, O. (1989). Factors influencing intentions of pregnant women to exercise after giving birth. *Public Health Reports*, 104, 188–195.

Goldberg, A.P. (1989). Aerobic and resistive exercise modify risk factors for coronary heart disease. *Medicine and Science in Sports and Exercise*, 21, 669–674.

Gondola, J.C. & Tuckman, B.W. (1982). Psychological mood states in 'average' marathon runners. *Perceptual and Motor Skills*, 55, 1295–1300.

Gotay, C.C. (1985). Why me? Attributions and adjustment by cancer patients and their mates at two stages in the disease process. *Social Science and Medicine*, 20, 825–831.

Gould, D. (1987). Understanding attrition in children's sport. In D. Gould & M. Weiss (Eds.). *Advances in Pediatric Sport Sciences: II. Behavourial Issues*. Champaign: Human Kinetics.

Gould, D. & Horn, T. (1984). Participation motivation in young athletes. In J. Silva & R. Weinberg (Eds.). *Psychological Foundations of Sport*. Champaign: Human Kinetics.

Graham, R.E., Dishman, R.K. & Holly, R.G. (1989). Estimates of Type A behaviour do not predict RPE. *Medicine and Science in Sports and Exercise*, 21 (2, Supplement), S14 (abstract).

Greenockle, K.M., Lee, A.A. & Lomax, R. (1990). The relationship between selected student characteristics and activity patterns in a required high school physical education class. *Research Quarterly for Exercise and Sport*, 61, 59–69.

Gregory, W.L. (1978). Locus of control for positive and negative outcomes. *Journal of Personality and Social Psychology*, 36, 840–849.

Greist, J.H., Eischens, R.R., Klein, M.H. & Faris, J.W. (1979a). Antidepressant running. *Psychiatric Annals*, 9, 134–140.

Greist, J.H., Klein, M.H., Eischens, R.R., Faris, J.W., Gurman, A.S. & Morgan, W.P. (1979b). Running as a treatment for depression. *Comprehensive Psychiatry*, 20, 41–54.

Greist, J.H., Klein, M.H., Eischens, R.R., Faris, J.W., Gurman, A.S. & Morgan, W.P. (1981). Running through your mind. In M.H. Sacks & M.L. Sachs (Eds.). *Psychology of Running*. Champaign: Human Kinetics.

Griffin, N.S. & Crawford, M.E. (1989). Measurement of movement confidence with a stunt movement confidence inventory. *Journal of Sport and Exercise Psychology*, 11, 26–40.

Griffin, N.S. & Keogh, J.F. (1982). A model of movement confidence. In J.A.S. Kelso & J.E. Clark (Eds.). *The Development of Movement Control and Co-ordination*. New York: Wiley.

Griffin, N.S., Keogh, J.F. & Maybee, R. (1984). Performer perceptions of movement confidence. *Journal of Sport Psychology*, 6, 395–407.

Grossman, A. (1984). Endorphins and exercise. *Clinical Cardiology*, 7, 255–260.

Grossman, A. & Sutton, J.R. (1985). Endorphins: What are they? How are they measured? What is their role in exercise? *Medicine and Science in Sports and Exercise*, 17, 74–81.

Gruber, J.J. (1986). Physical activity and self-esteem development in children: A meta-analysis. In G.A. Stull & H.M. Eckert (Eds.). *Effects of Physical Activity on Children*. Champaign: Human Kinetics and American Academy of Physical Education.

Hagberg, J.M. (1990). Exercise, fitness, and hypertension. In C. Bouchard, R.J. Shephard, T. Stephens, J.R. Sutton & B.D. McPherson (Eds.). *Exercise, Fitness and Health: A Consensus of Current Knowledge*. Champaign: Human Kinetics.

Haier, R.J., Quaid, K. & Mills, J. (1981). Naloxone alters pain perception after jogging. *Psychiatric Research*, 5, 231–232.

Hailey, B.J. & Bailey, L. (1982). Negative addiction in runners: A quantitative approach. *Journal of Sport Behaviour*, 5, 150–154.

Haisch, J., Rduch, G. & Haisch, I. (1985). Long-term effects of attribution therapy measures in the obese: Effects of attribution training on successful slimming and dropout rate in a 23-week weight reduction programme. *Psychotherapy, Medicine and Psychology*, 35, 133–140.

Hamilton, R. (1984). Education for life: An assessment of the role of a recreational programme in the rehabilitation of the day patients in a psychiatric hospital. *International Journal of Lifelong Education*, 3, 223–232.

Harber, V.J. & Sutton, J.R. (1984). Endorphins and exercise. *Sports Medicine*, 1, 154–171.

Hardy, C.J. & Rejeski, W.J. (1989). Not what, but how one feels: The measurement of affect during exercise. *Journal of Sport and Exercise Psychology*, 11, 304–317.

Hardy, C.J., Hall, E.G. & Prestholdt, P.H. (1986). The mediational role of social influence in the perception of exertion. *Journal of Sport Psychology*, 8, 88–104.

Harris, D.V. (1973). *Involvement in Sport*. Philadelphia: Lea & Febiger.

Harris, D.V. & Harris, B. (1984). *Athletes' Guide to Sport Psychology*. Champaign: Leisure Press.

Harrison, J.E. & Chow, R. (1990). Discussion: Exercise, fitness, osteoarthritis, and osteoporosis. In C. Bouchard, R.J. Shephard, T. Stephens, J.R. Sutton & B.D. McPherson (Eds.). *Exercise, Fitness and Health: A Consensus of Current Knowledge*. Champaign: Human Kinetics.

Harter, S. (1978). Effectance motivation reconsidered: Toward a developmental model. *Human Development*, 21, 34– 64.

Harter, S. (1981). A new self-report scale of intrinsic versus extrinsic orientation in the classroom: Motivational and informational components. *Developmental Psychology*, 17, 300–312.

Harter, S. (1982). The Perceived Competence Scale for children. *Child Development*, 53, 87–97.

Harter, S. (1983). Developmental perspectives on the self-system. In E.M. Hetherington (Ed.). *Handbook of Child Psychology. IV. Socialisation, Personality and Social Development*. New York: Wiley.

Harter, S. & Connell, J.P. (1984). A model of children's achievement and related self-perceptions of competence, control and motivational orientation. In J.G. Nicholls (Ed.). *Advances in Motivation and Achievement. III. The Development of Achievement Motivation*. Greenwich, CT: JAI Press.

Hartz, G.W., Wallace, W.L. & Cayton, T.G. (1982). Effect of aerobic conditioning upon mood in clinically depressed men and women: A preliminary investigation. *Perceptual and Motor Skills*, 55, 1217–1218.

Hatfield, B.D. & Landers, D.M. (1987). Psychophysiology in exercise and sport research: An overview. *Exercise and Sport Sciences Reviews*, 15, 351–387.

Hawley, L.M. & Butterfield, G.E. (1981). Letter to the editor. *New England Journal of Medicine*, 305, 1591–1592.

Haynes, R.B. (1976). A critical review of the 'determinants' of patient compliance with therapeutic regimes. In D.L. Sackett & R.B. Haynes (Eds.). *Compliance with Therapeutic Regimes*. Baltimore: Johns Hopkins University Press.

Health and Physical Education Project Newsletter (1986). A health focus in athletics: Some food for thought. *Health and Physical Education Project Newsletter*, 6, 1–2.

Health and Physical Education Project Newsletter (1987). A health focus in athletics: Throwing challenges. *Health and Physical Education Project Newsletter*, 10, 6–8.

Health-related Physical Activity in the National Curriculum (1990). Report of the British Association of Sports Sciences, Health Education Authority, and Physical Education Association joint working party. *British Journal of Physical Education*, 21, 225.

Heartbeat Wales (1987). *Exercise for Health: Health-related Fitness in Wales*. Heartbeat Report 23. Cardiff: Heartbeat Wales.

Heiby, E.M., Onorato, V.A. & Sato, R.A. (1987). Cross-validation of the Self-Motivation Inventory. *Journal of Sport Psychology*, 9, 394–399.

Heider, F. (1944). Social perception and phenomenal causality. *Psychological Review*, 51, 358–374.

Heider, F. (1958). *The Psychology of Interpersonal Relations*. New York: Wiley.

Hesso, R. & Sorenson, M. (1982). Physical activity in the treatment of mental disorders. *Scandinavian Journal of Social Medicine*, 29 (Supplement), 259–264.

Hewstone, M. (1983) (Ed.). *Attribution Theory: Social and Functional Extensions*. Oxford: Blackwell.

Hewstone, M. (1989). *Causal Attribution: From Cognitive Processes to Collective Beliefs*. Oxford: Blackwell.

Hewstone, M. & Antaki, C. (1988). Attribution theory and social explanations. In M. Hewstone, W. Stroebe, J-P. Codol & G.M. Stephenson (Eds.). *Introduction to Social Psychology*. Oxford: Blackwell.

H.M.I. (1989). *Physical Education from 5 to 16*. London: Her Majesty's Stationery Office.

Hochstetler, S.A., Rejeski, W.J. & Best, D.L. (1985). The influence of sex-role orientation on ratings of perceived exertion. *Sex Roles*, 12, 825–835.

Hodgdon, R.E. & Reimer, D. (1960). Some muscular strength and endurance scores of psychiatric patients. *Journal of the Association of Physical and Mental Rehabilitation*, 14, 38–44.

Horne, J.A. & Staff, C.H. (1983). Exercise and sleep: Body healing effects. *Sleep*, 6, 34–46.

Hovland, C.I. & Rosenberg, M.J. (1960) (Eds.). *Attitudes, Organisation and Change: An Analysis of Consistency among Attitude Components*. New Haven: Yale University Press.

Howlett, T.A., Tomlin, S., Ngahfoong, L. et al (1984). Release of β-endorphin and met-enkaphalin during exercise in normal women: Response to training. *British Medical Journal*, 288, 1950–1952.

Hughes, J.R. (1984). Psychological effects of habitual aerobic exercise: A critical review. *Preventive Medicine*, 13, 66–78.

Hunter, J.E., Schmidt, F.L. & Jackson, G.B. (1982). *Meta-analysis: Cumulating Research Findings Across Studies*. Beverly Hills: Sage.

Ingjer, F. & Dahl, H.A. (1979). Dropouts from an endurance training programme: Some histochemical and physiological aspects. *Scandinavian Journal of Sports Sciences*, 1, 20–22.

Iso-Ahola, S.E. (1980). *The Social Psychology of Leisure and Recreation*. Dubuque: Wm C. Brown.

Iso-Ahola, S.E. & Hatfield, B.D. (1985). *Psychology of Sports: A Social-Psychological Approach*. Dubuque: Wm C. Brown.

Iverson, D.C., Fielding, J.E., Crow, R.S. & Christenson, G.M. (1985). The promotion of physical activity in the United States population: The status of programmes in medical, worksite, community, and school settings. *Public Health Reports*, 100, 212–224.

Janz, N.K. & Becker, M.H. (1984). The Health Belief Model: A decade later. *Health Education Quarterly*, 11, 1–47.

Johnson, L. & Biddle, S.J.H. (1989). Persistence after failure: An exploratory study of 'learned helplessness' in motor performance. *British Journal of Physical Education Research Supplement*, 5, 7–10.

Jones, E.E. & Davis, K.E. (1965). From acts to dispositions: The attribution process in person perception. In L. Berkowitz (Ed.). *Advances in Experimental Social Psychology. Vol 2*. New York: Academic Press.

Jorgenson, C.B. & Jorgenson, D.E. (1979). Effects of running on perception of self and others. *Perceptual and Motor Skills*, 48, 242.

Juneau, M., Rogers, F., DeSantos, V., Yee, M., Evans, A. & Bohn, A. (1987). Effectiveness of self-monitored, home-based, moderate intensity exercise training in middle-aged men and women. *American Journal of Cardiology*, 60, 66–70.

Kaplan, R.M., Atkins, C.J. & Reinsch, S. (1984). Specific efficacy expectations mediate exercise compliance in patients with COPD. *Health Psychology*, 3, 223–242.

Kasl, S.V. & Cobb, S. (1966). Health behaviour, illness behaviour and sick-role behaviour. *Archives on Environmental Health*, 12, 246–266.

Kassin, S.M. & Lepper, M.R. (1984). Oversufficient and insufficient justification effects: Cognitive and behavioural development. In J.G. Nicholls (Ed.). *Advances in Motivation and Achievement. Vol 3*. London: JAI Press.

Kau, J.L. & Fischer, J. (1974). Self-modification of exercise behaviour. *Journal of Behaviour Therapy and Experimental Psychiatry*, 5, 213–214.

Kazdin, A.E. (1975). *Behaviour Modification in Applied Settings*. Illinois: Homewood.

Kazdin, A.E. (1978). Conceptual and assessment issues raised by self-efficacy theory. *Advances in Behaviour Research and Therapy*, 1, 177–186.

Keefe, F.J. & Blumenthal, J.A. (1980). The life fitness programme: A behavioural approach to making exercise a habit. *Journal of Behaviour Therapy and Experimental Psychiatry*, 11, 31–34.

Kelemen, M.H. (1989). Resistive training safety and assessment guidelines for cardiac and coronary prone patients. *Medicine and Science in Sports and Exercise*, 21, 675–677.

Kelley, H.H. (1967). Attribution theory in social psychology. In D. Levine (Ed.). *Nebraska Symposium on Motivation.* Lincoln: University of Nebraska Press.

Kelly, G.A. (1955). *The Psychology of Personal Constructs.* New York: Norton.

Kelly, G.A. (1963). *A Theory of Personality: The Psychology of Personal Constructs.* New York: Norton.

Kendzierski, D. (1990). Decision making versus decision implementation: An action control approach to exercise adoption and adherence. *Journal of Applied Social Psychology,* 20, 27–45.

Kendzierski, D. & LaMastro, V.D. (1988). Reconsidering the role of attitudes in exercise behaviour: A decision theoretic approach. *Journal of Applied Social Psychology,* 18, 737–759.

Kenney, E.A., Rejeski, W.J. & Messier, S.P. (1987). Managing exercise distress: The effect of broad spectrum intervention on affect, RPE, and running efficiency. *Canadian Journal of Sport Sciences,* 12, 97–105.

Kenyon, G.S. (1968). Six scales for assessing attitude toward physical activity. *Research Quarterly,* 39, 566–574.

Keogh, J.F., Griffin, N.S. & Spector, R. (1981). Observer perceptions of movement confidence. *Research Quarterly for Exercise and Sport,* 52, 465–473.

King, J.B. (1982). The impact of patients' perceptions of high blood pressure on attendance at screening: An attributional extension of the Health Belief Model. *Social Science and Medicine,* 16, 1079–1092.

King, J.B. (1983). Attribution theory and the Health Belief Model. In M. Hewstone (Ed.). *Attribution Theory: Social and Functional Extensions.* Oxford: Blackwell.

King, A.C. & Frederiksen, L.W. (1984). Low-cost strategies for increasing exercise behaviour: Relapse prevention training and social support. *Behaviour Modification,* 8, 3–21.

Kirschenbaum, D.S. (1987). Toward the prevention of sedentary lifestyles. In W.P. Morgan & S.E. Goldston (Eds.). *Exercise and Mental Health.* Washington: Hemisphere.

Kirschenbaum, D.S. & Wittrock, D.A. (1984). Cognitive-behavioural interventions in sport: A self-regulatory perspective. In J. Silva & R. Weinberg (Eds.). *Psychological Foundations of Sport.* Champaign: Human Kinetics.

Kirscht, J.P. (1988). The Health Belief Model and predictions of health actions. In D.S. Gochman (Ed.). *Health Behaviour: Emerging Research Perspectives.* New York: Plenum.

Klein, M.H., Griest, J.H., Gurman, A.S. et al (1985). A comparative outcome study of group psychotherapy vs. exercise treatments for depression. *International Journal of Mental Health,* 13, 148–177.

Knapp, D.N. (1988). Behavioural management techniques and exercise promotion. In R.K. Dishman (Ed.). *Exercise Adherence: Its Impact on Public Health.* Champaign: Human Kinetics..

Knight, P.O., Schocken, D.D. & Powers, P.S. (1987). Gender comparison in anorexia nervosa and obligatory running. *Medicine and Science in Sports and Exercise,* 9 (Supplement), S66. [abstract]

Kobasa, S.C. (1979). Stressful life events, personality and health: An enquiry into hardiness. *Journal of Personality and Social Psychology,* 37, 1–11.

Koplan, J.P., Siscovick, D.S. & Goldbaum, G.M. (1985). The risks of exercise: A public health view of injuries and hazards. *Public Health Reports,* 100, 189–195.

Kostrubala, T. (1976). *The Joy of Running*. New York: Lippincott.

Krantz, D.S., Grunberg, N.E. & Baum, A. (1985). Health psychology. *Annual Review of Psychology*, 36, 349–383.

Kraus, H. & Raab, W. (1961). *Hypokinetic disease*. Springfield: C.C. Thomas.

Kristeller, J.L. & Rodin, J. (1985). A three-stage model of treatment continuity: Compliance, adherence and maintenance. In A. Baum, S.E. Taylor & J.E. Singer (Eds.). *Handbook of Psychology and Health. IV. Social Psychological Aspects of Health*. Hillsdale, NJ: Erlbaum.

Kuhl, J. (1985). Volitional mediators of cognition-behaviour consistency: Self-regulatory processes and action versus state orientation. In J. Kuhl & J. Beckmann (Eds.). *Action Control: From Cognition to Behaviour*. New York: Springer-Verlag.

Laffrey, S.C. & Isenberg, M. (1983). The relationship of internal locus of control, value placed on health, perceived importance of exercise, and participation in physical activity during leisure. *International Journal of Nursing Studies*, 20, 187–196.

LaPorte, R.E., Montoye, H.J. & Caspersen, C.J. (1985). Assessment of physical activity in epidemiological research: Problems and prospects. *Public Health Reports*, 100, 131–146.

Lau, R.R. (1988). Beliefs about control and health behaviour. In D.S. Goschman (Ed.). *Health Behaviour: Emerging Research Perspectives*. New York: Plenum.

Lau, R.R. & Hartman, K.A. (1983). Common sense representations of common illnesses. *Health Psychology*, 2, 167–185.

Lawrence, P., Ponder, M. & LePage, Y. (1988). *A Study of Lifestyle and Health in Guernsey 1988*. Guernsey: States of Guernsey.

Lazarus, R.S. (1975). A cognitively oriented psychologist looks at biofeedback. *American Psychologist*, 30, 553–561.

Lazarus, R.S. & Folkman, S. (1984). *Stress, Appraisal and Coping*. New York: Springer-Verlag.

Lee, A.M., Carter, J.A. & Greenockle, K.M. (1987). Children and fitness: A pedagogical perspective. *Research Quarterly for Exercise and Sport*, 58, 321–325.

Lee, C. & Owen, N. (1985a). Reasons for discontinuing regular physical activity subsequent to a fitness course. *The ACHPER National Journal*, March, 7–9.

Lee, C. & Owen, N. (1985b). Behaviourally-based principles as guidelines for health promotion. *Community Health Studies*, 9, 131–138.

Lee, C. & Owen, N. (1986). Exercise persistence: Contributions of psychology to the promotion of regular physical activity. *Australian Psychologist*, 21, 427–466.

Lenney, E. (1977). Women's self-confidence in achievement situations. *Psychological Bulletin*, 84, 1–13.

Lepper, M.R. & Greene, D. (1975). Turning play into work: Effects of adult surveillance and extrinsic rewards on children's intrinsic motivation. *Journal of Personality and Social Psychology*, 31, 479–486.

Lepper, M.R., Greene, D. & Nisbett, R.E. (1973). Undermining children's intrinsic interest with extrinsic reward: A test of the 'overjustification' hypothesis. *Journal of Personality and Social Psychology*, 28, 129–137.

Levenson, H. (1974). Activism and powerful others: Distinctions with the concept of internal-external control. *Journal of Personality Assessment*, 38, 377–383.

Levenson, H. (1981). Differentiating among internality, powerful others and chance. In H.M. Lefcourt (Ed.). *Research with the Locus of Control Construct. Vol 1*. New York: Academic Press.

Levin, S.J. & Giminio, F.A. (1982). Psychological effects of aerobic exercise on schizophrenic patients. *Medicine and Science in Sports and Exercise*, 14, 116.

Lindsay-Reid, E. & Osborn, R.W. (1980). Readiness for exercise adoption. *Social Science and Medicine*, 14, 139–146.

Lion, L.S. (1978). Psychological effects of jogging: A preliminary study. *Perceptual and Motor Skills*, 47, 1215–1218.

Liska, A.E. (1984). A critical examination of the causal structure of the Fishbein/Ajzen attitude-behaviour model. *Social Psychology Quarterly*, 47, 61–74.

Locke, E.A. & Latham, G.P. (1985). The application of goal-setting to sports. *Journal of Sport Psychology*, 7, 205–222.

Locke, E.A., Latham, G.P. & Erez, M. (1988). The determinants of goal commitment. *Academy of Management Review*, 13, 23–39.

Long, B.C. & Haney, C.J. (1986). Enhancing physical activity in sedentary women: Information, locus of control and attitudes. *Journal of Sport Psychology*, 8, 8–24.

Lowery, B.J. & Jacobsen, B.S. (1985). Attributional analysis of chronic illness outcomes. *Nursing Research*, 34, 82–88.

MacConnie, S.E., Gilliam, T.B., Geenen, D.L. & Pels, A.E. (1982). Daily physical activity patterns of prepubertal children involved in a vigorous exercise programme. *International Journal of Sports Medicine*, 3, 202–207.

Mackinnon, L.T. (1989). Exercise and natural killer cells: What is the relationship? *Sports Medicine*, 7, 141–149.

Maehr, M.L. & Braskamp, L.A. (1986). *The Motivation Factor: A Theory of Personal Investment*. Lexington, Mass: Lexington Books.

Maehr, M.L. & Nicholls, J.G. (1980). Culture and achievement motivation: A second look. In N. Warren (Ed.). *Studies in Cross-cultural Psychology. Vol II*. New York: Academic Press.

Magill, R.A. (1989). *Motor Learning: Concepts and Applications*. Dubuque: Wm C. Brown.

Mahoney, M.J. & Mahoney, K. (1976). *Permanent Weight Control*. New York: Norton.

Maier, S.F. & Laudenslager, M. (1985). Stress and health: Exploring the links. *Psychology Today*, August, 44–49.

Maiman, L.A. & Becker, M.H. (1974). The Health Belief Model: Origins and correlates in psychological theory. *Health Education Monographs*, 2, 337–353.

Malina, R.M. (1988). Physical activity in early and modern populations: An evolutionary view. In R.M. Malina & H.M. Eckert (Eds.). *Physical Activity in Early and Modern Populations*. Champaign: Human Kinetics and The American Academy of Physical Education.

Malina, R.M. (1989). Children in the exercise sciences. *Research Quarterly for Exercise and Sport*, 60, 305–317.

Markoff, R.A., Ryan, P. & Young, T. (1982). Endorphins and mood changes in long distance running. *Medicine and Science in Sports and Exercise*, 14, 11–15.

Marlatt, G.A. (1985). Relapse prevention: Theoretical rationale and overview of the model. In G.A. Marlatt & J.R. Gordon (Eds.). *Relapse Prevention: Maintenance Strategies in the Treatment of Addictive Behaviours*. New York: Guilford Press.

Marlatt, G.A. & Gordon, J.R. (1985) (Eds.). *Relapse Prevention: Maintenance Strategies in the Treatment of Addictive Behaviours*. New York: Guilford Press.

Martens, R., Vealey, R.S. & Burton, D. (1990). *Competitive Anxiety in Sport*. Champaign: Human Kinetics.

Martin, J.E. (1981). Exercise management: Shaping and maintaining physical fitness. *Behavioural Medicine Advances*, 4, 3–5.

Martin, J.E. & Calfas, K.J. (1989). Is it possible to lower blood pressure with exercise? Efficacy and adherence issues. *Journal of Applied Sport Psychology*, 1, 109–131.

Martin, J.E. & Dubbert, P.M. (1982). Exercise applications and promotion in behavioural medicine. *Journal of Consulting and Clinical Psychology*, 50, 1004–1017.

Martin, J.E., Dubbert, P.M., Katell, A.D., Thompson, J.K., Raczynski, J.R. & Lake, M. (1984). Behavioural control of exercise: Studies 1 through 6. *Journal of Consulting and Clinical Psychology*, 52, 795–811.

Martinsen, E.W. (1987). Exercise and medication in the psychiatric patient. In W.P. Morgan & S.E. Goldston (Eds.). *Exercise and Mental Health*. Washington, DC: Hemisphere.

Martinsen, E.W. (1988). Exercise intervention studies in patients with anxiety and depressive disorders. In *Sport, Health, Psychology and Exercise Symposium proceedings*. London: The Sports Council/Health Education Authority.

Martinsen, E.W., Medhus, A. & Sandvik, L. (1985). Effects of aerobic exercise on depression: A controlled study. *British Medical Journal*, 291, 109.

Martinsen, E.W., Hoffart, A. & Solberg, O. (1988). Comparing aerobic and nonaerobic forms of exercise in the treatment of clinical depression: A randomised trial. In *Sport, Health, Psychology and Exercise Symposium proceedings*. London: The Sports Council/Health Education Authority.

Martinsen, E.W., Strand, J., Paulsson, G. & Kaggestad, J. (1989). Physical fitness level in patients with anxiety and depressive disorders. *International Journal of Sports Medicine*, 10, 58–61.

Massie, J.F. & Shephard, R.J. (1971). Physiological and psychological effects of training: A comparison of individual and gymnasium programmes, with a characterisation of the exercise 'dropout'. *Medicine and Science in Sports*, 3, 110–117.

Mathews, A. & Steptoe, A. (1988). *Essential Psychology for Medical Practice*. Edinburgh: Churchill Livingstone.

McAuley, E. & Gill, D.L. (1983). Reliability and validity of the Physical Self-Efficacy Scale in a competitive sport setting. *Journal of Sport Psychology*, 5, 410–418.

McAuley, E. & Tammen, V.V. (1989). The effects of subjective and objective competitive outcomes on intrinsic motivation. *Journal of Sport and Exercise Psychology*, 11, 84–93.

McAuley, E., Duncan, T. & Tammen, V.V. (1989a). Psychometric properties of the Intrinsic Motivation Inventory in a competitive sport setting: A confirmatory factor analysis. *Research Quarterly for Exercise and Sport*, 60, 48–58.

McAuley, E., Duncan,T. & Wraith, S.C. (1989b). Intrinsic motivation and exercise behaviour: A confirmatory factor analysis. Paper presented at North American Society for the Psychology of Sport and Physical Activity conference, Kent State University, Ohio, USA.

McCann, I.L. & Holmes, D.S. (1984). Influence of aerobic exercise on depression. *Journal of Personality and Social Psychology*, 46, 1142–1147.

McCaul, K.D., O'Neill, H.K. & Glasgow, R.E. (1988). Predicting the performance of dental hygiene behaviours: An examination of the Fishbein and Ajzen model and self-efficacy expectations. *Journal of Applied Social Psychology*, 18, 114–128.

McCready, M.L. & Long, B.C. (1985). Locus of control, attitudes toward physical activity, and exercise adherence. *Journal of Sport Psychology*, 7, 346–359.

McGuire, W.J. (1985). Attitudes and attitude change. In G. Lindzey & E. Aronson (Eds.). *Handbook of Social Psychology. Vol 2*. New York: Random House.

McIntosh, P. & Charlton, V. (1985). *The Impact of 'Sport for All' Policy*. London: The Sports Council.

McNair, D.M., Lorr, M. & Droppleman, L.F. (1971). *Profile of Mood States Manual*. San Diego: Educational and Industrial Testing Service.

McSherry, J.A. (1984). The diagnostic challenge of anorexia nervosa. *American Family Physician*, 29, 141–145.

McSwegin, P.J., Pemberton, C. & Petray, C. (1989). An educational plan. *Journal of Physical Education, Recreation and Dance*, 60(1), 32–34.

Mental Disorder Programme Planning Group (1985). *Mental Health in Focus*. London: Her Majesty's Stationery Office.

Mento, A.J., Steel, R.P. & Karren, R.J. (1987). A meta-analytic study of the effects of goal-setting on task performance: 1966–1984. *Organizational Behaviour and Human Decision Processes*, 39, 52–83.

Mercer, T.H. (1989). Being habitually active in leisure time: Today's best buy for public health. *British Journal of Physical Education*, 20, 137–144.

Mihalik, B.J., O'Leary, J.T., McGuire, F.A. & Dottavio, F.D. (1989). Sports involvement across the life span: Expansion and contraction of sports activities. *Research Quarterly for Exercise and Sport*, 60, 396–398.

Mihevic, P.M. (1982). Anxiety, depression and exercise. *Quest*, 33, 140–153.

Miller Lite (1983). *Miller Lite Report on American Attitudes Toward Sports*. Milwaukee: Miller Lite.

Mineka, S. & Hendersen, R.W. (1985). Controllability and predictability in acquired motivation. *Annual Review of Psychology*, 36, 495–529.

Montgomery, S.A. & Asberg, M. (1979). A new depression scale designed to be sensitive to change. *British Journal of Psychiatry*, 134, 382–389.

Moore, M. (1982). Endorphins and exercise: A puzzling relationship. *The Physician and Sportsmedicine*, 10, 111–119.

Morgan, W.P. (1969). A pilot investigation of physical working capacity in depressed and non-depressed psychiatric males. *Research Quarterly*, 40, 849–861.

Morgan, W.P. (1979a). Anxiety reduction following acute physical activity. *Psychiatric Annals*, 9, 141–147.

Morgan, W.P. (1979b). Negative addiction in runners. *The Physician and Sportsmedicine*, 7, 56–63; 67–70.

Morgan, W.P. (1980a). The trait psychology controversy. *Research Quarterly for Exercise and Sport*, 51, 50–76.

Morgan, W.P. (1980b). Test of champions: The iceberg profile. *Psychology Today.*, 14, 92–99; 101; 108.

Morgan, W.P. (1985). Affective beneficence of vigorous physical activity. *Medicine and Science in Sports and Exercise*, 17, 94–100.

Morgan, W.P. & Goldston, S.E. (1987) (Eds.). *Exercise and Mental Health*. Washington: Hemisphere.

Morgan, W.P. & O'Connor, P.J. (1988). Exercise and mental health. In R.K. Dishman (Ed.). *Exercise Adherence: Its Impact on Public Health*. Champaign: Human Kinetics.

Morgan, W.P. & Pollock, M.L. (1977). Psychological characterisation of the elite distance runner. *Annals of the New York Academy of Sciences*, 301, 382–403.

Morgan, W.P., Horstman, D.H., Cymerman, A. & Stokes, J. (1980). Exercise as a relaxation technique. *Primary Cardiology*, 6, 48–57.

Morris, J.N., Heady, J.A., Raffle, P.A.B., Roberts, C.G. & Parks, J.W. (1953).

Coronary heart disease and physical activity of work. *The Lancet*, ii, 1053–1057; 1111–1120.

Morris, J.N., Kagan, A., Pattison, D.C., Gardner, M. & Raffle, P.A.B. (1966). Incidence and prediction of ischaemic heart disease in London busmen. *The Lancet*, ii, 552–559.

Morris, J.N., Everett, M.G. & Semmence, A.M. (1987). Exercise and coronary heart disease. In D. Macleod, R. Maughan, M. Nimmo, T. Reilly & C. Williams (Eds.). *Exercise: Benefits, Limits and Adaptations*. London: Spon.

Morris, M., Steinberg, H., Sykes, E. & Salmon, P. (1988). Temporary deprivation from running produces 'withdrawal' syndrome. In *Sport, Health, Psychology and Exercise Symposium proceedings*. London: The Sports Council/Health Education Authority.

Moses, J., Steptoe, A., Mathews, A. & Edwards, S. (1989). The effects of exercise training on mental well-being in the normal population: A controlled trial. *Journal of Psychosomatic Research*, 33, 47–61.

Murdoch, F.A., & Mutrie, N. (1988). Short term intervention for withdrawal from benzodiazepines: A comparative study of group therapy plus exercise versus group therapy. Unpublished manuscript, Department of Physical Education and Sports Science, University of Glasgow, Scotland.

Mutrie, N. (1985). *Goal setting*. Coach Education Modules 1 and 2. Scottish Sports Council.

Mutrie, N. (1986). Exercise as a treatment for depression within a national health service. Unpublished doctoral dissertation, The Pennsylvania State University.

Mutrie, N. (1987). The psychological effects of exercise for women. In D. Macleod, R. Maughan, M. Nimmo, T. Reilly & C. Williams (Eds.). *Exercise: Benefits, Limits and Adaptations*. London: Spon.

Mutrie, N. & Grant, S. (1985). We live in testing times: Individual and group fitness tests at Glasgow University. Paper presented at the Scottish Universities Physical Education Association conference, Strathclyde University.

Mutrie, N. & Knill-Jones, R. (1985). Reasons for running: 1984 survey of the Glasgow People's Marathon. Paper presented at International Society of Sports Psychology World Congress, Copenhagen, Denmark.

Nachemson, A.L. (1990). Exercise, fitness, and back pain. In C. Bouchard, R.J. Shephard, T. Stephens, J.R. Sutton & B.D. McPherson (Eds.). *Exercise, Fitness and Health: A Consensus of Current Knowledge*. Champaign: Human Kinetics.

Nash, H.L. (1987). Do compulsive runners and anorectic patients share common bonds? *The Physician and Sportsmedicine*, 15, 162–167.

National Forum for Coronary Heart Disease Prevention (1988).*Coronary Heart Disease Prevention: Action in the UK 1984–1987*. London: Health Education Authority and National Forum for Coronary Heart Disease Prevention.

Naylor, J.C. & Ilgen, D.R. (1984). Goal-setting: A theoretical analysis of a motivational technology. *Research in Organisational Behaviour*, 6, 95–140.

Newton, M. & Mutrie, N. (1991). The psychological effects of exercise in cardiac rehabilitation. *Scottish Medical Journal*.

Nicholls, J.G. (1984). Achievement motivation: Conceptions of ability, subjective experience, task choice and performance. *Psychological Review*, 91, 328–346.

Nielson, A.B., Borsdorf, L.L. & Corbin, C.B. (1984). Commitment to specific and general physical activity. Paper presented at Olympic Scientific Congress, Eugene, Oregon.

Noland, M.P. (1989). The effects of self-monitoring and reinforcement on exercise adherence. *Research Quarterly for Exercise and Sport*, 60, 216–224.

Noland, M.P. & Feldman, R.H.L. (1984). Factors related to the leisure exercise behaviour of 'returning' women college students. *Health Education*, March/April, 32–36.

Noland, M.P. & Feldman, R.H.L. (1985). An empirical investigation of leisure exercise behaviour in adult women. *Health Education*, Oct/Nov, 29–34.

Nowlis, D. & Greenberg, N. (1979). Empirical description of effects of exercise on mood. *Perceptual and Motor Skills*, 49, 1001–1002.

Nutbeam, D. (1984). *The Dorset Get-Fit Campaign*. Positive Health technical report 4: Wessex Regional Health Authority.

O'Connell, J. & Price, J. (1982). Health locus of control of physical fitness programme participants. *Perceptual and Motor Skills*, 55, 925–926.

O'Connell, J.K., Price, J.H., Roberts, S.M., Jurs, S.G. & McKinley, R. (1985). Utilising the Health Belief Model to predict dietary and exercising behaviour of obese and non-obese adolescents. *Health Education Quarterly*, 12, 343–351.

Oldridge, N.B. (1982). Compliance and exercise in primary and secondary prevention of coronary heart disease: A review. *Preventive Medicine*, 11, 56–70.

Oldridge, N.B. (1984). Compliance and dropout in cardiac exercise rehabilitation. *Journal of Cardiac Rehabilitation*, 4, 166–177.

Oldridge, N.B. (1988). Compliance with exercise in cardiac rehabilitation. In R.K. Dishman (Ed.). *Exercise Adherence: Its Impact on Public Health*. Champaign: Human Kinetics.

Oldridge, N.B. & Jones, N.L. (1983). Improving patient compliance in cardiac rehabilitation: Effects of written agreement and self-monitoring. *Journal of Cardiac Rehabilitation*, 3, 257–262.

Oldridge, N.B. & Spencer, J. (1985). Exercise habits and perceptions before and after graduation or dropout from supervised cardiac rehabilitation. *Journal of Cardiopulmonary Rehabilitation*, 5, 313–319.

O'Leary, A. (1985). Self-efficacy and health. *Behaviour Research and Therapy*, 23, 437–451.

Olson, J.M. & Zanna, M.P. (1981). *Promoting Physical Activity: A Social Psychological Perspective*. Report prepared for the Ministry of Culture and Recreation, Toronto, Canada.

Olson, J.M. & Zanna, M.P. (1982). *Predicting Adherence to a Programme of Physical Exercise: An Empirical Study*. Report prepared for Ontario Ministry of Tourism and Recreation, Toronto, Canada.

Orwin, A. (1981). 'The running treatment': A preliminary communication on a new use for an old therapy (physical activity) in the agoraphobic syndrome. In M.H. Sacks & M.L. Sachs (Eds.). *Psychology of Running*. Champaign: Human Kinetics.

Ossip-Klein, D.J., Doyne, E.J., Bowman, E.D., Osborn, K.M., McDougall-Wilson, I.B. & Neimeyer, R.A. (1989). Effects of running and weight lifting on self-concept in clinically depressed women. *Journal of Consulting and Clinical Psychology*, 57, 158–161.

Paffenbarger, R.S. (1988). Contributions of epidemiology to exercise science and cardiovascular health. *Medicine and Science in Sports and Exercise*, 20, 426–438.

Paffenbarger, R.S. & Hyde, R.T. (1988). Exercise adherence, coronary heart disease and longevity. In R.K. Dishman (Ed.). *Exercise Adherence: Its Impact on Public Health*. Champaign: Human Kinetics.

Paffenbarger, R.S., Wing, A.L. & Hyde, R.T. (1978). Physical activity as an index of heart attack risk in college alumni. *American Journal of Epidemiology*, 108, 161–175.

Paffenbarger, R.S., Hyde, R.T., Wing, A.L. & Hsieh, C.C. (1986). Physical activity, all-cause mortality, and longevity of college alumni. *New England Journal of Medicine*, 314, 605–613.

Paffenbarger, R.S., Hyde, R.T. & Wing, A.L. (1990). Physical activity and physical fitness as determinants of health and longevity. In C. Bouchard, R.J. Shephard, T. Stephens, J.R. Sutton & B.D. McPherson (Eds.). *Exercise, Fitness and Health: A Consensus of Current Knowledge*. Champaign: Human Kinetics.

Palenzuela, D.L. (1988). Refining the theory and measurement of expectancy of internal versus external control of reinforcement. *Personality and Individual Differences*, 9, 607–629.

Parcel, G.S., Simons-Morton, B.G., O'Hara, N.M., Baranowski, T., Kolbe, L.J. & Bee, D.E. (1987). School promotion of healthful diet and exercise behaviour: An integration of organisational change and social learning theory interventions. *Journal of School Health*, 57(4), 150–156.

Pargman, D. & Baker, M.C. (1980). Running high: Enkaphalin indicated. *Journal of Drug Issues*, 10, 341–349.

Pate, R.R. (1988). The evolving definition of physical fitness. *Quest*, 40, 174–179.

Patton, R.W., Corry, J.M., Gettman, L.R. & Graf, J.S. (1986). *Implementing Health/Fitness Programs*. Champaign: Human Kinetics.

Paxton, S.J., Trinder, J. & Montgomery, I. (1983). Does aerobic fitness affect sleep? *Psychophysiology*, 20, 320–324.

Pender, N.J. & Pender, A.R. (1986). Attitudes, subjective norms and intentions to engage in health behaviours. *Nursing Research*, 35, 15–18.

Perkins, K.A., Rapp, S.R., Carlson, C.R. & Wallace, C.E. (1986). A behavioural intervention to increase exercise among nursing home residents. *Gerontology*, 26, 479–481.

Perry, C.L., Klepp, K.I., Halper, A. et al. (1987). Promoting healthy eating and physical activity patterns among adolescents: A pilot study of 'Slice of Life'. *Health Education Research*, 2, 93–103.

Peterson, C. & Seligman, M.E.P. (1984). Causal explanations as a risk factor for depression: Theory and evidence. *Psychological Review*, 91, 347–374.

Physical Education Association (1987). *Report of a Commission of Enquiry: Physical Education in Schools*. London: PEA.

Pill, R. & Stott, N.C.H. (1985). Choice or chance: Further evidence on ideas of illness and responsibility for health. *Social Science and Medicine*, 20, 981–991.

Pitts, F.N. & McClure, J.N. (1967). Lactate metabolism in anxiety neurosis. *New England Journal of Medicine*, 277, 1329–1336.

Platt, J.R. (1964). Strong inference. *Science*, 146, 347–353.

Pollatschek, J.L. & O'Hagan, F.J. (1989). An investigation of the psycho-physical influences of a quality daily physical education programme. *Health Education Research: Theory and Practice*, 4, 341–350.

Powell, K.E. (1988). Habitual exercise and public health: An epidemiological view. In R.K. Dishman (Ed.). *Exercise Adherence: Its Impact on Public Health.* Champaign: Human Kinetics.

Powell, K.E. & Dysinger, W. (1987). Childhood participation in organised school sports and physical education as precursors of adult physical activity. *American Journal of Preventive Medicine,* 3, 276–281.

Powell, K.E., Spain, K.S., Christenson, G.M. & Mollenkamp, M.P. (1986). The status of the 1990 objectives for physical fitness and exercise. *Public Health Reports,* 101, 15–21.

Powell, K.E., Thompson, P.D., Caspersen, C.J. & Kendrick, J.S. (1987). Physical activity and the incidence of coronary heart disease. *Annual Review of Public Health,* 8, 253–287.

Prapavessis, H. & Carron, A.V. (1988). Learned helplessness in sport. *The Sport Psychologist,* 2, 189–201.

Prentice-Dunn, S. & Rogers, R.W. (1986). Protection Motivation Theory and preventive health: Beyond the Health Belief Model. *Health Education Research: Theory and Practice,* 1, 153–161.

Prosser, G., Carson, P., Gelson, A. et al (1978). Assessing the psychological effects of an exercise training programme for patients following myocardial infarction: A pilot study. *British Journal of Medical Psychology,* 51, 95–102.

Prosser, G., Carson, P., Phillips, R et al. (1981). Morale in coronary patients following an exercise programme. *Journal of Psychosomatic Research,* 25, 587–593.

Prosser, G., Carson, P. & Phillips, R. (1985). Exercise after myocardial infarction: Long-term rehabilitation effects. *Journal of Psychosomatic Research,* 29, 535–540.

Ramlow, J., Kriska, A. & LaPorte, R.E. (1987). Physical activity in the population: The epidemiologic spectrum. *Research Quarterly for Exercise and Sport,* 58, 111–113.

Rees, D.W. (1985). Health beliefs and compliance with alcoholism treatment. *Journal of Studies on Alcohol,* 46, 517–524.

Rees, D. W. & Farmer, R. (1985). Health beliefs and attendance for specialist alcoholism treatment. *British Journal of Psychiatry,* 147, 317–319.

Rees, J. (1988). Keep-fit women 'risk addiction and illness'. *The Daily Telegraph,* October 11th.

Reid, D.W. & Ware, E.E. (1973). Multidimensionality of internal–external control: Implications for past and future research. *Canadian Journal of Behavioural Science,* 5, 264–271.

Reiter, M.A. (1981). Effects of a physical exercise programme on selected mood states in a group of women over age 65. *Dissertation Abstracts International,* 42(5), 1974A.

Rejeski, W.J. (1981). The perception of exertion: A social psychophysiological integration. *Journal of Sport Psychology,* 3, 305–320.

Rejeski, W.J. (1985). Perceived exertion: An active or passive process? *Journal of Sport Psychology,* 7, 371–378.

Rejeski, W.J. & Brawley, L.R. (1983). Attribution theory in sport: Current status and new perspectives. *Journal of Sport Psychology,* 5, 77–99.

Rejeski, W.J. & Brawley, L.R. (1988). Defining the boundaries of sport psychology. *The Sport Psychologist,* 2, 231–242.

Rejeski, W.J. & Kenney, E.A. (1988). *Fitness Motivation: Preventing Participant Dropout.* Champaign: Life Enhancement Publications.

Rejeski, W.J. & Sanford, B. (1984). Feminine-typed females: The role of affective schema in the perception of exercise intensity. *Journal of Sport Psychology*, 6, 197–207.

Reuter, M.A. (1979). The effect of running on individuals who are clinically depressed. Unpublished Master's thesis, The Pennsylvania State University.

Riddle, P.K. (1980). Attitudes, beliefs, behavioural intentions and behaviours of women and men toward regular jogging. *Research Quarterly for Exercise and Sport*, 51, 663–674.

Riggs, C.E. (1981). Endorphins, neurotransmitters, and/or neuromodulators and exercise. In M.H. Sacks & M.L. Sachs (Eds.). *Psychology of Running*. Champaign: Human Kinetics.

Rippetoe, P.A. & Rogers, R.W. (1987). Effects of components of Protection Motivation Theory on adaptive and maladaptive coping with a health threat. *Journal of Personality and Social Psychology*, 52, 596–604.

Robbins, J.M. & Joseph, P. (1985). Experiencing exercise withdrawal: Possible consequences of therapeutic and mastery running. *Journal of Sport Psychology*, 7, 23–39.

Roberts, G.C. (1984). Toward a new theory of motivation in sport: The role of perceived ability. In J. Silva & R.S. Weinberg (Eds.). *Psychological Foundations of Sport*. Champaign: Human Kinetics.

Robertson, & Mutrie, N. (1989). Factors in adherence to exercise. *Physical Education Review*, 12, 138–146.

Rodin, J. (1978). Somatopsychics and attribution. *Personality and Social Psychology Bulletin*, 4, 531–540.

Rogers, R.W. (1983). Cognitive and physiological processes in fear appeals and attitude change: A revised theory of protection motivation. In J.R. Cacioppo & R.E. Petty (Eds.). *Social Psychology: A Source Book*. New York: Guilford Press.

Rosen, L.W. & Hough, D.D. (1988). Pathogenic weight control behaviours of female college gymnasts. *The Physician and Sportsmedicine*, 16(9), 11–14.

Rosen, L.W., McKeag, D.B., Hough, D.D. & Curley, V. (1986). Pathogenic weight control behaviour in female athletes. *The Physician and Sportsmedicine*, 14(1), 79–86.

Rosenstock, I.M. (1974). Historical origins of the Health Belief Model. *Health Education Monographs*, 2, 328–335.

Rosenstock, I.M. & Kirscht, J.P. (1979). Why people seek health care. In G.C. Stone, F. Cohen & N.E. Adler (Eds.). *Health Psychology: A Handbook*. San Francisco: Jossey Bass.

Roth, D.L. & Holmes, D.S. (1985). Influence of physical fitness in determining the impact of stressful life events on physical and psychological health. *Psychosomatic Medicine*, 47, 164–173.

Rotter, J.B. (1954). *Social Learning and Clinical Psychology*. Englewood Cliffs, NJ: Prentice-Hall.

Rotter, J.B. (1966). Generalised expectancies for internal versus external control of reinforcement. *Psychological Monographs*, 80 (Whole No. 609), 1–28.

Rotter, J.B. (1975). Some problems and misconceptions related to the construct of internal versus external control of reinforcement. *Journal of Consulting and Clinical Psychology*, 43, 56–67.

Rotter, J.B. (1979). Comments on section IV: Individual differences and perceived control. In L.C. Perlmuter & R.A. Monty (Eds.). *Choice and Perceived Control*. Hillsdale, NJ: Erlbaum.

Russell, D. (1982). The Causal Dimension Scale: A measure of how individuals perceive causes. *Journal of Personality and Social Psychology*, 42, 1137–1145.

Ryan, A.J. (1984). Exercise and health: Lessons from the past. In H.M. Eckert & H.J. Montoye (Eds.). *Exercise and Health*. Champaign: Human Kinetics and The American Academy of Physical Education.

Ryan, R.M. (1982). Control and information in the interpersonal sphere: An extension of Cognitive Evaluation Theory. *Journal of Personality and Social Psychology*, 43, 736–750.

Ryckman, R.M., Robbins, M.A., Thornton, B. & Cantrell, P. (1982). Development and validation of a Physical Self-Efficacy Scale. *Journal of Personality and Social Psychology*, 42, 891–900.

Sachs, M.L. (1981). Running addiction. In M.H. Sacks & M.L. Sachs (Eds.). *Psychology of Running*. Champaign: Human Kinetics.

Sachs, M.L. (1984). The runner's high. In M.L. Sachs & G.W. Buffone (Eds.). *Running as Therapy*. Lincoln, Nebraska: University of Nebraska Press.

Safrit, M.J., Hooper, L.M., Ehlert, S.A., Costa, M.G. & Patterson, P. (1988). The validity generalisation of distance run tests. *Canadian Journal of Sports Sciences*, 13, 188–196.

Sallis, J.F. (1987). A commentary on 'Children and fitness: A public health perspective'. *Research Quarterly for Exercise and Sport*, 58, 326–330.

Sallis, J.F. & Hovell, M.F. (1990). Determinants of exercise behaviour. *Exercise and Sport Sciences Reviews*, 18, 307–330.

Sallis, J.F., Haskell, W., Fortmann, S., Vranizan, K., Taylor, C.B. & Solomon, D. (1986). Predictors of adoption and maintenance of physical activity in a community sample. *Preventive Medicine*, 15, 331–341.

Saltzer, E.B. (1982). The Weight Locus of Control (WLOC) Scale: A specific measure for obesity research. *Journal of Personality Assessment*, 46, 620–628.

Saris, W.H.M. (1986). Habitual physical activity in children: Methodology and findings in health and disease. *Medicine and Science in Sports and Exercise*, 18, 253–263.

Scanlan, T.K. & Lewthwaite, R. (1986). Social psychological aspects of competition for male youth sport participants. IV. Predictors of enjoyment. *Journal of Sport Psychology*, 8, 25–35.

Schafer, W. (1978). *Stress, Distress and Growth*. Davis, Ca: Responsible Action.

Scherf, J. & Franklin, B.A. (1987). Exercise compliance: A data documentation system. *Journal of Physical Education, Recreation and Dance*, 58, 26–28.

Schifter, D.E. & Ajzen, I. (1985). Intention, perceived control and weight loss: An application of the Theory of Planned Behaviour. *Journal of Personality and Social Psychology*, 49, 843–851.

Schlackmans (1986). *Women's Fitness and Exercise Classes. Vol I. Summary and Conclusions*. London: Schlackmans.

Schmidt, R.A. (1986). *Motor Control and Learning*. Champaign: Human Kinetics.

School Sport Forum (1988). *Sport and Young People: Partnership and Action*. London: Sports Council.

Schull, W.J. (1990). Heredity, fitness, and health. In C. Bouchard, R.J. Shephard, T. Stephens, J.R. Sutton & B.D. McPherson (Eds.). *Exercise, Fitness and Health: A Consensus of Current Knowledge*. Champaign: Human Kinetics.

Schunk, D.H. (1981). Modelling and attributional effects on children's achievement: A self-efficacy analysis. *Journal of Educational Psychology*, 73, 93–105.

Schunk, D.H. (1982). Effects of effort attributional feedback on children's perceived self-efficacy and achievement. *Journal of Educational Psychology*, 74, 548–556.

Schunk, D.H. (1983). Ability versus effort attributional feedback: Differential effects on self-efficacy and achievement. *Journal of Educational Psychology*, 75, 848–856.

Schunk, D.H. (1984). Sequential attributional feedback and children's achievement behaviours. *Journal of Educational Psychology*, 76, 1159–1169.

Schutz, R.W., Smoll, F.L., Carre, F.A. & Mosher, R.E. (1985). Inventories and norms for children's attitudes toward physical activity. *Research Quarterly for Exercise and Sport*, 56, 256–265.

Schwartz, G.E., Davidson, R.J. & Goleman, D.J. (1978). Patterning of cognitive and somatic processes in the self-regulation of anxiety: Effects of meditation versus exercise. *Psychosomatic Medicine*, 40, 321–328.

Sechrist, K.R., Walker, S.N. & Pender, N.J. (1987). Development and psychometric evaluation of the exercise benefits/barriers scale. *Research in Nursing and Health*, 10, 357–365.

Sechrist, W. (1983). Causal attribution and personal responsibility for health and disease. *Health Education*, 14(2), 51–54.

Seefeldt, V. & Vogel, P. (1987). Children and fitness: A public health perspective – A response. *Research Quarterly for Exercise and Sport*, 58, 331–333.

Seligman, M.E.P. (1975). *Helplessness: On Depression, Development and Death*. San Francisco: W.H. Freeman.

Selye, H. (1956). *The Stress of Life*. New York: McGraw-Hill.

Serfass, R.C. & Gerberich, S.G. (1984). Exercise for optimal health: Strategies and motivational considerations. *Preventive Medicine*, 13, 79–99.

Sforzo, G.A. (1988). Opioids and exercise: An update. *Sports Medicine*, 7, 109–124.

Shephard, R.J. (1985). Motivation: The key to fitness compliance. *The Physician and Sportsmedicine*, 13(7), 88–101.

Shephard, R.J. (1986). *Economic Benefits of Enhanced Fitness*. Champaign: Human Kinetics.

Shephard, R.J. (1988). Exercise adherence in corporate settings: Personal traits and programme barriers. In R.K. Dishman (Ed.). *Exercise Adherence: Its Impact on Public Health*. Champaign: Human Kinetics.

Shephard, R.J. (1989a). Current perspectives on the economics of fitness and sport with particular reference to worksite programmes. *Sports Medicine*, 7, 286–309.

Shephard, R.J. (1989b). Exercise and lifestyle change. *British Journal of Sports Medicine*, 23, 11–22.

Shephard, R.J., Jequier, J.C., Lavallee, H., La Barre, R. & Rajii, M. (1980). Habitual physical activity: Effects of sex, milieu, season and required activity. *Journal of Sports Medicine and Physical Fitness*, 20, 55–66.

Sherer, M., Maddux, J.E., Mercandante, B. & Prentice-Dunn, S. (1982). The Self-Efficacy Scale: Construction and validation. *Psychological Reports*, 51, 663–671.

Sherin, K. (1983). Aerobic exercise: Can you answer the questions your patients ask? *Postgraduate Medicine*, 73, 157–159; 162–164.

Sidney, K.H., Niinimaa, V. & Shephard, R.J. (1983). Attitudes towards exercise and sports: Sex and age differences and changes with endurance training. *Journal of Sports Sciences*, 1, 195–210.

Silva, J. & Weinberg, R.S. (1984) (Eds.). *Psychological Foundations of Sport*. Champaign: Human Kinetics.

Simons-Morton, B.G., O'Hara, N.M., Simons-Morton, D.G. & Parcel, G.S. (1987).

Children and fitness: A public health perspective. *Research Quarterly for Exercise and Sport*, 58, 295–302.

Simons-Morton, B.G., O'Hara, N.M., Simons-Morton, D.G. & Parcel, G.S. (1988a). Children and fitness: A public health perspective – Reaction to the reactions. *Research Quarterly for Exercise and Sport*, 59, 177–179.

Simons-Morton, B.G., Parcel, G.S., O'Hara, N.M., Blair, S.N. & Pate, R.R. (1988b). Health-related physical fitness in childhood: Status and recommendations. *Annual Review of Public Health*, 9, 403–425.

Sinyor, D., Schwartz, S.G., Peronnet, F., Brisson, G. & Seraganian, P. (1983). Aerobic fitness level and reactivity to psychosocial stress: Physiological, biochemical and subjective measures. *Psychosomatic Medicine*, 45, 205–217.

Siscovick, D.S. (1990). Risks of exercising: Sudden cardiac death and injuries. In C. Bouchard, R.J. Shephard, T. Stephens, J.R. Sutton & B.D. McPherson (Eds.). *Exercise, Fitness and Health: A Consensus of Current Knowledge*. Champaign: Human Kinetics.

Siscovick, D.S., Weiss, N.S., Fletcher, R.H. & Lasky, T. (1984). The incidence of primary cardiac arrest during vigorous exercise. *New England Journal of Medicine*, 311, 874–877.

Slenker, S., Price, J., Roberts, S. & Jurs, S. (1984). Joggers versus nonexercisers: An analysis of knowledge, attitudes and beliefs about jogging. *Research Quarterly for Exercise and Sport*, 55, 371–378.

Slenker, S., Price, J. & O'Connell, J. (1985). Health locus of control of joggers and nonexercisers. *Perceptual and Motor Skills*, 61, 323–328.

Smedslund, J. (1978). Bandura's theory of self-efficacy: A set of common sense theorems. *Scandinavian Journal of Psychology*, 19, 1–14.

Smith, E.L., Smith, K.A. & Gilligan, C. (1990). Exercise, fitness, osteoarthritis, and osteoporosis. In C. Bouchard, R.J. Shephard, T. Stephens, J.R. Sutton & B.D. McPherson (Eds.). *Exercise, Fitness and Health: A Consensus of Current Knowledge*. Champaign: Human Kinetics.

Smith, G.T. (1985). *Measurement of Health*. London: Office of Health Economics.

Smith, R. (1988). Gymnastics with a health focus. *Health and Physical Education Project Newsletter*, 19, 1–3.

Smith, R.A. (1989). Fitness testing in a private health club: A case study. *British Journal of Physical Education*, 20(2), 72–73.

Smith, R.A. & Biddle, S.J.H. (1990a). Attitudes and health-related exercise: Review and critique. Paper presented at AIESEP World Congress, Loughborough University, England.

Smith, R.A. & Biddle, S.J.H. (1990b). Exercise adherence in the commercial sector. Paper presented at European Health Psychology Society 4th annual conference, University of Oxford, England.

Sonstroem, R.J. (1978). Physical estimation and attraction scales: Rationale and research. *Medicine and Science in Sports*, 10, 97–102.

Sonstroem, R.J. (1982a). Exercise and self-esteem: Recommendations for expository research. *Quest*, 33, 124–139.

Sonstroem, R.J. (1982b). Attitudes and beliefs in the prediction of exercise participation. In R.C. Cantu & W.J. Gillespie (Eds.). *Sports Medicine, Sports Science: Bridging the Gap*. Lexington, Mass: Collamore Press.

Sonstroem, R.J. (1984). Exercise and self-esteem. *Exercise and Sport Sciences Reviews*, 12, 123–155.

Sonstroem, R.J. (1988). Psychological models. In R.K. Dishman (Ed.). *Exercise Adherence: Its Impact on Public Health.* Champaign: Human Kinetics.

Sonstroem, R.J. & Kampper, K.P. (1980). Prediction of athletic participation in middle school males. *Research Quarterly for Exercise and Sport,* 51, 685–694.

Sonstroem, R.J. & Morgan, W.P. (1989). Exercise and self-esteem: Rationale and model. *Medicine and Science in Sports and Exercise,* 21, 329–337.

Sonstroem, R.J. & Walker, M. (1973). Relationship of attitudes and locus of control to exercise and physical fitness. *Perceptual and Motor Skills,* 36, 1031–1034.

Sparkes, A.C. (1989). Health-related fitness: An example of innovation without change. *British Journal of Physical Education,* 20(2), 60–63.

Spielberger, C.D. (1987). Stress, emotions and health. In W.P. Morgan & S.E. Goldston (Eds.). *Exercise and Mental Health.* Washington: Hemisphere.

Spielberger, C.D., Gorsuch, R.L. & Lushene, R. (1970). *State-Trait Anxiety Inventory Manual.* Palo Alto: Consulting Psychologists Press.

Spitzer, R.L., Endicott, J. & Robins, E. (1978). Research diagnostic criteria: Rationale and reliability. *Archives of General Psychiatry,* 35, 773–782.

Sports Council & Health Education Authority (1988). *Children's Exercise, Health and Fitness: Fact Sheet.* London: Sports Council and Health Education Authority.

Stahlberg, D. & Frey, D. (1988). Attitudes I: Structure, measurement and functions. In M. Hewstone, W. Stroebe, J-P. Cobol & G. Stephenson (Eds.). *Introduction to Social Psychology.* Oxford: Blackwell.

Steinberg, H. & Sykes, E.A. (1985). Introduction to symposium on endorphins and behavioural processes: Review of literature on endorphins and exercise. *Pharmacology, Biochemistry and Behaviour,* 23, 857–862.

Steinberg, H., Sykes, E. & Morris, M. (1988). Exercise addiction: The opiate connection. In *Sport, Health, Psychology and Exercise Symposium proceedings.* London: The Sports Council/Health Education Authority.

Steinhardt, M.A. & Carrier, K.M. (1989). Early and continued participation in a work-site health and fitness programme. *Research Quarterly for Exercise and Sport,* 60, 117–126.

Steinhardt, M.A. & Dishman, R.K. (1989). Reliability and validity of expected outcomes and barriers for habitual physical activity. *Journal of Occupational Medicine,* 31, 536–546.

Stephens, T. (1987). Secular trends in adult physical activity: Exercise boom or bust? *Research Quarterly for Exercise and Sport,* 58, 94–105.

Stephens, T. (1988). Physical activity and mental health in the United States and Canada: Evidence from four population surveys. *Preventive Medicine,* 17, 35–47.

Stephens, T., Jacobs, D.R. & White, C.C. (1985). A descriptive epidemiology of leisure-time physical activity. *Public Health Reports,* 100, 147–158.

Steptoe, A. & Bolton, J. (1988). The short-term influence of high and low intensity physical exercise on mood. *Psychology and Health,* 2, 91–106.

Steptoe, A. & Cox, S. (1988). Acute effects of aerobic exercise on mood. *Health Psychology,* 7, 329–340.

Steptoe, A., Moses, J., Edwards, S. & Mathews, A. (1988). Effects of aerobic conditioning on mental well-being and reactivity to stress. In *Sport, Health, Psychology and Exercise Symposium proceedings.* London: The Sports Council/Health Education Authority.

Stewart, K.J. (1989). Introduction to the symposium: Resistive weight training: A new approach to exercise for cardiac and coronary disease prone populations.

Medicine and Science in Sports and Exercise, 21, 667–668.

Stoeckle, J.D. & Barsky, A.J. (1980). Attributions: Uses of social science knowledge in the 'doctoring' of primary care. In L. Eisenberg & A. Kleinman (Eds.). *The Relevance of Social Science for Medicine*. London: D. Reidel.

Strecher, V.J., DeVellis, B.E., Becker, M.H. & Rosenstock, I.M. (1986). The role of self-efficacy in achieving health behaviour change. *Health Education Quarterly*, 13, 73–92.

Strickland, B.R. (1978). Internal-external expectancies and health-related behaviours. *Journal of Consulting and Clinical Psychology*, 46, 1192–1211.

Strickland, B.R. (1979). Internal-external expectancies and cardiovascular functioning. In L.C. Perlmuter & R.A. Monty (Eds.). *Choice and Perceived Control*. Hillsdale, NJ: Erlbaum.

Stroebe, W. & Jonas, K. (1988). Attitudes II: Strategies of attitude change. In M. Hewstone, W. Stroebe, J-P. Cobol & G. Stephenson (Eds.). *Introduction to Social Psychology*. Oxford: Blackwell.

Summers, J.J., Sargent, G.I., Levey, A.J. & Murray, K.D. (1982). Middle-aged, non-elite marathon runners: A profile. *Perceptual and Motor Skills*, 52, 963–969.

Summers, J.J., Machin, V.J. & Sargent, G.I. (1983). Psychosocial factors related to marathon running. *Journal of Sport Psychology*, 5, 314–331.

Sutherland, R., Armstrong, G., Wilson, J., Henderson, S., Aitchison, T. & Grant, S. (1990). A physiological evaluation of university fitness sessions. Paper presented at the Scottish Universities Physical Education Association conference, Glasgow.

Taylor, C.B., Bandura, A., Ewart, C.E., Miller, N.H. & DeBusk, R.F. (1985). Exercise testing to enhance wives' confidence in their husbands' cardiac capabilities soon after clinically uncomplicated acute myocardial infarction. *American Journal of Cardiology*, 55, 635–638.

Thompson, C.E. & Wankel, L.M. (1980). The effects of perceived activity choice upon frequency of exercise behaviour. *Journal of Applied Social Psychology*, 10, 436–443.

Thompson, J.K., Jarvie, G.J., Lahey, B.B. & Cureton, K.J. (1982). Exercise and obesity: Etiology, physiology and intervention. *Psychological Bulletin*, 91, 55–79.

Thow, M. & Newton, M. (1990). The Gartnavel experience in health promotion 1986. *Physiotherapy*, 76(1), 2–6.

Tieman, J.G., Dishman, R.K. & Holly, R.G. (1989). Public self-consciousness does not predict RPE. *Medicine and Science in Sports and Exercise*, 21, (2, Supplement), S14 [abstract].

Tirrell, B.E. & Hart, L.K. (1980). The relationship of health beliefs and knowledge to exercise compliance in patients after coronary bypass. *Heart and Lung*, 9, 487–493.

Tooman, M.E. (1982). The effect of running and its deprivation on muscle tension, mood and anxiety. Unpublished Master's thesis, The Pennsylvania State University.

Tooman, M.E., Harris, D.V. & Mutrie, N. (1985). The effect of running and its deprivation on muscle tension, mood and anxiety. Paper presented at the International Society of Sports Psychology World Congress, Copenhagen, Denmark.

Triandis, H.C. (1977). *Interpersonal Behaviour*. Monterey: Brooks/Cole.

Trotter, R.J. (1984). Rethinking the high in runner's high. *Psychology Today*, May 8.

Tucker, L.A., Cole, G.E. & Friedman, G.M. (1986). Physical fitness: A buffer against stress. *Perceptual and Motor Skills*, 63, 955–961.

Vallerand, R.J. (1987). Antecedents of self-related affects in sport: Preliminary evidence on the intuitive-reflective appraisal model. *Journal of Sport Psychology*, 9, 161–182.

Vallerand, R.J., Deci, E.L. & Ryan, R.M. (1987). Intrinsic motivation in sport. *Exercise and Sport Sciences Reviews*, 15, 389–425.

Valois, P., Desharnais, R. & Godin, G. (1988). A comparison of the Fishbein and Ajzen and the Triandis attitudinal models for the prediction of exercise intention and behaviour. *Journal of Behavioural Medicine*, 11, 459–472.

van Doornen, L.J.P., de Geus, E.J.C. & Orlebeke, J.F. (1988). Aerobic fitness and the physiological stress response: A critical evaluation. *Social Science and Medicine*, 26, 303–307.

Vealey, R.S. (1986a). Conceptualisation of sport – confidence and competitive orientation: Preliminary investigation and instrument development. *Journal of Sport Psychology*, 8, 221–246.

Vealey, R.S. (1986b). Imagery training for performance enhancement. In J.M. Williams (Ed.). *Applied Sport Psychology*. Palo Alto: Mayfield.

Vogel, P.G. (1986). Effects of physical education programmes on children. In V. Seefeldt (Ed.). *Physical Activity and Well-being*. Reston, VA: American Alliance of Health, Physical Education, Recreation and Dance.

Vranic, M. & Wasserman, D. (1990). Exercise, fitness, and diabetes. In C. Bouchard, R.J. Shephard, T. Stephens, J.R. Sutton & B.D. McPherson (Eds.). *Exercise, Fitness and Health: A Consensus of Current Knowledge*. Champaign: Human Kinetics.

Wales, D.N. (1985). The effects of tempo and disposition in music on perceived exertion, brain waves, and mood during aerobic exercise. Unpublished Master's thesis, The Pennsylvania State University.

Wallace, P.G. & Haines, A.P. (1984). General practitioner and health promotion: What patients think. *British Medical Journal*, 289, 534–536.

Wallston, B.S. & Wallston, K.A. (1978). Locus of control and health: A review. *Health Education Mongraphs*, 6, 107–117.

Wallston, B.S. & Wallston, K.A. (1985). Social psychological models of health behaviour: An examination and integration. In A. Baum, S.E. Taylor & J.E. Singer (Eds.). *Handbook of Psychology and Health. IV. Social Psychological Aspects of Health*. Hillsdale, NJ: Erlbaum.

Wallston, B.S., Wallston, K.A., Kaplan, G.D. & Maides, S.A. (1976). Development and validation of the Health Locus of Control (HLC) Scale. *Journal of Consulting and Clinical Psychology*, 44, 580–585.

Wallston, K.A. & Wallston, B.S. (1981). Health locus of control scales. In H. Lefcourt (Ed.). *Research with the Locus of Control Construct. Vol 1*. New York: Academic Press.

Wallston, K.A., Wallston, B.S. & DeVellis, R. (1978). Development of the multidimensional health locus of control (MHLC) scales. *Health Education Monographs*, 6, 160–170.

Walter, S.D. & Hart, L.E. (1990). Application of epidemiological methodology to sports and exercise science research. *Exercise and Sport Sciences Reviews*, 18, 417–448.

Wankel, L.M. (1984). Decision-making and social-support strategies for increasing exercise involvement. *Journal of Cardiac Rehabilitation*, 4, 124–135.

Wankel, L.M. (1985). Personal and situational factors affecting exercise involvement:

The importance of enjoyment. *Research Quarterly for Exercise and Sport*, 56, 275–282.

Wankel, L.M. (1988). Exercise adherence and leisure activity: Patterns of involvement and interventions to facilitate regular activity. In R.K. Dishman (Ed.). *Exercise Adherence: Its Impact on Public Health*. Champaign: Human Kinetics.

Wankel, L.M. & Kreisel, P.S.J. (1985). Factors underlying enjoyment of youth sports: Sport and age group comparisons. *Journal of Sport Psychology*, 7, 51–64.

Wankel, L.M. & Thompson, C.E. (1977). Motivating people to be physically active: Self-persuasion vs. balanced decision-making. *Journal of Applied Social Psychology*, 7, 332–340.

Wankel, L.M., Yardley, J.K. & Graham, J. (1985). The effects of motivational interventions upon the exercise adherence of high and low self-motivated adults. *Canadian Journal of Applied Sports Science*, 10, 147–156.

Wanzel, R.S. & Danielson, R.R. (1977). Improve adherence to your fitness programme. *Recreation Management*, July pp. 16–19; August pp. 38–41; September pp. 34–37.

Ward, A. & Morgan, W.P. (1984). Adherence patterns of healthy men and women enrolled in an adult exercise programme. *Journal of Cardiac Rehabilitation*, 4, 143–152.

Warshaw, L.J. (1979). *Managing Stress*. Reading, Mass: Addison-Wesley.

Weber, J. & Wertheim, E.H. (1989). Relationships of self-monitoring, special attention, body fat percentage, and self-motivation to attendance at a community gymnasium. *Journal of Sport and Exercise Psychology*, 11, 105–114.

Weinberg, R.S. (1984). The relationship between extrinsic rewards and intrinsic motivation in sport. In J. Silva & R.S. Weinberg (Eds.). *Psychological Foundations of Sport*. Champaign: Human Kinetics.

Weinberg, R.S., Hughes, H.H., Critelli, J.W., England, R. & Jackson, A. (1984). Effects of pre-existing and manipulated self-efficacy on weight loss in a self-control programme. *Journal of Research in Personality*, 18, 352–358.

Weiner, B. (1979). A theory of motivation for some classroom experiences. *Journal of Educational Psychology*, 71, 3–25.

Weiner, B. (1980). *Human Motivation*. New York: Holt, Rinehart & Winston.

Weiner, B. (1986). *An Attributional Theory of Motivation and Emotion*. New York: Springer-Verlag.

Weiss, M.R., Bredemeier, B.J. & Shewchuk, R.M. (1985). An intrinsic/extrinsic motivation scale for the youth sport setting: A confirmatory factor analysis. *Journal of Sport Psychology*, 7, 75–91.

Wells, N. (1985). *Back Pain*. London: Office of Health Economics.

Wells, N. (1987). *Coronary Heart Disease: The Need for Action*. London: Office of Health Economics.

White, A. & Coakley, J.J. (1986). *Making Decisions: The Response of Young People in the Medway Towns to the 'Ever Thought of Sport?' Campaign*. London: Greater London and South East Region Sports Council.

Whitehead, J.R. & Corbin, C.B. (1988). Multidimensional scales for the measurement of locus of control of reinforcements for physical fitness behaviours. *Research Quarterly for Exercise and Sport*, 59, 108–117.

Whitehead, J.R. & Corbin, C.B. (1989). Youth fitness testing: The effects of positive and negative feedback on intrinsic motivation. Paper presented at North American Society for the Psychology of Sport and Physical Activity conference, Kent State University, Ohio, USA.

Whitehead, J.R., Pemberton, C.L. & Corbin, C.B. (1990). Perspectives on the physical fitness testing of children: The case for a realistic educational approach. *Pediatric Exercise Science*, 2, 111–123.

Widmeyer, W.N., Brawley, L.R. & Carron, A.V. (1985). *The Measurement of Cohesion in Sports Teams: The Group Environment Questionnaire*. London, Ontario: Sports Dynamics.

Wier, L.T. & Jackson, A.S. (1989). Factors affecting compliance in the NASA/Johnson Space Centre fitness programme. *Sports Medicine*, 8, 9–14.

Wilbur, C.S. & Garner, D. (1984). Marketing health to employees: The Johnson and Johnson 'Live for Life' programme. In L.W. Frederiksen, L.J. Solomon & K.A. Brehony (Eds.). *Marketing Health Behaviour: Principles, Techniques and Applications*. New York: Plenum.

Wilbur, C.S., Hartwell, T.D. & Piserchia, P.V. (1986). The Johnson and Johnson 'Live for Life' programme: Its organisation and evaluation plan. In M.F. Cataldo & T.J. Coates (Eds.). *Health and Industry: A Behavioural Medicine Perspective*. New York: John Wiley.

Wilkes, R.L. & Summers, J.J. (1984). Cognitions, mediating variables, and strength performance. *Journal of Sport Psychology*, 6, 351–359.

Williams, J.G. & Eston, R.G. (1989). Determination of the intensity dimension in vigorous exercise programmes with particular reference to the use of the rating of perceived exertion. *Sports Medicine*, 8, 177–189.

Williams, L.R.T., Hughes, J.R. & Martin, C. (1982). Effects of daily physical education on children's attitudes toward physical activity. *New Zealand Journal of Health, Physical Education and Recreation*. 15(2), 31–35.

Wilson, V.E., Morley, M.C. & Bird, E.I. (1980). Mood profile of marathon runners, joggers and non-exercisers. *Perceptual and Motor Skills*, 50, 117–118.

Wood, D.T. (1977). The relationship between state anxiety and physical activity. *American Corrective Therapy Journal*, 31 (3), 67–69.

World Health Organization (1986). *Targets for Health for All*. Copenhagen: WHO.

Wurtele, S.K. (1986). Self-efficacy and athletic performance: A review. *Journal of Social and Clinical Psychology*, 4, 290–301.

Wurtele, S.K. & Maddux, J.E. (1987). Relative contributions of Protection Motivation Theory components in predicting exercise intentions and behaviour. *Health Psychology*, 6, 453–466.

Wurtele, S.K., Roberts, M.C. & Leeper, J.D. (1982). Health beliefs and intentions: Predictors of return compliance in a tuberculosis detection drive. *Journal of Applied Social Psychology*, 12, 128–136.

Wysocki, T., Hall, G., Iwata, B. & Riordan, M. (1979). Behavioural management of exercise: Contracting for aerobic points. *Journal of Applied Behaviour Analysis*, 12, 55–64.

Yates, A., Leehey, K. & Shisslak, C.M. (1983). Running: An analogue of anorexia? *New England Journal of Medicine*, 308, 251–255.

Young, R.J. (1979). The effect of regular exercise on cognitive functioning and personality. *British Journal of Sports Medicine*, 13, 110–117.

Young, R.J. & Ismail, A.H. (1977). Comparison of selected physiological and personality variables in regular and non-regular adult male exercisers. *Research Quarterly*, 48, 617–622.

Zankel, J.T. & Field, J.M. (1959). Physical fitness index in psychiatric patients. *Journal of the Association for Physical and Mental Rehabilitation*, 13, 50–51.

Subject Index

Printing: Mercedesdruck, Berlin
Binding: Buchbinderei Lüderitz & Bauer, Berlin